ASSESSING ADOLESCENT PSYCHOPATHOLOGY

Assessing Adolescent Psychopathology: MMPI-A/MMPI-A-RF, Fourth Edition provides updated recommendations for researchers and clinicians concerning the MMPI-A, the most widely used objective personality test with adolescents, and also introduces the MMPI-A-Restructured Form (MMPI-A-RF), the newest form of the MMPI for use with adolescents. Further, this fourth edition includes comprehensive information on both MMPI forms for adolescents, including descriptions of the development, structure, and interpretive approaches to the MMPI-A and the MMPI-A-RF. This text provides extensive clinical case examples of the interpretation of both tests, including samples of computer based test package output, and identifies important areas of similarities and differences between these two important tests of adolescent psychopathology.

Robert P. Archer, PhD, ABPP, is the Frank Harrell Redwood Distinguished Professor and Director of Psychology in the Department of Psychiatry and Behavioral Sciences at the Eastern Virginia Medical School in Norfolk, Virginia. He is a co-author of the MMPI-A, and the lead author for the MMPI-A-RF. He was the founding editor of the journal *Assessment* and is the President-Elect of the Society of Personality Assessment.

ASSESSING ADOLESCENT PSYCHOPATHOLOGY

MMPI-A/MMPI-A-RF, Fourth Edition

Robert P. Archer

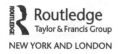

Routledge
Taylor & Francis Group

NEW YORK AND LONDON

Fourth edition published 2017
by Routledge
711 Third Avenue, New York, NY 10017

and by Routledge
2 Park Square, Milton Park, Abingdon, Oxon, OX14 4RN

Routledge is an imprint of the Taylor & Francis Group, an informa business

First edition published by Lawrence Erlbaum Associates 1992
Third edition published by Routledge 2005

Library of Congress Cataloging in Publication Data
Names: Archer, Robert P.
Title: Assessing adolescent psychopathology : MMPI-A, MMPI-A-RF
    / Robert P. Archer, Eastern Virginia Medical School. Other titles:
    MMPI-A | MMPI-A-RF
Description: Fourth edition. | New York, NY : Routledge, 2016. Includes
    bibliographical references and index.
Identifiers: LCCN 2015050124 | ISBN 9781138830875 (alk. paper) |
    ISBN 9781138830868 (alk. paper) | ISBN 9781315737010 (alk. paper)
Subjects: LCSH: Minnesota Multiphasic Personality Inventory for
    Adolescents. | Adolescent psychopathology—Diagnosis.
Classification: LCC RJ503.7.M56 A73 2016 DDC 616.8900835—dc23
LC record available at http://lccn.loc.gov/2015050124

ISBN: 978-1-138-83087-5 (hbk)
ISBN: 978-1-138-83086-8 (pbk)
ISBN: 978-1-315-73701-0 (ebk)

Typeset in Bembo
by Swales & Willis Ltd, Exeter, Devon, UK

To Mr. David Elkins and Ms. Scheryl Chadwick with much gratitude for all their efforts in creating this fourth edition.

CONTENTS

PREFACE TO THE FOURTH EDITION

The first edition of *MMPI-A: Assessing Adolescent Psychopathology* was published in August 1992 to coincide with the original release of the MMPI-A manual and test materials for this instrument. This new and fourth edition coincides with the publication of the MMPI-A-RF, for the first time providing test users with choices concerning the form of the MMPI they utilize to evaluate adolescent psychopathology. The purpose of the current revision is to update and incorporate the rapidly expanding literature on the MMPI-A, and to introduce readers to the structure and uses of the MMPI-A-RF. This fourth edition continues to include chapters on the critical issues of adolescent development and psychopathology, as well as providing a comprehensive review of the development, administration, and scoring procedures for both the MMPI-A and the MMPI-A-RF. The objective of this volume is to expand the coverage of the MMPI-A to include the newest literature on this established test instrument, while also providing the reader with useful and practical information concerning the development and utilization of the MMPI-A-RF. In describing both instruments, it is my hope that sufficient information is provided to guide clinical uses of these tests and also stimulate future research efforts with both of these inter-related instruments.

I would like to note several individuals who were invaluable in the creation of this fourth edition. Mr. David Elkins, Research Associate at the Eastern Virginia Medical School, has been a central resource and colleague, not only in the development of this text, but in all of my research efforts since 1992. Additionally, I wish to express my sincere appreciation to Ms. Scheryl Chadwick, who has handled all of the demands of her position as the Program Coordinator of our Psychology Internship Training Program at EVMS, while also providing the timely and extensive manuscript preparation connected with this edition.

I would also like to express my thanks to Beverly Kaemmer at the University of Minnesota Press for all of her help and assistance in providing me with the materials necessary for the revision. It has been my privilege to work with three outstanding psychologists in the development of the MMPI-A-RF, the most memorable and enjoyable collaborative experience of my career. Dr. Richard Handel is my colleague and member of our faculty at the Eastern Virginia Medical School, and it was very natural for us to extend our collaboration on numerous MMPI-A and MMPI-2 research projects to the task of development of the MMPI-A-RF. Dr. Yossef Ben-Porath of Kent State University and Dr. Auke Tellegen of the University of Minnesota are towering figures in the field of Personality Assessment, and it was indeed a rare privilege to be able to work with, and to learn from them, in the development of the MMPI-A-RF. Further, I would like to sincerely thank the individuals who served as reviewers for the original proposal for the fourth edition: Dr. Randolph Arnau in the Psychology Department at the University of Southern Mississippi, Dr. Radhika Krishnamurthy in the Psychology Department at Florida Institute of Technology, and Dr. Brian Wald, a Clinical and Forensic Psychologist in private practice in Virginia Beach, Virginia. Finally, I would like to express my deepest gratitude for the support and longstanding patience of my wife, Dr. Linda R. Archer, and my daughter, Dr. Elizabeth W. Wheeler, for their support on this, and all my previous, MMPI projects.

This fourth edition marks a particularly exciting period of development in the assessment of adolescent psychopathology with the MMPI. It is my hope that this text will be helpful to test users in discerning the relative advantages and limitations of both the MMPI-A and MMPI-A-RF and the implications of their choices for test administration, scoring, and interpretation. From 1942 until the publication of the MMPI-A in 1992, the original form of the MMPI was widely used with adolescents, resulting in a number of benefits as well as problems when adolescents were evaluated on an instrument designed primarily for adults. From 1992 until the present, the MMPI-A has been an effective means of distinguishing various forms of psychopathology among adolescents, with its own set of strengths and liabilities. With the publication of this fourth edition, test users will now have the opportunity to evaluate the newest member of the MMPI family of instruments and this test (much like the MMPI and MMPI-A) will be found to have its own strengths and weaknesses in dealing with this complex and crucially important clinical and research area of the psychological assessment of adolescents.

1

ADOLESCENT DEVELOPMENT AND PSYCHOPATHOLOGY

The development of the Minnesota Multiphasic Personality Inventory-Adolescent (MMPI-A) and, most recently, the Minnesota Multiphasic Personality Inventory-Adolescent-Restructured Form (MMPI-A-RF) have substantially assisted in deriving interpretive comments relevant to and appropriate for adolescents, but using these specialized forms of the MMPI does not substitute for an awareness of salient developmental issues. Thus, the purpose of this chapter is to provide a brief overview of adolescent development and psychopathology, with particular attention focused on ways in which developmentally related issues may affect MMPI-A and MMPI-A-RF interpretation practices.

Developmental Tasks During Adolescence

Achenbach (1978) suggested that an understanding of psychopathology in children and adolescents must be firmly grounded in the study of normal development. Human development is a continuous process, but there may be critical periods in our development during which adaptational success or failure heavily influences the course of later development in the life cycle. Adolescence clearly is one of these critical developmental transitions. Holmbeck and Updegrove (1995) have observed that adolescence is "characterized by more biological, psychological, and social role changes than other life stages except infancy" (p. 16). As noted by Petersen and Hamburg (1986), the number and extent of changes that occur simultaneously during adolescence present major challenges to the development of mature and effective coping strategies. Ineffective coping strategies may contribute to a variety of problem behaviors during adolescent development. Further, failures in adolescent development may result in psychopathology manifested during later life stages.

Three major areas of changes and challenges that face the individual during adolescence are reviewed here, including physiological processes, cognitive processes, and psychological and emotional challenges.

Physiological/Sexual Maturation

Kimmel and Weiner (1985) defined puberty as "the process of becoming physically and sexually mature and developing the adult characteristics of one's sex" (p. 592). Petersen (1985) noted several characteristics of puberty that are important in understanding adolescent development. Puberty is a universal experience that may, however, be delayed, or in some cases even prevented by the occurrence of physical disease or traumatic psychological events. Paikoff and Brooks-Gunn (1991) noted that the timing of puberty has been shown to vary as a function of the adolescent's health status, nutrition, ethnicity, genetic inheritance, exercise level, and stress experiences. They observed that the parent–child relationship is typically affected by pubertal development, with decreases in time spent with parents and submissiveness to parental decisions typically found during early adolescence. Further, Petersen stressed that puberty is a process, rather than an isolated temporal event. This process involves changes that result in a sexually immature child achieving full reproductive potential. These physical changes are typically manifested in the growth of underarm and pubic hair, maturation of genitalia, and the first menstruation in girls. Often, the clearest signs of adolescent development are physical changes associated with the onset of puberty.

Fundamental physical changes, in terms of endocrinological, biochemical, and physiological processes, occur during adolescence. For example, Stone and Church (1957) noted that an individual is expected to increase 25% in height and 100% in weight during this developmental stage. Additionally, there is a marked increase in pituitary activity leading to increased production of hormones by the thyroid, adrenal, and other glands that are centrally involved in sexual maturation.

There are notable differences in the rate of physical maturation between boys and girls, and there are also very wide individual variations in sexual maturation within genders. Figures 1.1 and 1.2 show varying degrees of sexual maturation for boys aged $14^{3/4}$ and girls aged $12^{3/4}$, and the velocity of growth in height by year of life. The data in Fig. 1.1 for pubertal development illustrate both the earlier maturation of females in relation to males, and the wide differences in pubertal development within genders at identical chronological ages. To the extent that pubertal development is precocious or significantly delayed, stress may occur that can be reflected in lower self-esteem or self-concept for the adolescent during this period. A monograph by the American Psychological Association (APA, 2002) provided data indicating that the current course of pubertal development for American adolescents is occurring substantially earlier than the guideposts originally provided by Tanner in the late 1960s for his British sample of adolescents. For example, the average age of menarche for girls in the United States is now around 12.5, and for boys the onset of puberty involving the enlargement of the testes occurs at around age 11.5, with the first ejaculation typically occurring between the ages of 12 and 14. A survey of 17,000 healthy girls between the ages of 3 and 12 who were participating in office visits with their pediatricians found that 6.7% of White girls and 27.2% of African-American girls showed some signs of puberty as early as age 7, e.g., pubic hair or breast development (Herman-Giddens et al., 1997; Kaplowitz & Oberfield, 1999). A description of

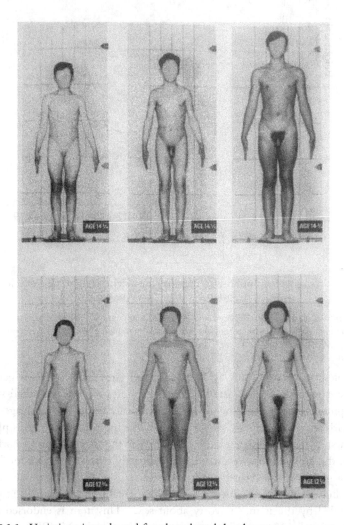

FIGURE 1.1   Variations in male and female pubertal development.

Source: Tanner, 1969. Copyright © by W.B. Saunders Company. Reproduced with permission.

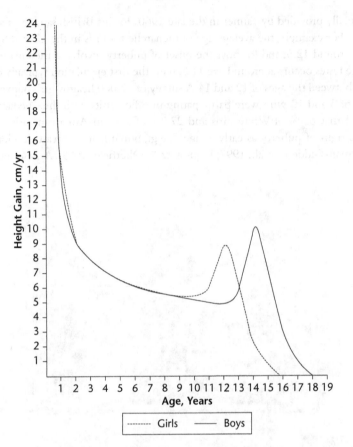

FIGURE 1.2 Standards from birth to maturity for height, weight, height velocity, and weight velocity: British children, 1965, Part I.

Source: Archives of Disease in Childhood, 41, 454–471. Copyright © by the Archives of Disease in Childhood. Reprinted with permission from BMJ Publishing Group Ltd. Reproduced from Tanner, J. M., Whitehouse, R. H., & Takaishi, M. (1966).

the adolescent growth spurt by Hoffmann and Greydanus (1997) is generally consistent with the earlier data by Tanner in indicating that the rapid skeletal developments which mark the growth spurt usually begin at around ages 10 to 12 in girls and around ages 12 to 14 for boys. The most dramatic rate of physical growth, shown in Fig. 1.2, tends to occur between the ages of 12 and 15, with the peak of the growth curve occurring approximately two years earlier for females than for males.

An illustration of the influence of developmental forces on MMPI responses is provided by the item, "I worry about sex." This item is endorsed in the *true* direction by 13% of adult female respondents in the MMPI-2 normative sample (Butcher, Dahlstrom, Graham, Tellegen and Kaemmer, 1989), and 15% of adult men. In contrast to adult samples, however, this item was endorsed as true by 37% of adolescent females and 30% of adolescent males in the MMPI-A normative sample (Butcher et al. 1992). The higher rate of endorsement of this item in the critical direction by the 14- to 18-year-old teenagers probably reflects the higher level of stress for adolescents related to issues of sexual maturation as well as sexual identity.

Cognitive Maturation and Brain Development

Adolescence may also be defined in terms of changes that occur in cognitive processes and brain development. White (2009) recently observed that as the adolescent begins the physical changes associated with puberty, the brain also undergoes dramatic changes with profound implications for development and psychopathology. White notes that some of the most intriguing of these changes occur in the frontal lobe area of the brain, a region associated with critical roles in decision-making and higher-order cognitive functioning. Frontal lobe gray matter volume reaches a peak around age 11 for girls and 12 for boys, at which point the brain begins the process of reducing brain volume and "pruning" synaptic connections into a configuration that will carry the individual through the adult years. These changes occurring in the frontal lobes during adolescence reflect a refinement of brain circuitry allowing for increased efficiency of functioning. Albert, Chein, and Steinberg (2013) have noted research findings that suggest that adolescent risk-taking behaviors derive, at least in part, from the maturational gap that occurs during early adolescence in terms of brain development. As the cognitive control system of the brain matures over the period of adolescence, teenagers grow correspondingly in their capacity to inhibit risk-taking and exercise self-regulation and control. Bonnie and Scott (2013) have noted that neuroscience has played an increasingly important role in juvenile justice policy concerning questions of whether and when adolescent offenders should be punished as adults. They noted three recent court opinions emphasizing reduced culpability of adolescents because of developmental immaturities, in part supported by neuroscience research. These decisions include Roper v. Simmons (2005) in which the Supreme Court rejected the death penalty for adolescents, and Graham v. Florida (2010) and Miller v. Alabama (2012) which rejected life sentences without parole for juveniles, based heavily on neuroscience research on the role of brain development on behavioral control.

The work of Piaget and his colleagues offers an approach to understanding these cognitive changes, with the final stage of cognitive development in Piaget's (1975) paradigm unfolding during adolescence. Specifically, Piaget postulated that during early adolescence, the individual typically makes the transition from Concrete Operations to the Formal Operations stage, the latter characterized by the capacity to manipulate ideas and concepts. According to Piaget (1975), "The adolescent is an individual who is capable . . . of building and understanding ideas or abstract theories and concepts. The child does not build theories" (p. 105). Thus, the adolescent is able to discern the real from the ideal, and to become passionately engaged by abstract concepts and notions. Adolescents begin to think of their world in new ways, including the ability to "think about thinking." Related to these changes in cognitive skills, Elkind (1978, 1980) argued that as adolescents become capable of thinking about their thoughts, they may also become excessively concerned with how they are perceived by others. This preoccupation includes an exaggerated view of the uniqueness of their own experiences, and the amount of time devoted by others to their appraisal. Elkind labeled the egocentric tendency of adolescents to believe that their behavior is intensely scrutinized by others as "the imaginary audience" (Elkind & Bowen, 1979).

Part of this self-absorption and belief in the uniqueness of one's own experiences may be reflected in the endorsement rate differences between adults and adolescents for the following abbreviated item, which is a member of scales *Pt* and *Sc*:

"Have strange thoughts."
(Endorsed true by 15% of MMPI-2 adult males and 10% of adult females, vs. 45% of boys in the MMPI-A normative sample and 46% of MMPI-A teenage girls.)

and to the following abbreviated item, a member of scales *Pd*, *Pa*, and *Sc*:

"Am misunderstood."
(Endorsed true by 9% of adult men and 9% of adult women in the MMPI-2 normative sample, vs. 25.6% of adolescent boys and 37.4% of adolescent girls in the MMPI-A normative sample.)

and to the following abbreviated item, a member of the *Mf* and *Si* scales:

"Don't mind not being better looking."
(Endorsed true by 77% and 59% of the MMPI-2 male and female normative samples, respectively, vs. 49% of adolescent boys and 38% of adolescent girls in the MMPI-A normative sample.)

Psychological Development

Finally, a host of psychological and emotional tasks, including the processes of individuation, the formation of ego identity, and ego maturation, are accomplished during adolescence. Blos (1967) discussed individuation as a process involved with the development of relative independence from family relationships, the weakening of infantile object ties, and an increased capacity to assume a functional role as a member of adult society. Blos defined and described this task as similar to the more primitive struggle for individuation in the attainment of object constancy that occurs toward the end of the third year of life. Thus, the early adolescent has marked ambivalence concerning issues of independence versus dependence, particularly in terms of their relationships to their parents. This ambivalence is likely to be seen in rapid and marked attitudinal and behavioral changes by the adolescent (e.g., one moment protesting any parental involvement or supervision and the next moment regressing to marked dependency on mother or father).

Erikson (1956) described ego identity formation during adolescence as the assembly of converging identity elements that occur at the end of childhood, achieved through a process of *normative crises*. Ego identity was viewed by Erikson as including the conscious sense of individual identity as well as an unconscious striving for a continuity of personal character. In this process of ego formation, the ego integrates previous childhood identifications into a new totality, which lays the foundation of the adult personality. Positive resolution of this issue leads to a sense of *ego identity*, or continuity in one's self-definition. Negative resolution of this challenge could result in *ego diffusion*, or uncertainty about who one is and what one will become in the future. This failure to achieve ego identity was related to the diagnostic category of identity problem (313.82) as described in the American Psychiatric Association's (1994) *Diagnostic and statistical manual of mental disorders* (DSM-IV). Marcia (1966) further defined Erikson's concept of ego identity in terms of two variables: commitment (whether or not the individual has accepted a set of values) and crisis (whether or not the individual has experienced an inner struggle in arriving at personal acceptance of a set of values). These two variables combine to yield four identity statuses in Marcia's model: *diffusion* (no commitment, no crisis); *foreclosure* (commitment without crisis); *moratorium* (crisis without commitment); and *achievement* (commitment after crisis). Marcia argued that these categories, in the order given, represent developmental levels of increasingly advanced maturation.

The process of individuation is most clearly noted during early phases of adolescence, whereas the process of identity formation and consolidation is typically manifested during later stages of adolescence. As a result of these processes, adolescents will typically modify the way in which they interact and relate to others. Specifically, adolescents begin to increase their involvement with peers, while decreasing their immediate identification with family members. Further, the early stages of individuation may result in an increase in conflict with parents, as the adolescent attempts preliminary definitions of the self, based on identifying the ways in which their feelings, thoughts, and attitudes may differ from those of their parents.

Loevinger (1976) articulated a concept of ego development in reference to the frameworks of meaning that individuals impose on their life experiences. Within Loevinger's model, the concept of ego development is a dimension of individual differences, as well as a developmental sequence of increasingly complex functioning in terms of impulse control, character development, interpersonal relationships, and cognitive complexity. At the three lowest levels of ego development, collectively grouped into the *preconformist* stage, the individual may be described as impulsive, motivated by personal gain in the avoidance of punishment, and oriented to the present rather than the past or future. Cognitive styles are stereotyped and concrete, and interpersonal relationships are opportunistic, exploitive, and demanding. During the second broad stage of development, referred to as the *conformist* stage, the individual begins to identify his or her welfare with that of the social group. The individual places emphasis on conformity to socially approved norms and standards and on issues of social acceptability in terms of attitudes and behaviors. As the individual enters the *postconformist* stages of development, self-awareness, cognitive complexity, and interpersonal style become increasingly complex and a balance is achieved between autonomy and interdependence. The maturational stages described by Loevinger do not refer to specific age groups, but she noted that higher stages of ego development would rarely be achieved by adolescents. Loevinger's view of development is very comprehensive and served as a basis for the development of the MMPI-A Immaturity (*IMM*) scale described in Chapter 6.

The following five MMPI abbreviated items illustrate substantial differences in endorsement frequency between adults in the MMPI-2 normative sample and adolescents in the MMPI-A normative sample:

"Rarely quarrel with family."

(Endorsed true by 78% of adult women and 79% of adult men, vs. 38% of adolescent girls and 46% of adolescent males.)

"Habits of some family members very irritating."

(Endorsed true by 66% of adult women and 48% of adult men, vs. 79% of adolescent girls and 67% of adolescent boys.)

"Most of family sympathetic."

(Endorsed true by 53% of adult women and 56% of adult men, vs. 31% of adolescent girls and 37% of adolescent boys.)

"Occasionally hate family members I love."

(Endorsed true by 44% of adult women and 32% of adult men, vs. 72% of adolescent girls and 59% of adolescent boys.)

"Judged unfairly by family."

(Endorsed true by 14% of adult women and 11% of adult men, vs. 43% of adolescent females and 40% of adolescent males.)

These differences in item endorsement patterns between adults and adolescents may be meaningfully viewed in reference to the adolescents' struggles

TABLE 1.1 Items Showing the Largest Differences for Boys in Percentage Endorsement as True Between the Adult (MMPI-2) Normative Sample and the Adolescent (MMPI-A and MMPI-A-RF) Normative Sample

MMPI-A/MMPI-A-RF		% Endorsement as True	
Item No.	Item Content	MMPI-2	MMPI-A
3/125	Feel rested in morning.*	68	35
79/201	Rarely quarrel with family.*	79	46
82/NA	Like loud parties.	45	75
128/130	Like to pick fights.*	16	48
137/92	Been unjustly punished.*	9	42
162/94	When bored, stir things up.*	43	73
208/NA	Often dream about things that shouldn't be talked about.	28	63
296/NA	Have strange thoughts.	15	45
307/139	Obsessed by terrible words.*	9	39
371/239	Too unsure of future to make plans.*	12	42

Source: Abbreviated items reproduced with permission. MMPI®–A Booklet of Abbreviated Items. Copyright © 2005 by the Regents of the University of Minnesota. MMPI-A-RF Test Booklet. Copyright © 2016 by the Regents of the University of Minnesota. Reproduced with the permission of the University of Minnesota Press. All rights reserved. "Minnesota Multiphasic Personality Inventory" and "MMPI" are trademarks owned by the University of Minnesota.

with individuation from the family and the tasks of identity formation and ego maturation. Tables 1.1 and 1.2 provide information on abbreviated items that show at least a 20% endorsement rate difference between adolescents and adults, separated by gender, as noted in the normative data for the MMPI-2, MMPI-A, and MMPI-A-RF for items retained in the latter test form.

The Effects of Maturation on MMPI Response Patterns

The preceding paragraphs discussed the implications of maturation for item-level response patterns. Maturational effects can also be demonstrated at the scale-level, particularly in relation to scales *F*, *Pd*, *Sc*, and *Ma*. These scales have traditionally shown substantial differences in mean values obtained from adolescent and adult samples (Archer, 1984, 1987b). For example, Fig. 1.3 presents the mean raw score values for normal adolescent and adult males and females with their responses and scores on the MMPI-2 60-item *F* scale with findings presented separately by chronological age. As shown in this figure, mean raw score values on *F* continue to decrease as the chronological age of the groups increases. It is most reasonable to interpret these differences as a reflection of maturational processes rather than levels of psychopathology. Thus, MMPI scales are subject to profound maturational effects that may serve to obscure or confound the interpretation of psychopathology based on test scores. In this regard, Achenbach (1978) commented that:

TABLE 1.2 Items Showing the Largest Differences for Girls in Percentage Endorsement as True Between the Adult (MMPI-2) Normative Sample and the Adolescent (MMPI-A and MMPI-A-RF) Normative Samples

MMPI-A/MMPI-A-RF		% Endorsement as True	
Item No.	Item Content	MMPI-2	MMPI-A/MMPI-A-RF
3/125	Feel rested in morning.*	66	29
21/177	Uncontrolled laughing and crying.*	18	64
79/201	Rarely quarrel with family.*	78	37
81/NA	Want to do harmful things.	16	53
82/NA	Like loud parties.	39	80
114/NA	Like collecting plants.	79	43
123/NA	Actions dictated by others.	26	62
162/94	When bored, stir things up.*	43	80
205/NA	Often very restless.	24	62
208/NA	Often dream about things that shouldn't be talked about.	27	65
235/NA	Often strangers look at me critically.	25	65
296/NA	Have strange thoughts.	10	46

Source: Abbreviated items reproduced with permission. MMPI®–A Booklet of Abbreviated Items. Copyright © 2005 by the Regents of the University of Minnesota. MMPI-A-RF Test Booklet. Copyright © 2016 by the Regents of the University of Minnesota. Reproduced with the permission of the University of Minnesota Press. All rights reserved. "Minnesota Multiphasic Personality Inventory" and "MMPI" are trademarks owned by the University of Minnesota.

> An often overlooked complication of the search for individual differences in children is that developmental differences account for significant variance in almost every measurable behavior. One consequence is that measurements repeated on the same subjects more than a few weeks apart are likely to differ as a function of development, even if the subjects show stability with respect to their rank ordering within their cohort. A second consequence is that unless all subjects in a sample are at the same developmental level with respect to the behavior in question, individual differences in the behavior may in fact reflect differences in developmental level rather than trait-like characteristics. A third consequence is that covariation among several measures may merely reflect the variance that they all share with development rather than an independent trait.
>
> (p. 765)

This phenomenon is certainly not limited to adolescent populations, and Colligan, Osborne, Swenson, and Offord (1983) and Colligan and Offord (1992) showed substantial age and maturational effects on standard MMPI scales studied across a broad range of age groups. Figures 1.4 and 1.5, for example, present cross-sectional changes in mean values on Scale 1 and on Scale 9, respectively,

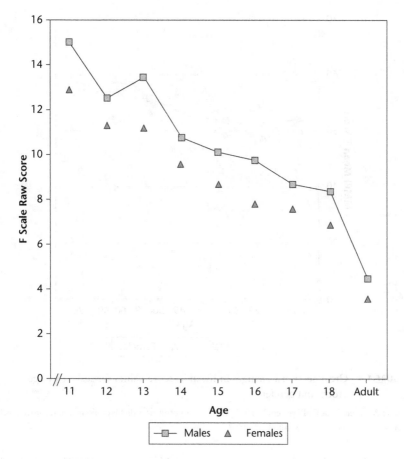

FIGURE 1.3   Mean MMPI-2 *F* scale raw score values for male and female
adolescents and adults.

for males and females across age categories ranging from 18/19 to 70+. Similarly,
Pancoast and Archer (1992) reported substantial differences in mean MMPI profiles for large samples of adolescents, college students, and adults when the mean
values of all three groups are plotted on the standard reference point of adult
norms, as shown in Fig. 1.6. Archer (2005) has concluded that given the fluid
nature of symptomatology during adolescence, long-term predictions based on
MMPI-A findings are ill-advised and that test results are best conceptualized as
reflecting an adolescent's functioning at a moment in time.

Thus far, maturational influences have been discussed in relation to chronological age, but, as is seen later during the description of the development of the
Immaturity scale for the MMPI-A, maturational effects can be clearly demonstrated on MMPI response patterns when chronological age is held constant and
maturity is measured more directly.

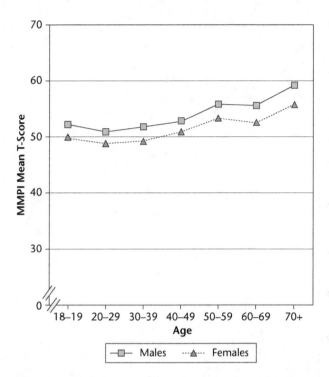

FIGURE 1.4 Cross-sectional changes in mean T-score values for scale *1* by age group and gender.

Source: Adapted from Colligan et al., 1983. Used with permission of Mayo Foundation for Medical Education and Research. All rights reserved.

Another method of examining maturational influences on MMPI scale-level data, which examined patterns of adolescent responses on the Harris–Lingoes subscales profiled on standard adult norms, was provided in research by Pancoast and Archer (1988). Harris and Lingoes (1955) rationally divided six of the MMPI clinical scales (*2, 3, 4, 6, 8,* and *9*) into subscales based on items that appeared logically similar in content. As is discussed later, the Harris–Lingoes subscales are frequently used in clinical practice to determine which content areas of a standard clinical scale were critically endorsed in producing an overall T-score elevation on the parent or standard scale. Adult norms for these subscales have been developed, and adolescent norms are available for the Harris–Lingoes subscales of the MMPI and the MMPI-A. In the Pancoast and Archer study, adolescent values were examined on adult norms in order to evaluate the ways in which adolescent response patterns might differ from those typically found for normal adults. These mean data are based on the adolescent normative data collected by Colligan and Offord (1989) at the Mayo Foundation, and a smaller sample of adolescents collected in Virginia in 1987. Figure 1.7 presents findings

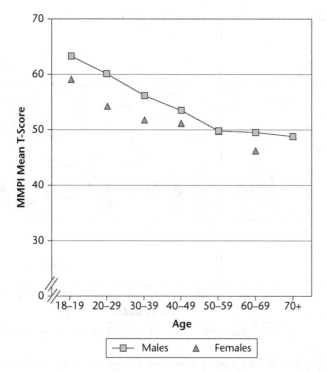

FIGURE 1.5   Cross-sectional changes in mean T-score values for scale *9* by age group and gender.

Source: Adapted from Colligan et al., 1983. Used with the permission of Mayo Foundation for Medical Education and Research. All rights reserved.

for the Harris–Lingoes MMPI subscales on adult norms for MMPI scales *D*, *Hy*, and *Pd*. Results show a general trend for subscales related to the *Pd* scale to show more extreme elevations than subscales related to scales *D* or *Hy*. Although most of the subscales for *Pd* are elevated, the highest elevation occurs for Pd_1 (Familial Discord), which deals with a struggle against familial controls and the perception of marked family conflict. In contrast, there is no elevation for Pd_3 (Social Imperturbability), which deals with denial of social anxiety and the experience of discomfort in social situations. Thus, although normal adolescents' experiences typically involve substantial degrees of family conflict, this struggle appears to be restricted primarily to familial issues and does not include a generalized social discomfort (Pd_3), nor does it necessarily include general conflicts with authority as measured by Pd_2 (Authority Conflicts).

Figure 1.8 presents Harris–Lingoes findings for the remaining three MMPI scales (*Pa*, *Sc*, and *Ma*). Findings from these scales also reveal an interpretable subscale pattern. For *Pa*, the highest subscale is Pa_1 (Persecutory Ideas), which primarily deals with the externalization of responsibility for one's problems and

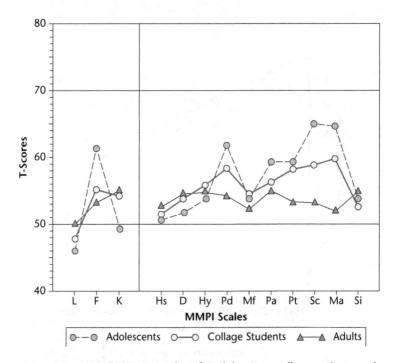

FIGURE 1.6   Mean MMPI T-score values for adolescents, college students, and adults as shown on adult non K-corrected norms.

Source: Pancoast and Archer, 1992. Copyright © by John Wiley & Sons, Inc. Reprinted with permission.

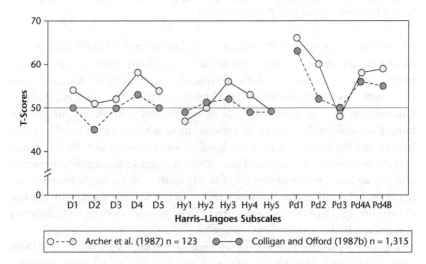

FIGURE 1.7   Harris–Lingoes subscale T-score values for adolescents based on adult norms: Subscales for *D*, *Hy*, and *Pd*.

Source: Pancoast and Archer, 1988. Copyright © by Lawrence Erlbaum Associates. Reprinted with permission.

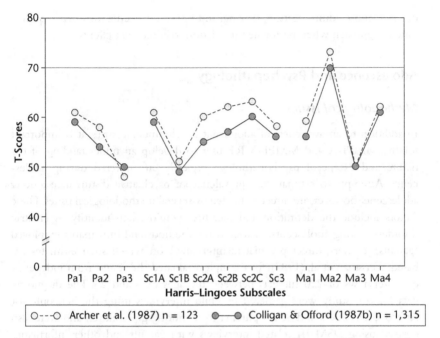

FIGURE 1.8   Harris–Lingoes subscale T–score values for adolescents based on adult norms: Subscales for *Pa*, *Sc*, and *Ma*.

Source: Pancoast and Archer, 1988. Copyright © by Lawrence Erlbaum Associates. Reprinted with permission.

the perception of being treated unfairly and punished by others. On the *Sc* scale, the highest subscale is Sc_2c (Lack of Ego Mastery, Defective Inhibition), which deals with feelings of restlessness, hyperactivity, and not being in control of one's impulses. On the *Ma* scale, the elevated Ma_2 (Psychomotor Acceleration) subscale relates to restlessness, excitement, and pressure for action. Overall, the Harris–Lingoes subscale pattern suggests that the normal adolescent, as evaluated by adult norms or standards, is typically preoccupied with the familial struggle for independence, focused on the perception of family conflicts, and that there is a driven, restless, and excited quality to this developmental experience that often involves a sense of being confined or misunderstood.

In summary, the use of the MMPI-A or MMPI-A-RF with adolescents requires a developmental perspective to understand and interpret test findings. This chapter so far has briefly discussed the dramatic physiological/sexual maturational changes, changes in cognitive processes, and some of the psychological challenges that occur during adolescence. These processes contribute to the observed differences between adults and adolescents in MMPI response patterns on the item, scale, and profile level. Recognition of the influence of these maturational and developmental factors was a major factor in the decision to create specialized forms of the MMPI for the assessment of adolescents, i.e., the MMPI-A and the MMPI-A-RF. A focal point of this book is to accurately discriminate and describe those administration, scoring, and interpretive situations that require a unique approach when performed in relation to adolescent clients.

Adolescence and Psychopathology

Methodological Issues

In addition to an awareness of adolescent developmental issues, it is important for the MMPI-A and MMPI-A-RF user to develop an understanding of the nature and extent of psychopathology typically encountered during adolescence. Attempts to estimate the prevalence of psychiatric disturbance among adolescents, however, are directly affected by several methodological issues. These factors include the definition and measures employed to identify psychiatric disorders among adolescents, as well as the methods and informants employed (parents, teachers, direct psychiatric interviews) on which such estimates are based. Weissman et al. (1987), for example, evaluated the results from independent interviews of 220 subjects between the ages of 6 and 23. The diagnostic data for this study were gathered by child interviews using the Schedule for Affective Disorders and Schizophrenia for School-Age Children and were also derived using DSM-III-related interviews with parents and other informants. The authors noted that considerable discrepancies were found between parents' and children's reports on the nature and degree of the child's psychopathology. They found that children's self-reports or self-descriptions produced evidence of considerably more psychopathology than did the descriptions of the child provided by their parents. Similar findings have also been reported by Reich and Earls (1987) when parental interview results are compared with the results of structured interview techniques used directly with children and adolescents, such as the Diagnostic Interview for Children and Adolescents (DICA). Further, an investigation by Rosenberg and Joshi (1986) found a significant relationship between the degree of marital discord and discrepancies within parental reports of child behavior problems. These researchers reported that the greater the marital difficulty, the greater the difference in adults' ratings of child behavior difficulties on the Achenbach and Edelbrock (1983) Child Behavior Checklist (CBCL). Williams, Hearn, Hostetler, and Ben-Porath (1990) compared structured interview findings on the Diagnostic Interview Schedule for Children (DISC) with self-report measures of psychopathology that included the MMPI. In addition, subjects' parents completed the Achenbach and Edelbrock CBCL, and teachers completed the teacher form of the CBCL. Findings indicated substantial levels of disagreement between these measures in the identification of psychologically disturbed subjects. Cantwell, Lewinsohn, Rohde, and Seeley (1997) evaluated the degree of agreement between parent and adolescent reports of major psychiatric disorders in adolescents from ages 14 through 18 inclusive. A total of 281 parent-adolescent pairs were interviewed separately regarding psychopathological symptoms using a version of the K-SADS (Kaufman et al., 1997) structured interview. Kappa values for parent-adolescent agreement ranged widely by disorder, from .19 for alcohol abuse/dependence to .79 for conduct disorder, with an average Kappa of .42 across all diagnostic categories. Parent-adolescent agreement was not found to be influenced by adolescent's gender, age, parental educational level, age of the onset of the disorder, or the severity of the disorder. Cantwell and his colleagues concluded, similar to earlier researchers, that adolescent self-reports tended to produce higher estimates of psychopathology than did parental reports, particularly for diagnoses that may be classified as internalizing disorders such as major depression or anxiety disorders. In contrast, externalizing disorders such as conduct disorders and oppositional-defiant disorder produced relatively high rates of agreement, and it appeared viable to base estimates of these latter disorders on the consensual reports of adolescents and their parents. Thus, it is clear that our estimates of adolescent psychopathology relate not only to how diagnostic questions are asked, but to whom such questions are addressed. A comprehensive review by Reyes and Kazdin (2005) also underscores that no single measure of psychopathology provides the "gold standard" by which to measure psychopathology in children. Further, these authors underscore the importance of the context in which information concerning a child's functioning is collected (e.g., for purposes of treatment-planning, child custody evaluation, or juvenile justice issues). In this view, the context in which informant data are collected is a significant influence on discrepancies that may occur between sources of information. Despite these methodological problems and limitations, it appears possible to offer some general conclusions concerning the overall prevalence of psychiatric disorders during adolescence, as well as some meaningful observations concerning the form of these disorders.

Prevalence Findings

One of the most widely cited studies on the prevalence of child and adolescent psychiatric disorders is the "Isle of Wight" study reported by Rutter, Graham, Chadwick, and Yule (1976) and summarized by Graham and Rutter (1985). In the Isle of Wight study, a total population of over 2,000 British 14- and 15-year-olds were screened using questionnaires administered to parents and teachers to identify those adolescents with "deviant" adjustment patterns. Adolescents for whom deviant scores were produced on either questionnaire, along with a group of randomly selected control subjects, were then given individual psychiatric assessments involving direct interviews with parents, teachers, and the adolescent. All assessments were conducted in a blind fashion in terms of interviewer's knowledge of the adolescent's membership in the deviant or control groups. The authors estimated that the one year period prevalence rate for psychiatric disorder in their sample was 21%. In general, psychiatric conditions appeared to occur with a slightly higher frequency during adolescence, in contrast to data available for middle childhood. Certain psychiatric conditions, however, did show substantial increases during adolescence, including the occurrence of affective disorders and depressive conditions. Along with the increase in depression, there was also a dramatic increase in the frequency of attempted and completed suicide.

In the United States, Gould, Wunsch-Hitzig, and Dohrenwend (1981) reported that the median prevalence rate for clinical maladjustment among children and adolescents was 11.8%, based on a review of 25 prevalence studies conducted between 1928 and 1975. The majority of these studies employed teachers' reports as a means of identifying psychiatrically disturbed children. Brandenburg, Friedman, and Silver (1989) noted that more recent epidemiologic field studies of child and adolescent psychopathology have employed diverse methods of case definition and have more frequently used a multi-method, multi-stage approach to case identification. Based on a review of eight recent studies, these authors placed the prevalence estimate of psychiatric disorder in children and adolescents at 14% to 20%. More recently, Breton et al., (1999) used the DISC to evaluate 12- to 14-year-old adolescents and their parents in the Quebec Child Mental Health Survey (QCMHS). Similar to earlier studies, these authors found that parents and adolescents had the highest rate of agreement for disruptive or externalizing disorders, and the lowest rate of agreement for the report of internalizing disorders. The overall six months' prevalence rate of psychopathology reported for the 2,400 children and adolescents in this study was 15.8%. Romano, Tremblay, Vitaro, Zoccolillo, and Pagani (2001) examined psychological functioning in a community sample of 1,201 adolescents aged 14 through 17, inclusive. Each of the adolescents and their mothers were administered the DISC to obtain prevalence estimates of DSM-III-R disorders and the amount of perceived impairment associated with each of these disorders. Adolescent females were found to report the highest prevalence of psychiatric disorders (15.5%), in contrast to the prevalence rate of 8.5% reported by male adolescents. Compared to their male counterparts, female adolescents reported significantly higher rates of internalizing disorders, including anxiety and depressive disorders. In contrast, the six-month prevalence of externalizing disorders among male adolescents was significantly higher. Roberts, Attkisson, and Rosenblatt (1998) reviewed 52 studies conducted between 1963 and 1996 that provided estimates of the overall prevalence of child and adolescent psychiatric disorders. Roberts and colleagues noted that while the prevalence estimates for psychopathology among adolescents varied widely, the median prevalence estimate was 15%, with little evidence that the prevalence of psychopathology was significantly changing across time. Roberts, Roberts, and Chan (2009) recently reported the one-year prevalence of psychiatric disorders and associated risk factors among adolescents in a sample of 3,134 youth-parent dyads followed across a one-year period. Incident rates were 2.8% for anxiety, 1.5% for mood disorders, 1.2% for attention-deficit/hyperactivity disorder, 2.9% for substance abuse/dependence disorders, and a total of 7.5% for one or more DSM-IV disorders. The most consistent factors related to the incidence of psychopathology involved stress indicators, particularly family stress variables. Costello, Copeland, and Angold (2012) reviewed research reporting the prevalence of psychiatric disorders for children, adolescents, and young adults in studies published since 1997. Their overall estimate, consistent with results from earlier studies, was that roughly one adolescent in five manifests a psychiatric disorder. Kazdin (2000) noted evidence of some gender differences in the rate and expression of psychopathology. For example, the prevalence of depression and eating disorders is much higher for females than males in the adolescent age grouping. Zahn-Waxler, Shirtcliff, and Marceau (2008) have also reported gender-related differences with early-onset disorders such as conduct disorders and autism showing a higher male prevalence, whereas adolescent-onset disorders such as anxiety and depression reflect a markedly higher female prevalence. The authors noted that boys and girls show gender differences in the types, rates, co-morbidities, antecedents, correlates, and trajectories for these disorders.

Beyond these prevalence studies of general psychopathology, several studies have attempted to identify the relative prevalence of specific types of psychiatric symptomatology or disorder within adolescent samples. Kashani et al. (1987) utilized both child and parent structured interviews to determine the prevalence of psychiatric disorder among 150 adolescents selected in a community sample. Roughly 41% were found to have at least one DSM-III diagnosis, and 19% were judged to have a diagnosis *and* to be functionally impaired to a degree indicating the need for psychiatric treatment. The three most common diagnoses found in this total sample were anxiety disorder (8.7%), conduct disorder (8.7%), and depression (combined categories of major depression and dysthymic disorder) with a frequency of 8%.

Kashani and Orvaschel (1988) randomly selected 150 adolescents between the ages of 14 and 16 from a roster of 1,703 students in a midwestern public school system. In this study of anxiety disorders during adolescence, both children and their parents were interviewed in their homes using the standard and parental interview forms of the DICA. Interview results were videotaped and scored by three trained raters with established interrater reliability. Additionally, participants received several objective personality assessment instruments related to self-concept, affect, and coping. Seventeen percent of this sample were found to meet the criteria for one or more forms of psychiatric disorder, and 8.7% were identified as positive cases of anxiety disorder. The most frequently occurring anxiety disorder in this sample was overanxious disorder. Results of this study tend to support the view that anxiety disorders are a major form of psychopathology in adolescent populations. In other research, Hillard, Slomowitz, and Levi (1987) studied 100 adult and 100 adolescent admissions to a university hospital psychiatric emergency service. The authors reported that adolescents were less likely to receive diagnoses of personality disorders or psychoses, but were more likely to receive diagnoses involving conduct disorder and adjustment disorder. Further, self-destructive ideation or behavior was present in 40% of the adolescents seen in the emergency room visits.

Lewinsohn, Hops, Roberts, Seeley, and Andrews (1993) reported findings from the Oregon Adolescent Depression Project (OADP), a large-scale community-based investigation of the epidemiology of depression and other psychiatric disorders in a population of approximately 10,200 students in nine high schools in two urban communities in west central Oregon. The authors presented data on the prevalence of psychiatric disorders in the 14 to 18 age range, which coincidentally corresponds to the age grouping employed in the MMPI-A normative sample. Additionally, an important characteristic of this study was that it relied exclusively on diagnostic information provided by adolescents in structured interview techniques and standardized questionnaires. Overall, findings from this study indicated that 11.2% of girls and 7.8% of boys met the criterion for a psychiatric diagnosis based on interview findings. Among these psychiatric diagnoses, major depression, unipolar depression, anxiety disorders, and substance abuse disorders were particularly prevalent. In general, female students were more likely than male students to receive diagnoses of unipolar depression, anxiety disorders, eating disorders, and adjustment disorders, whereas boys were more likely to receive a diagnosis of disruptive behavior disorder. Lewinsohn, Klein, and Seeley (1995) followed up this research by evaluating the self-reports of 1,709 adolescents between the ages of 14 and 18 on the SADS (Endicott & Spitzer, 1978) to specifically focus on the prevalence and clinical characteristics of bipolar and manic disorder. The lifetime prevalence of bipolar disorder in this Oregon sample (primarily bipolar disorder and cyclothymia) was approximately 1%. Costello and colleagues (Costello et al., 1996) found a three-month prevalence rate for any DSM-III-R Axis I disorder of 20.3% in a sample of 9-, 11-, and 13-year-old boys and girls in the southeastern United States. The more common diagnoses were anxiety disorders (5.7%), enuresis (5.1%), tic disorders (4.2%), conduct disorders (3.3%), oppositional-defiant disorders (2.7%), and hyperactivity (1.9%).

The issue of suicidal ideation and behavior has received special focus in a number of studies of adolescence. Friedman, Asnis, Boeck, and DiFiore (1987), for example, investigated 300 high school students who were anonymously surveyed regarding their experiences with suicidal ideation and behaviors. Roughly 53% of this sample stated that they had thought about killing themselves but did not actually try, and 9% of the total sample stated that they had attempted suicide at least once. These findings indicated that suicidal ideation is relatively common among adolescents, but also suggested that actual suicide attempts were disturbingly frequent. In this regard, Kimmel and Weiner (1985) noted that suicide is the third most common cause of death for adolescents aged 15 to 19, with the suicide rate particularly marked for White male adolescents. Further, the rate of adolescent suicide has nearly doubled between 1960 and 1975, and about 10% of adolescents seen in mental health clinics, and more than

25% of those admitted to psychiatric units in general hospitals, have threatened or attempted suicide (Kimmel & Weiner, 1985). Boys appear four times more likely than girls to actually kill themselves, whereas girls appear three times more likely to make a suicide attempt. Within the MMPI-A normative sample, 21% of boys and 38% of girls responded true to abbreviated Item 177, "Think about killing self."

The age-specific U.S. mortality rate for suicide occurring in 1990 was 0.8 per 100,000 for 10- to 14-year-olds, and 3.7 per 100,000 for adolescents in the 15- to 19-year-old age grouping (Center for Disease Control and Prevention (CDC), 2007). The CDC (2007) reported a suicide mortality rate in 2004 of 1.7 per 100,000 for 10- to 14-year-olds, and 12.6 per 100,000 for adolescents ages 15 to 19, inclusive. In this latter age grouping, boys were four times more likely than girls to commit suicide, while girls were twice as likely to attempt suicide. Later data (CDC, 2009b) show that these gender disparities have remained constant.

In 2011, a national survey of adolescents (CDC, 2012) in 9th through 12th grade found that 15.8% of these adolescents reported the occurrence of suicidal ideation during the 12 months preceding the survey. Further, 12.8% of all students reported they had made a plan concerning how they would attempt suicide during this period, and 7.8% reported one or more actual suicide attempts. Finally, 2.4% of the students reported a suicide attempt that resulted in an injury or medical problem requiring medical evaluation and/or treatment (CDC, 2012). In addition, some important demographic patterns have emerged from national studies on mortality rates. For example, for the period 2005 through 2009, American Indian and Alaskan Native adolescents are more likely than adolescents from other ethnic backgrounds to commit suicide.

Several general conclusions seem possible from these and other investigations of psychopathology during adolescence. First, the majority of adolescents do not show evidence of psychopathology that would result in psychiatric diagnosis. The rate of psychopathology during adolescence appears "only slightly higher than that found earlier in childhood or later in life" (Petersen & Hamburg, 1986, p. 491). There is evidence that the frequency and severity of depression does increase during adolescence, and there is a marked increase in both suicide attempts and suicide fatalities during this period of development. Several disorders tend to make their first appearance during adolescence, including anorexia nervosa, bipolar illness, bulimia, obsessive-compulsive disorder, schizophrenia, and substance abuse, although other disorders, such as enuresis and encopresis, become less frequent (Burke, Burke, Regier, & Rae, 1990; Graham & Rutter, 1985). Although the rate of anxiety disorders and conduct disorders may show little change during adolescence, the expression of symptoms related to these disorders does change. The rate of specific phobic disorders appears to decrease during adolescence, whereas conduct disorders more frequently involve violence (Graham & Rutter, 1985; Petersen & Hamburg, 1986).

The "Storm and Stress" Model and Psychopathology

G. Stanley Hall (1904), considered by many to be the father of child psychology in the United States, was the formulator of the *Sturm und Drang* or Storm and Stress model of adolescent development. This view, consistent with that of Anna Freud (1958), postulates that adolescence is typically accompanied by emotional upheavals and behavioral turbulence. Anna Freud postulated that adolescents who did not demonstrate turbulent features of adjustment were at risk for the development of serious psychopathological symptoms in adulthood. Freud's formulation of this view is represented in her statement that "the upholding of a steady equilibrium during the process [of adolescence] is, in itself, abnormal" (p. 275). Freud's view of adolescent development may be best illustrated by the following quotation:

> I take it that it is normal for an adolescent to behave for a considerable length of time in an inconsistent and unpredictable manner; to fight his impulses and to accept them; to ward them off successfully and to be overrun by them; to love his parents and to hate them; to revolt against them and to be dependent on them; to be deeply ashamed to acknowledge his mother before others and, unexpectedly, to desire heart-to-heart talks with her; to thrive on imitation and identification with others while searching unceasingly for his own identity; to be more idealistic, artistic, generous, unselfish than he will ever be again, but also the opposite - self-centered, egoistic, calculating. Such fluctuations between extreme opposites would be deemed highly abnormal at any other time of life. At this time they may signify no more than that an adult structure of personality takes a long time to emerge, that the ego of the individual in question does not cease to experiment and is in no hurry to close down on possibilities.
>
> (p. 276)

Blos (1962) also felt that the psychiatric symptoms typically presented during adolescence were often ill-defined, unstable, and transitory in nature and did not signify stable markers of psychiatric illness. Similarly, Erikson (1956) proposed that the adolescent's struggles for self-definition frequently resulted in deviations from expected or normal behavior, which he termed *identity diffusion* or *identity confusion*, and differentiated from stable psychopathology.

Many have objected to the Storm and Stress view of adolescent development, particularly the implication that normal adolescent development is characterized by substantial turbulence and lability. Bandura (1964), for example, argued that many adolescents establish more trusting and relaxed relations with their parents during adolescence while also increasing contact with peer groups. Thus, the shifting away from the nuclear family to the peer group is not necessarily and inevitably a source of family tension. Offer and Offer (1975) investigated suburban male adolescents and found that, although transient episodes of non-disabling depression and anxiety were common, only 20% of adolescents demonstrated moderate to severe symptomatology. This estimate, as we have seen, is generally consistent with reports of the prevalence of significant psychopathology in adolescent populations. Further, these investigators also found that 20% of their sample did not appear to experience any significant turmoil during their adolescent development and were able to successfully cope with the wide variety of challenges it presented. Most recently, Casey and Caudle (2013) cautioned against the over-generalization that all adolescents experience similar degrees of storm and stress. They noted that adolescents' ability to exercise self-control, reflected in the capacity to suppress inappropriate emotions, desires and actions, varies widely and is a reflection of behavioral and genetic factors that influence the brain's ability to adapt to changing environmental demands

Rutter et al. (1976) examined the concept of adolescent turmoil within the context of their findings in the Isle of Wight study of 14- and 15-year-olds. These authors concluded that parent-child alienation was not a feature common to adolescents in general but, rather, appeared restricted to adolescents who already showed signs of psychiatric problems. On the other hand, "inner turmoil," which was defined by the researchers as feelings of misery and self-depreciation, appeared to be frequently associated with adolescence. The authors concluded that

> adolescent turmoil is a fact, not a fiction, but its psychiatric importance has probably been overestimated in the past. Certainly it would be most unwise to assume that adolescents will grow out of their problems to a greater extent than do younger children.

> (p. 55)

In their review of the literature on adolescent psychopathology, Weiner and Del Gaudio (1976) offered the following three conclusions: First, psychiatric symptoms are not a normal feature of adolescence; second, boundaries between normal and abnormal adolescence may be drawn despite inherent difficulties; and third, rather than a passing phase, psychological disturbance during adolescence typically requires treatment for remission. This concept has also been expressed by Kimmel and Weiner (1985) in their statement that

> by and large, people remain basically the same in how they think, handle interpersonal relationships, and are perceived by others. For better or worse, adults tend to display many of the same personality characteristics and same relative level of adjustment they did as adolescents.

> (p. 449)

Viewed within the context of our data on the prevalence of psychiatric disorders during adolescence, the debate surrounding the stability of adolescent symptomatology appears to center on the distinction between psychopathology as defined by DSM-5 categories, and terms such as *Turbulence* and *Storm and Stress*. Incidence estimates of psychopathology during adolescence appear to fall within a reasonably stable range of 12% to 22% (Costello, Copeland, & Angold, 2012; National Institute of Mental Health, 1990; Powers, Hauser, & Kilner, 1989). The adolescents identified in these studies do, in fact, appear to suffer from stable psychiatric disorders that would not be expected to remit without active and effective treatment. For example, it is estimated that almost half of children or adolescents receiving conduct disorder diagnoses will become antisocial adults, and that untreated depression and anxiety disorders during adolescence often persist into adulthood (National Institute of Mental Health, 1990). Further, a study by Hofstra, Van der Ende, and Verhulst (2002) also demonstrated a continuity between child and adult psychopathology in a sample of 1,578 children and adolescents selected from the Dutch general population and followed up 14 years later. These authors found that childhood behavior and emotional problems were related to psychiatric diagnoses in adulthood. The strongest associations between specific childhood problem areas and adult diagnoses were found for social problems in girls which were generally predictive of the occurrence of DSM disorders. Rule-breaking behavior in boys was also predictive of later mood disorder and/or disruptive disorders in adulthood. On the other hand, many more adolescents go through a period of turbulence and lability during adolescent development that would *not* qualify as a DSM-defined disorder, but is commonly associated with accomplishing the mastery of the various adaptational challenges presented during this developmental period. Although it is clear that the dividing line between these two groups is frequently blurred and difficult to discern, it serves little purpose to view these groups as homogeneous in terms of the severity of their symptoms or implications for long-term adjustment. It might be expected that MMPI-A and/or MMPI-A-RF test results should prove to be a substantial value to the clinician in rendering this important diagnostic distinction.

Stability of Adolescents' MMPI/MMPI-A Features

Whether adolescent symptomatology is stable or transitory, it appears relatively clear that those features and characteristics measured by the MMPI or MMPI-A in the assessment of adolescents serve to accurately describe the teenager at the moment of testing (e.g., Archer, 2005). Adolescents' test scores often do not, however, provide the types of data necessary to make accurate long-term predictions concerning psychopathology or personality functioning. The MMPI-A and MMPI-A-RF are best used as methods of deriving an overall estimate and current description of adolescent psychopathology, rather than as a method of making long-range predictions regarding future adjustment.

An illustration of the variability inherent in adolescent personality structure may be found in data reported by Hathaway and Monachesi (1963) in their classic study of adolescents' MMPI response patterns. These authors evaluated

15,300 Grade 9 children within Minnesota school systems between 1948 and 1954, and retested a subset of 3,856 of these students in Grade 12 during the 1956–57 school year. Examining adolescents who were tested in both the 9th and 12th grade, Hathaway and Monachesi found test-retest correlation coefficients ranging from the low to mid .30s on scales such as *Pd* and *Pa*, to values in the high .50s and low .60s for scale *Si*. Hathaway and Monachesi concluded that these correlations underscored the degree of change that may occur within an adolescent's MMPI profile, reflecting the fluid nature of adolescents' overall personality organizations. Hathaway and Monachesi noted, however, that the stability of an adolescent's profile tends to increase when T-score values are substantially elevated in the initial testing. Thus, clinically elevated profile characteristics may be subject to less change than marginally elevated profile features. Even in clinical or preclinical adolescent populations, however, substantial change often occurs in MMPI profile features. Similar to the Hathaway and Monachesi results, Lowman, Galinsky, and Gray-Little (1980) reported that relatively pathological MMPI profiles of eighth graders in a rural county in North Carolina were generally not predictive of level of psychological disturbance or achievement for this sample at young adulthood.

Hathaway and Monachesi (1963) indicated that MMPI profiles produced by an adolescent often change across time because of the "transient organization of the personality" during adolescence. They noted that such psychometric changes, rather than indicating difficulties in test construction, indicate the sensitivity of instruments such as the MMPI to the ongoing change in maturational process. These phenomena do, however, limit the utility of tests such as the MMPI when such instruments are applied in a long-range predictive, rather than descriptive, manner.

Summary

This chapter has provided a brief review of adolescent development and issues related to developmental psychopathology during this maturational stage. As is discussed in the following chapters, the MMPI-A and MMPI-A-RF present a variety of features that facilitate the accurate identification and description of psychopathology among adolescents. For example, both test instruments represent modifications of the original MMPI to improve item clarity and relevance for adolescents, and incorporate new scales of psychopathology of particular relevance to adolescents such as the Conduct Disorders, School Problems, and Immaturity scales on the MMPI-A and the Negative School Attitudes, Conduct Problems, and Negative Peer Influence scales on the MMPI-A-RF. As stressed throughout this chapter, however, these instruments improve the assessment of adolescent psychopathology when employed by clinicians who are sensitive to the developmental issues of this unique population.

2

DEVELOPMENT OF THE MMPI, MMPI-A, AND MMPI-A-RF

Development of the MMPI

Work on the instrument that was to become the Minnesota Multiphasic Personality Inventory (MMPI) was begun in 1937 by Stark R. Hathaway, a psychologist, and J. C. McKinley, a neuropsychiatrist. The test authors were stimulated to develop a "personality inventory" based on their pursuit of several objectives. First, they had noticed that a large proportion of patients presenting for medical treatment manifested "one or more complaints that turn out to be psychoneurotic in nature" (McKinley & Hathaway, 1943, p. 161). The two test authors sought to develop an instrument that would be useful in identifying and describing these patients in a manner that was more efficient and effective than the psychiatric interview techniques traditionally used for psychological evaluations of medical patients. Apparently, Hathaway also believed that such an instrument might assist researchers in attempting to evaluate the efficacy of new treatment interventions by allowing for the systematic matching and evaluation of treatment groups. For example, Hathaway (1964), in reference to the use of insulin therapy, which was prevalent in the 1930s, noted:

> There was no way that our hospital staff could select a group of patients for the new treatment who would be surely comparable in diagnosis and severity of illness to those from some other setting. It became an obvious possibility that one might devise a personality test which, like intelligence tests, would somehow stabilize the identification of the illness and provide an estimate of its severity. Toward this problem the MMPI research was initiated.
>
> (p. 205)

Finally, Hathaway was also interested in the development of a personality assessment instrument that could assess changes in symptomatology across time. Further, when such a measure was administered at various stages of the treatment process, it would provide the clinician with an index of therapeutic change. In this regard, Hathaway (1965) stated that the MMPI was designed to serve as an

> objective aid in the routine psychiatric case workup of adult patients and as a method of determining the severity of the condition. As a corollary to this, the inventory was expected to provide an objective estimate of psychothera-peutic effect and other changes in the severity of their conditions over time.
> (p. 463)

As noted by Colligan et al. (1983), the first published reference to the MMPI project was listed as a footnote to a 1939 paper (Hathaway, 1939). The MMPI was initially referred to as the "Medical and Psychiatric Inventory," later titled the "Multiphasic Personality Schedule" in a 1940 paper by Hathaway and McKinley, and finally designated the Minnesota Multiphasic Personality Inventory in the 1943 publication of the instrument through the University of Minnesota Press. Hathaway and McKinley had initial difficulty in finding a publisher for the MMPI, and Hathaway noted that "Dr. McKinley and I had faith sufficient to carry us through several rejections before the University of Minnesota Press finally undertook publication" (cited in Dahlstrom & Welsh, 1960, p. vii). Despite this humble beginning, the MMPI has become the most widely used objective personality assessment instrument across a wide variety of clinical settings (Lees-Haley, Smith, Williams, & Dunn, 1996; Lubin, Larsen, & Matarazzo, 1984; Lubin, Larsen, Matarazzo, & Seever, 1985; Lubin, Wallis, & Paine, 1971; Piotrowski & Keller, 1989, 1992). Butcher (1987a) estimated that over 10,000 books and articles have been produced on the MMPI and Butcher and Owen (1978) reported that 84% of all research on personality inventory instruments has been focused on the MMPI. Butcher and Williams (2000) noted that by 1989 there were over 140 MMPI translations in 46 countries.

Historical Context

In their development of the MMPI, Hathaway and McKinley were sensitive to many of the problems that existed in the personality inventories of that era. For example, the Woodworth Personal Data Sheet (1920) was a 169-item, self-rating scale designed to detect neurotic maladjustment used in screening draftees during World War I. Respondents answered *yes* or *no* to the series of questions, and the total number of positive answers was used to determine whether the individual was referred for additional psychiatric interview. Following the development of the Woodworth Personal Data Sheet, several other rationally developed questionnaires were created, including the Bell Adjustment Inventory (Bell, 1934), and the Bernreuter Personality Inventory (Bernreuter, 1933). Rational scale construction involves the selection of items that logically or rationally appear to measure important areas. The selection of these items is based on the developer's theory, clinical experience, and intuition. A fundamental assumption inherent in this test construction method was that the items actually measured what the authors assumed they measured. Over time, however, it became clear that items selected exclusively on a rational basis were not always indicative of deviant behavior, and that test subjects did not always respond accurately and honestly to test instruments. As noted by Greene (1980), critical studies and reviews appeared by several authors, including Landis and Katz (1934) and Super (1942) that strongly criticized the effectiveness of these rationally derived personality inventories. For example, test scores produced by normal subjects and subjects in clinical settings were often found to show little difference on these measures.

Hathaway and McKinley were also aware of the rudimentary efforts to develop validity scales as employed in the Humm–Wadsworth Temperament Scale (Humm & Wadsworth, 1935). This symptom checklist measure contained a "no count" score consisting of the number of items or symptoms denied (i.e., not endorsed by the subject) in responding to the instrument. Thus, a high no count score was seen as reflective of a subject who was excessively guarded or defensive, whereas a very low no count score might indicate a tendency to exaggerate or overreport symptoms. Additionally, Hathaway and McKinley began work on the MMPI following Strong's (1927, 1943) use of criterion groups in the development of a vocational or occupational-interest inventory (i.e., the Strong Vocational Interest Blank). Thus, Hathaway and McKinley had available a model of scale construction that stood in contrast to the rational development procedures that had typically been used for personality measures. They were also motivated by the need for the creation of an inventory that would be of practical use in clinical settings. By the late 1930s, much of personality assessment was seen as irrelevant by applied psychologists, as acknowledged by Hathaway (1965) in his comment that "it was so widely accepted that personality inventories were valueless that some program directors did not feel that any course work in their nature and interpretation was worth the effort" (p. 461).

Development Methods for the Original MMPI

Greene (2011) dramatically noted that "Out of the psychiatric wilderness of the early 1930s appeared two men, Stark Hathaway and J. C. McKinley, who, under the banner of empiricism, waged a new battle for the scientific advancement of personality assessment" (p. 5). Numerous descriptions of the developmental procedures used in the creation of the MMPI have been extensively documented by authors including Colligan et al. (1983), Dahlstrom, Welsh, and Dahlstrom (1972, 1975), Friedman, Webb, and Lewak (1989), Friedman, Lewak, Nichols, and Webb (2001), Graham (2000), and Greene (2000). The procedures employed by Hathaway and McKinley are therefore only briefly summarized in this text.

A salient feature of Hathaway and McKinley's approach to the creation of the MMPI was their use of the *criterion keying* method, or the empirical method of inventory construction. Indeed, the MMPI is usually cited as the outstanding example of this test construction method (e.g., Anastasi, 1982). In the criterion keying approach, items are presented to two or more groups of subjects. One subject group serves as a criterion group that manifests a defining diagnosis or characteristic that the test is meant to measure, and there are one or more comparison groups that do not manifest the trait or characteristic under study. Responses of the criterion and comparison groups are compared, and items are then selected for inventory membership that empirically demonstrate significant differences in response frequency. As noted by Friedman et al. (2001), scales constructed utilizing this methodology are usually named after the criterion group. For example, if the criterion group consisted of clinically depressed patients, the scale would probably be labeled a *Depression scale*. Further, scoring is usually accomplished by assigning one point to each item answered in the direction that is more frequently endorsed by criterion subjects. Additionally, the higher an individual scores on this type of measure, the more items he or she has answered in a direction consistent with that of the criterion group members.

Much as earlier researchers did, Hathaway and McKinley began their construction of the MMPI by generating an extensive pool of items from which various scales might be constructed. Specifically, they created nearly 1,000 self-referenced statements inspired from a wide variety of sources, including psychiatric examination forms, psychiatric textbooks, previously published scales of personality and social attitudes, and their own clinical experience (Hathaway & McKinley, 1940). They then reduced this list to 504 items by deleting items that duplicated content, or that the authors subjectively felt had relatively little significance or value. Thus, the authors used a subjective and rational method to create the initial item pool. To simplify the task of identifying item duplication, Hathaway and McKinley constructed 25 content categories for the original MMPI item pool, which are shown in Table 2.1. In addition to the items shown in Table 2.1, 55 items were subsequently added "primarily related to masculinity-femininity" (McKinley & Hathaway, 1943, p. 162) and 9 items were apparently deleted (Colligan et al., 1983), resulting in the creation of a final pool of 550 items. These items were then employed to construct scales by comparing the item responses of normal individuals against those of psychiatric patients who held membership in relatively homogeneous clinical criterion groups.

Normative Groups

The normal criterion group primarily used in developing the MMPI consisted of individuals ($N = 724$) who were visiting friends or relatives receiving treatment at the University of Minnesota Hospital. These subjects, ages 16 years and

TABLE 2.1 Content Categories of the Original 504 MMPI Items as Determined by Hathaway and McKinley

No.	Category	Number of Items
1	General health	9
2	General neurologic	19
3	Cranial nerves	11
4	Motility and coordination	6
5	Sensibility	5
6	Vasomotor, trophic, speech, secretory	10
7	Cardiorespiratory	5
8	Gastrointestinal	11
9	Genitourinary	6
10	Habits	20
11	Family and marital	29
12	Occupational	18
13	Educational	12
14	Sexual attitudes	19
15	Religious attitudes	20
16	Political attitudes—law and order	46
17	Social attitudes	72
18	Affect, depressive	32
19	Affect, manic	24
20	Obsessive, compulsive	15
21	Delusions, hallucinations, illusions, ideas of reference	31
22	Phobias	29
23	Sadistic, masochistic	7
24	Morale	33
25	Items to "indicate whether the individual is trying to place himself in an improbably acceptable or unacceptable light"	15

Source: From Colligan, Osborne, Swenson, and Offord (1983). Adapted with permission of Mayo Foundation for Medical Education and Research. All rights reserved.

older, were approached in the halls or waiting rooms of the hospital and invited to participate in the research project if preliminary screening indicated that they were not receiving treatment for any psychiatric or medical illness. The overall age, gender, and marital status of this University of Minnesota group was reported to be comparable to the 1930 United States Census findings (Hathaway & McKinley, 1940). Dahlstrom et al. (1972) described the Minnesota normative sample as follows:

> In 1940, such a Minnesota normal adult was about thirty-five years old, was married, lived in a small town or rural area, had had eight years of general schooling, and worked at a skilled or semiskilled trade (or was married to a man with such an occupational level).

(p. 8)

In addition, Hathaway and McKinley collected data from two other samples of "normals." One of these samples consisted of 265 high school graduates who were coming to the University of Minnesota Testing Bureau for college counseling and guidance, and 265 individuals who were contacted through the local Works Progress Administration (WPA), a federally funded employment project. This latter group consisted of skilled workers who were "all white-collar workers and were used as controls for urban background and socioeconomic level" (Dahlstrom & Welsh, 1960, p. 46).

Colligan et al. (1983) noted that the original normative data collected by Hathaway and McKinley are no longer available. However, a subsample of these data, referred to as the Minnesota normal "purified" sample, was developed by Hathaway and Briggs (1957). The Hathaway and Briggs sample consists of 225 males and 315 females drawn from the general Minnesota normal sample. These data have been preserved and were the basis for the development of Appendix K in the MMPI-2 Manual (Butcher et al., 1989). Appendix K provides T-score values, based on the purified sample of the original Hathaway/McKinley norms, for MMPI-2 Basic scales.

Clinical Scales

The clinical criterion groups utilized by Hathaway and McKinley defined the eight MMPI Basic Scales and consisted of carefully selected psychiatric patients in the following diagnostic categories: Hypochondriasis (scale *1*), Depression (scale *2*), Hysteria (scale *3*), Psychopathic Deviate (scale *4*), Paranoia (scale *6*), Psychasthenia (scale *7*), Schizophrenia (scale *8*), and Hypomania (scale *9*). Detailed descriptions of these clinical criterion groups were provided by Colligan et al. (1983), Dahlstrom and Dahlstrom (1980), Dahlstrom et al. (1972), and Greene (1980, 2000). In addition, a group consisting of "homosexual invert males" was employed by Hathaway and McKinley in the development of the Masculinity–Femininity scale (scale *5*). Finally, the Social Introversion–Extroversion scale, developed by Drake (1946), was eventually added as the 10th Basic Scale of the MMPI (scale *Si*). The *Si* scale remains the only standard scale that was developed outside of the original Hathaway group, and the only scale for which a psychiatric criterion group was not obtained (Colligan et al., 1983).

Validity Scales

In addition to the 10 standard clinical scales, Hathaway and McKinley also developed 4 validity scales for the MMPI, the purpose of which was to detect deviant test-taking attitudes or response sets. These measures included the Cannot Say or (*?*) scale, which was simply the total number of MMPI items that were either omitted or endorsed as both true and false, and the *L* or Lie scale, which consisted of 15 rationally derived items that present common human faults or foibles. The *L* scale was designed to detect crude attempts to present oneself in an unrealistically favorable manner. The *F* scale was composed of 64 items that were selected because they were endorsed in a particular direction by 10% or fewer of the Minnesota normal group. Hathaway and McKinley (1943) suggested that high scores on the *F* scale would imply that the clinical scale profile was invalid because the subject was careless, unable to comprehend the items, or that extensive scoring errors had occurred. The T-score conversion values for *F*, like those for the Cannot Say scale and scale *L*, were arbitrarily assigned by McKinley and Hathaway rather than based on a linear transformation of raw score data from the Minnesota normal sample.

The final validity scale developed for the MMPI was the *K* scale. The *K* scale was developed by selecting 25 male and 25 female psychiatric patients who produced normal-range clinical scale values (i.e., T-score values ≤ 69 on all clinical scales). These subjects, therefore, could be considered to be false negatives (Meehl & Hathaway, 1946). The profiles of these false-negative patients were compared with the responses of the Minnesota normal cases, that is, true negatives. Item analysis revealed 22 items that discriminated the "true- and false-negative profiles in their item endorsements by at least 30%" (Dahlstrom et al., 1972, p. 124). Eight additional items were eventually added to the *K* scale to aid in the accurate discrimination of depressed and schizophrenic patients from subjects in the normative group. The main function of the *K* scale was to improve the discriminative power of the clinical scales in detecting psychopathology, and varying proportions of the *K* scale raw score total have traditionally been added to scales *1*, *4*, *7*, *8*, and *9* when using the *K*-correction procedure with adult respondents. The standard validity and clinical scales are discussed in more detail in later chapters of this book dealing with validity assessment and clinical interpretation strategies.

Important Features

Before leaving the topic of the development of the original form of the MMPI, two general points should be made regarding characteristics of the instrument that have largely contributed to its popularity among clinical practitioners. First, as discussed by Graham (2012), it rapidly became apparent following the publication of the MMPI that its interpretation was considerably more complex than was initially anticipated. Rather than producing an elevated score on a single clinical scale, many psychiatric patients produced multiple elevations involving several scales. Thus, for example, depressed patients often produced elevations on the Depression scale, but also obtained high scores on other standard clinical scales of this instrument. According to Graham, this phenomenon resulted from several factors, including a high degree of intercorrelation among the MMPI standard scales. Indeed, a variety of approaches have been used with MMPI data over the past 40 years in attempts to yield useful diagnostic information. No approach has produced more than modest correspondence between MMPI-derived diagnoses and psychiatric diagnoses based on clinical judgment or standard diagnostic interviews (e.g., Pancoast, Archer, & Gordon, 1988).

For these reasons, the MMPI has come to be used in a manner different from that originally envisioned by Hathaway and McKinley, particularly in terms of profile interpretation. Specifically, the usefulness of the particular scale labels or names has been deemphasized, a practice reflected in the tendency of MMPI interpreters to refer to MMPI scales by their numbers rather than criterion group labels (e.g., references to scale 7 rather than to the Psychasthenia scale). Accompanying this change, numerous researchers have set about establishing the meaning of clinical scales through extensive clinical correlate research. In this research approach, the actual extra test correlates of the MMPI scales are identified through empirical research efforts based on careful studies of individuals who produce certain patterns of MMPI scale elevations. The net impact of this shift in interpretive focus has been that the MMPI is standardly used as a *descriptive* instrument, and that this descriptive capacity of the MMPI is based on the accumulation of numerous research studies concerning the test characteristics of specific MMPI configuration groups. As noted by Graham (2012):

> Thus, even though the MMPI was not particularly successful in terms of its original purpose (differential diagnosis of clinical groups believed in the 1930s to be discrete psychiatric types), the test can be used to generate descriptions of and inferences about individuals (normal persons and patients) on the basis of their scores. It is this behavioral description approach to the utilization of the test in everyday practice that has led to its great popularity among practicing clinicians.
>
> (p. 6)

It should also be noted that this approach to the interpretation of the MMPI has linked the usefulness of the test not to aspects of its original psychometric construction, but rather to the massive accumulation of research literature that has been developed for this test instrument. Thus, the major clinical value of the MMPI lies in what we have come to know about what test results "mean."

A second important feature of the MMPI concerns the development of a broad variety of validity scales and indices through which the consistency and accuracy of the clients' self-reports can be evaluated. The MMPI was among the first personality assessment instruments to strongly emphasize the use of validity scales to assist in determining the interpretability of clinical test findings. Thus, the MMPI interpreter can estimate the degree to which test findings are influenced by a number of factors related to the respondents' willingness and capacity to respond in a valid manner. This feature, in turn, has allowed the extension of the MMPI to assessment issues not originally envisioned by Hathaway and McKinley. These latter tasks have included the psychological screening of individuals in personnel and forensic settings, situations that differ substantially from those of the typical psychological treatment setting. Beyond the original four validity scales, numerous other MMPI measures have been subsequently developed to assess issues related to technical profile validity (e.g., the Carelessness scale and the Test-Retest Index). Many of these have been reviewed extensively by Greene (1989a, 2000).

MMPI-2

The MMPI was updated and restandardized, resulting in the release of the MMPI-2 in 1989 (Butcher et al., 1989), 46 years after the original publication of the instrument. The revision involved a modernization of the content and language of test items, the elimination of objectionable items, and the creation of new scales, including a series of 15 Content scales (Archer, 1992; Nichols, 1992). The development of the MMPI-2 also involved the collection of a nationally representative normative data sample of 2,600 adult men and women throughout the United States. The MMPI-2 contains 567 items that heavily overlap with items from both the original form of the MMPI and the adolescent form of the MMPI (MMPI-A). Several comprehensive guides to the MMPI-2 are now available (Butcher, 2005; Graham, 2012; Greene, 2011; Nichols, 2001), and a text has been specifically devoted to a description of the MMPI-2 Content scales (Butcher, Graham, Williams, & Ben-Porath, 1990). In addition, a research base has been developed for the interpretation of MMPI-2 profile codes (e.g., Archer, Griffin, & Aiduk, 1995; Graham, Ben-Porath, & McNulty, 1999). It should be specifically noted, however, that the MMPI-2 was designed and normed for individuals who are 18 years of age or older. Adolescent norms were *not* developed for the MMPI-2, nor was it intended for use in the assessment of adolescents.

The Use of the MMPI With Adolescents

The application of the MMPI to adolescent populations for both clinical and research purposes occurred early in the development of this instrument. Although the MMPI was originally intended for administration to individuals who were 16 years of age or older, Dahlstrom et al. (1972) noted that the test could be used effectively with "bright children as young as 12" (p. 21). The delineation of age 12 as the lower limit for administration of the MMPI was probably related to the estimate that a sixth-grade reading level was a prerequisite for understanding the MMPI item pool (Archer, 1987b).

Early Applications

The first research application of the MMPI with adolescents appears to have been made by Dora Capwell in 1941, two years before the formal publication of the MMPI in 1943. Capwell (1945a) demonstrated the ability of the MMPI to accurately discriminate between groups of delinquent and non-delinquent adolescent girls based on *Pd* scale elevation. Further, the MMPI *Pd* scale differences between these groups were maintained in a follow-up study that reevaluated

MMPI profiles 4 to 15 months following the initial MMPI administration (Capwell, 1945b). Early studies by Monachesi (1948, 1950) also served to provide validity data concerning the *Pd* scale by demonstrating that delinquent boys scored significantly higher on this measure than normal male adolescents. In addition, the 1950 study by Monachesi included a sample of incarcerated female delinquents who produced findings that replicated the earlier reports of Capwell. Following these initial studies, the MMPI was used with adolescents in various attempts to predict, diagnose, and plan treatment programs for delinquent adolescents (e.g., Ball, 1962; Hathaway & Monachesi, 1951, 1952). Pursuing this research topic, Hathaway and Monachesi eventually collected the largest MMPI dataset ever obtained on adolescents, in a longitudinal study of the relationship between MMPI findings and delinquent behaviors.

Hathaway and Monachesi administered the MMPI to 3,971 Minnesota ninth-graders during the 1947–1948 school year in a study that served as a prelude to the collection of a larger sample, termed the *statewide sample*. The statewide sample was collected during the spring of 1954, when Hathaway and Monachesi tested 11,329 ninth-graders in 86 communities in Minnesota. Their combined samples involved approximately 15,000 adolescents, including a wide sample of Minnesota children from both urban and rural settings. In addition to the MMPI, subjects' school records were obtained and teachers were asked to indicate which students they felt were most likely either to have psychiatric or legal difficulty. Hathaway and Monachesi also gathered information concerning test scores on such instruments as intelligence tests and the Strong Vocational Interest Blank. The MMPI was then repeated on a sample of 3,976 of these children when they reached 12th grade during the 1956–1957 school year.

Follow-up data were obtained by field workers in the children's community area, who searched files of public agencies, including police and court records. The authors continued to acquire biographical information on members of this sample until the mid-1960s (e.g., Hathaway, Reynolds, & Monachesi, 1969) and other researchers performed follow-up studies on various subsections of the sample (e.g., Hanson, Gottesman, & Heston, 1990). A summary of the early findings from this investigation was published in a 1963 book by Hathaway and Monachesi entitled *Adolescent personality and behavior: MMPI patterns of normal, delinquent, dropout, and other outcomes*.

Hathaway and Monachesi (1953, 1961, 1963) undertook the collection of this massive dataset in order to implement a longitudinal/prospective study that would identify personality variables related to the onset of delinquency. Rather than retroactively identifying a group of delinquent adolescents based on psychosocial histories, they chose to follow adolescents longitudinally to *predict* involvement in antisocial or delinquent behaviors. Thus, Hathaway and Monachesi hoped to identify MMPI predictors that could serve as indicators of risk factors associated with the later development of delinquent behaviors. Monachesi and Hathaway (1969) summarized their results as follows:

Scales *4*, *8*, and *9*, the excitatory scales, were found to be associated with high delinquency rates. When profiles were deviant on these scales, singly or in combination, delinquency rates were considerably larger than the overall rate. Thus, it was found that boys with the excitatory MMPI scale codes (where scales *4*, *8*, and *9* in combination were the most deviant scales in the profile) had a delinquency rate of 41.9% in contrast to the overall rate of 34.6%. Again, scales *0*, *2*, and *5* are the suppressor scales and were the dominant scales in the profiles of boys with low delinquency rates (27.1% as against 34.6%). The variable scales *1*, *3*, *6*, and *7* were again found to have little relationship with delinquency. Of great interest is the fact that some of these relationships are even more marked for girls. In this case, the MMPI data are so closely related to delinquency that it was found that girls with the excitatory code profile had a delinquency rate twice as large as the overall rate. Again, the more deviant scores on scales *4*, *8*, and *9*, the higher the delinquency rate. Girls with inhibitor or suppressor scale scores have lower delinquency rates than the overall rate.

(p. 217)

Systematic follow-up and extensions of this work, usually based on further analyses of the Minnesota statewide sample, have provided relatively consistent support for the concept that elevations on scales *Pd*, *Sc*, and *Ma* serve an *excitatory* function. Higher scores on these scales are predictive of higher rates of "acting out" or delinquent behavior in adolescent samples (e.g., Briggs, Wirt, & Johnson, 1961; Rempel, 1958; Wirt & Briggs, 1959). Findings by Briggs et al. indicated that the accuracy of prediction to delinquent behaviors increased when MMPI data were combined with data regarding the family history of severe disease or death. Specifically, Briggs et al. found that when elevations on excitatory scales were combined with positive histories for family trauma, the frequency of delinquent behavior was twice that of the general population. Similarly, Rempel reported that he could accurately identify 69.5% of a delinquent sample based on analysis of MMPI scales. When MMPI data were combined with school record data in a linear regression procedure, the accurate identification rate for delinquent boys rose to 74.2%. Huesmann, Lefkowitz, and Eron (1978) found that a simple linear summation of the sums of scales *Pd*, *Ma*, and *F* served as the best predictor of delinquent and aggressive behavior in a sample of 426 nineteen-year-old adolescents. This procedure was effective in predicting concurrent incidents of aggression and delinquency as well as retroactively accounting for significant proportions of variance in the ratings of aggressiveness for subjects at age 9.

The research by Hathaway and Monachesi has proved to be very valuable in several ways. First, this research established that the MMPI could usefully predict at least one broad area of important behavior displayed by adolescents: delinquency. Second, the results of their investigation also provided a body of crucial information concerning differences in item endorsement for male versus female adolescents, for adolescents versus adults, and also identified important longitudinal test-retest differences in item endorsement patterns occurring between middle and late adolescence. Third, the data collected by Hathaway and Monachesi provided a major component of the traditionally used adolescent norms later developed by Marks and Briggs (1972), and have also served as the exclusive data source for another set of adolescent norms developed by Gottesman, Hanson, Kroeker, and Briggs (published in Archer, 1987b). Further, Hathaway and Monachesi empirically established the clinical correlates of high and low scores for each of the 10 standard clinical scales, separately for each gender. Finally, this project has provided an extraordinarily rich source of data in follow-up investigations of the original Hathaway and Monachesi subjects, spanning topics from the prediction of juvenile delinquency to the personality precursors of schizophrenia (e.g., Hanson et al., 1990).

Development of Adolescent Norms and Codetype Correlates

The most frequently used adolescent norms for the original MMPI were derived by Marks and Briggs in 1967 and first published in Dahlstrom et al. (1972, pp. 388–399). These norms have also been published in several other texts, including Marks, Seeman, and Haller (1974, pp. 155–162) and Archer (1987b, pp. 197–213, 1997a, pp. 343–360). The Marks and Briggs adolescent norms were based on the responses of approximately 1,800 normal adolescents, and reported separately for males and females at age groupings of 17, 16, 15, and a category of 14 and below. The sample sizes used to create these norms ranged from 166 males and 139 females at age 17, to 271 males and 280 females at ages 14 and below.

The Marks and Briggs adolescent norms were based on responses of 720 adolescents selected from the data collected by Hathaway and Monachesi (1963) in the Minnesota statewide sample, combined with additional data from 1,046 adolescents collected during 1964 and 1965 in six states: Alabama, California, Kansas, Missouri, North Carolina, and Ohio. Marks et al. (1974) reported that this sample consisted of White adolescents who were not receiving treatment for emotional disturbance at the time of their MMPI evaluation. Much of the research that has been performed on the use of the MMPI with adolescent populations has been based on the Marks and Briggs normative set.

Like the original Minnesota adult norms, the norms developed by Marks and Briggs converted raw scores to T-scores using the standard linear transformation procedure. T-scores were therefore determined by taking the nearest integer value of T through the use of the following formula:

$$T = 50 + \frac{10(X_i - M)}{SD}$$

In this formula, M and SD represent the mean and standard deviation of the raw scores for a particular scale based on the normative distribution of subjects in the appropriate age category and gender, and Xi is equal to the raw score value earned by a particular subject. Also, similar to the Minnesota normal adult sample, the adolescent norms were based on White respondents.

There were several distinguishing features to the adolescent norms developed by Marks and Briggs (1972). First, Marks and Briggs did not develop a K-correction procedure for use with their adolescent norms. Marks et al. (1974) listed several reasons for this decision. They noted that the original K-weights were developed on a small sample of adults and their applicability and generalizability to adolescents was questionable. Further, they cited research findings indicating that K-correction procedures with adolescents reduced, rather than increased, relationships to external criteria. Additionally, the normative data reported by Marks and Briggs included the scores from all respondents, without screening out subjects based on validity criteria related to scores on L, F, or K. Thus, all profiles were utilized in this dataset, regardless of validity scale values. The most extensive description of the adolescent norms developed by Marks and Briggs is provided in the Marks et al. (1974) text entitled *The actuarial use of the MMPI with adolescents and adults.*

In addition to adolescent norms, the Marks et al. (1974) text also contained actuarial-based personality descriptors for a series of 29 MMPI high-point codetypes. The main subject pool utilized by Marks and his colleagues to derive these codetype descriptors involved 834 adolescents between the ages of 12 and 18. These adolescents were evaluated after receiving at least 10 hours of psychotherapy between 1965 and 1970. They were described as White teenagers who were not "mentally deficient or retarded" (p. 138). Marks et al. also reported that they later added an additional sample of 419 adolescents who received psychiatric services in the years 1970 to 1973. Adolescents in their samples completed the MMPI and a personal data form that included a self-description adjective checklist and questions covering such topics as attitudes toward self, attitudes toward others, motivational needs, and areas of conflict. The study also employed 172 therapists from 30 states, who provided descriptive ratings on the adolescents. According to Marks et al. (1974):

> Of the 172 psychotherapists who provided patient ratings, 116 were either Board certified psychiatrists, Ph.D. level clinical psychologists, or M.S.W. level social workers with two additional years of therapy experience. These "experienced" therapists rated 746 patients or 90% of the cases; an additional 24 therapists who were either third- or fourth-year clinical psychology interns, third-year psychiatric residents, or recent M.S.W. graduates rated 83 patients or 10% of the cases.
>
> (p. 139)

Clinician ratings involved multiple instruments, including a case data schedule, an adjective checklist, and a Q-sort of personality descriptors.

Therapists' ratings were based on available evidence, including case records, chart notes, and psychological test findings, excluding MMPI results.

Taken together, the preliminary codetype pool available to Marks et al. consisted of 2,302 descriptors that were potentially relevant to adolescents' experiences. The authors then selected from these potential correlates or descriptors 1,265 descriptors that were deemed to be relevant for both male and female respondents, which occurred with sufficient frequency to allow for statistical analyses, and which offered information that was clinically relevant in terms of patient description. Data from adolescents were then grouped into descriptive categories related to 29 high-point codetypes with an average sample size of 13.4 respondents per codetype. Descriptors were developed that differentiated between *high* and *low* profiles (profiles above and below the median two-point codetype elevation for that grouping, respectively), as well as between two-point code reversals (e.g., *2-4* in contrast to *4-2* codes). A detailed discussion of the codetype procedures used in this correlate study is presented in Marks et al. (1974) and in Archer (1987b).

The Marks et al. (1974) clinical correlate study was crucial in providing clinicians with the first correlate information necessary to interpret adolescents' codetype patterns. Further, the information provided by Marks et al. was sufficiently comprehensive, and flexible in terms of application, that their system was capable of classifying a large proportion of adolescent profiles typically obtained in clinical settings. The Marks et al. actuarial data descriptions for adolescents represented a substantial improvement over the Hathaway and Monachesi (1961) text, *An atlas of juvenile MMPI profiles*, which was composed of 1,088 MMPI codes representing individual profile configurations from their sample of Minnesota ninth-graders. Each profile was accompanied by a short case history and a brief description of that subject's most salient personality features. Clinicians using this atlas identified the cases with profiles most similar to the one produced by their patient, and read the accompanying case description. The clinicians had to derive their own summary of personality features commonly found for the codetype, without the assistance of statistical evaluations to identify the most relevant descriptors for the codetype in general.

Later Contributions (1975–1991) Based on the MMPI

After the publication of the text by Marks et al. (1974), substantial work was done in applying the MMPI to adolescents. This work was summarized by Archer (1984, 1987b), Archer and Krishnamurthy (2002), Butcher and Williams (2000), and by Colligan and Offord (1989). Specifically, Archer reviewed the numerous studies indicating that adolescent response patterns should be evaluated exclusively with reference to adolescent norms, in contrast to the application of adult norms. Colligan and Offord (1989) noted research done with adolescent samples in the areas of medical evaluation, school adjustment, and juvenile delinquency.

Of particular interest is the work that has been done subsequent to Marks et al. (1974) in the areas of adolescent norm development and clinical correlates.

In addition to the adolescent norms developed by Marks and Briggs (1972), adolescent MMPI norms for the traditional MMPI instrument were developed by Gottesman, Hanson, Kroeker, and Briggs (published in Archer, 1987b), and by Colligan and Offord (1989) at the Mayo Clinic. The norms developed by Gottesman and his colleagues represent a comprehensive analysis of the approximately 15,000 ninth-grade adolescents tested between 1948 and 1954, and the approximately 3,500 12th graders tested during 1956 and 1957 by Hathaway and Monachesi in their statewide sample. The sample sizes, validity criteria, raw score, and T-score data for this project were reported in Archer, 1987b, Appendix C. In addition to standard scale data, Gottesman et al. provided T-score conversions for a variety of MMPI special scales, including Barron's (1953) Ego Strength scale, MacAndrew's (1965) Alcoholism scale, Welsh's (1956) Anxiety and Repression scales, the Wiggins (1969) Content scales, and the special scales developed by Rosen (1962) for differential diagnosis of psychiatric patients.

Colligan and Offord (1989) also collected normative data for the original form of the MMPI based on the responses of 691 girls and 624 boys between the ages of 13 and 17, inclusive. In collecting these data during the mid-1980s, the authors randomly sampled from 11,930 households in Minnesota, Iowa, and Wisconsin that were within a 50-mile radius of the Mayo Clinic, which is located in Rochester, Minnesota. Telephone interviews established that slightly more than 10% of these households contained adolescents within the appropriate age groups, and after excluding adolescents with potentially handicapping disabilities, 1,412 adolescents were targeted for evaluation. MMPI materials were then mailed to these households, resulting in return rates of 83% for female adolescents and 72% for male adolescents. Colligan and Offord found little evidence of significant differences in mean raw score values across age groups, and therefore the final norms are based on normalized T-score conversions for 13- through 17-year-olds, with conversions presented separately by gender. Colligan and Offord (1991) also provided K-corrected T-score values for these norms.

In addition to the work that has been done on adolescent normative values, several investigations were also conducted that examined the clinical correlates of single-scale and two-point codetypes based on the traditional Marks and Briggs adolescent norms. Archer, Gordon, Giannetti, and Singles (1988), for example, examined descriptive correlates of single-scale high-point elevations for scales 2, 3, 4, 8, and 9 in a sample of 112 adolescent inpatients. Clinical descriptors were collected for subjects based on their psychometric self-reports and patient ratings by parents, nursing staff, and individual psychotherapists. In general, findings from this study produced correlate patterns that were highly similar to those reported for basic MMPI scales in the adult literature. Using a similar methodology, Archer, Gordon, Anderson, and Giannetti (1989) also investigated the clinical correlates of the MacAndrew Alcoholism scale, Welsh's Anxiety and Repression scales, and Barron's Ego Strength scale in a sample of 68 adolescent inpatients. Results from this study also indicated patterns of clinically relevant descriptors that were largely consistent with findings derived from studies of adult respondents. Ball, Archer, Struve, Hunter, and Gordon (1987) found evidence of subtle, but detectable, neurological differences between adolescent psychiatric inpatients with and without elevated scale *1* values. Further, Archer and Gordon (1988) found that scale *8* elevations were an effective and sensitive indicator of the presence of schizophrenic diagnoses in a sample of adolescent inpatients.

Williams and Butcher (1989a) also examined single-scale correlates in a sample of 492 boys and 352 girls primarily evaluated in either substance abuse or psychiatric inpatient units. Standard scale values were investigated in relationship to data derived from psychiatric records and parental and treatment staff ratings and reports. Similar to Archer et al. (1988), the authors concluded that single-scale descriptors found for these adolescents were consistent with those reported in adult studies. Additionally, Williams and Butcher (1989b) investigated code-type correlates for this sample of 844 adolescents and found that although some of the codetype descriptors reported by Marks et al. (1974) were replicated in this study, other descriptor patterns were not supported. Studies by Lachar and Wrobel (1990) and by Wrobel and Lachar (1992) examined the issue of gender differences in correlate patterns and found evidence of substantially different correlate patterns for male and female adolescents, underscoring the possibility of important gender differences in MMPI clinical correlates for adolescents.

Several researchers have also examined the effects of using both adolescent and adult norms in terms of profile elevation and configuration. Specifically, studies by Archer (1984), Ehrenworth and Archer (1985), Klinge, Lachar, Grissell, and Berman (1978), Klinge and Strauss (1976), and Lachar, Klinge, and Grissell (1976) examined the effects of using adolescent and adult norms in profiling responses of male and female adolescents admitted to inpatient psychiatric services. These studies have consistently shown that the degree of psychopathology displayed by adolescent respondents tends to be more pronounced when adult norms are employed, particularly on scales *F*, *4*, and *8*. Finally, factor analytic studies have been reported based on scale-level data by Archer (1984), and by Archer and Klinefelter (1991) on both the item and scale-level. In general, the results of these studies produced factor patterns that are reasonably consistent with those that have been typically derived from factor analytic findings in adult samples.

Frequency of Use of the MMPI in Adolescent Assessments

As we have seen, research attention was heavily focused on the use of the MMPI in adolescent populations. Until the early 1990s, however, no surveys of test usage were specifically targeted with practitioners who worked mainly with adolescents. Therefore, the relative popularity of instruments such as the MMPI among such practitioners remained unclear. In addressing this issue, Archer, Maruish, Imhof, and Piotrowski (1991) asked psychologists how frequently they used each of 67 instruments in their assessment of adolescent clients. The results for these assessment instruments were evaluated based on total number of "mentions" as well as tabulated with adjustments for frequency of test usage. The MMPI was the third most frequently mentioned assessment instrument with adolescents (behind the Wechsler scales and the Rorschach), and the sixth most frequently employed instrument when scores were adjusted for frequency of use (following the Wechsler, Rorschach, Bender-Gestalt, Thematic Apperception Test (TAT), and Sentence Completion). The MMPI was the most frequently employed objective personality assessment instrument with teenagers when either total mentions or weighted scores were evaluated.

Respondents were also asked to indicate those instruments used in their standard test batteries with adolescents, with the results of this question shown in Fig. 2.1. As shown in this figure, the Wechsler IQ measures and the Rorschach were the most frequently reported tests included within standard batteries. The MMPI ranked fifth and was included by roughly half of the survey respondents. In contrast, the only other objective personality assessment included in Fig. 2.1 is the Millon Adolescent Personality Inventory (Millon, Green, & Meagher, 1977), which was included in only 17% of the standard test batteries reported by the respondents. Overall, the results of the survey by Archer, Maruish, et al. (1991) indicated that the MMPI, consistent with surveys of test use in adult

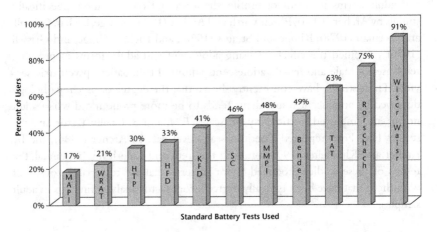

FIGURE 2.1 Most frequently used psychological instruments in "standard batteries" with adolescents.

populations (e.g., Lubin et al., 1985) was the most frequently used objective personality assessment instrument in evaluations of adolescents.

Development of the MMPI-A

Despite the past popularity of the MMPI, researchers and clinicians expressed concerns regarding several aspects of the use of the MMPI to assess teenagers. For example, Archer, Maruish, et al. (1991) asked survey respondents to indicate their perceptions concerning the major advantages and disadvantages of using the MMPI with adolescents. Major advantages reported included the comprehensive and accurate nature of clinically relevant descriptors, the relative ease of administration and scoring, and the extensive adolescent research data base available for this instrument. Forty-nine percent of respondents, however, indicated that they felt the test was too long, 20% of respondents had concerns regarding inadequate or outdated adolescent norms, 18% felt that the reading level of the original MMPI was too high, and 17% of respondents objected to the use of inappropriate or outdated language in the item pool. Consistent with most of the survey respondents' views, Table 2.2 summarizes a variety of factors pointing to the need for revision of the original test instrument.

Serious concerns were expressed regarding the nature of the adolescent norms available for the original MMPI. Specifically, the Marks and Briggs (1972) adolescent norms were based on data samples collected in the late 1940s through mid-1960s on White adolescents. This adolescent dataset was therefore substantially dated, and dramatically limited in terms of ethnic representation. Pancoast and Archer (1988) examined the adequacy of the traditional adolescent norms in an analysis of normal adolescent samples collected between 1947 and 1965,

TABLE 2.2 Factors Contributing to the Development of the MMPI-A

I	Need for contemporary norms
	A. Current norms
	B. National sample
	C. Ethnic representation
II	Need for revision of item pool
	A. Elimination of offensive items
	B. Elimination of items inappropriate for adolescents
	C. Rewritten items to simplify wording or sentence structure
	D. Inclusion of new items of specific relevance for adolescents
III	Need for creation of scales to assess adolescent problem areas
	A. New supplementary scales including the Immaturity scale
	B. Several new content scales including School Problems and Conduct Problems
IV	Need to standardize MMPI assessment practices for adolescents
	A. Confusion regarding appropriate norms
	B. Confusion regarding interpretation practices
	C. Fostering interest in special scale use

and normal adolescent samples collected in the decade following 1975. Findings supported the adequacy of the traditional adolescent norms for evaluations of samples of normal adolescents collected between 1947 and 1965. This interval of time coincides with the data collection period for the adolescent samples used in the Marks and Briggs (1972) norms. MMPI patterns produced by more contemporary samples of adolescents, however, were elevated above the Marks and Briggs mean values on most clinical scales. These findings suggest that the traditional adolescent norms may not provide an accurate normative baseline, in terms of mean fit, for evaluations of contemporary adolescents.

There were also criticisms of some of the item content of the original MMPI as inappropriate or offensive in the assessment of teenagers. Most clinicians who used the traditional form with teenagers were probably aware that an item concerning "drop the handkerchief" had little meaning for today's adolescents, and that questions concerning "deportment" were not readily understood by many adolescents. Similarly, questions such as "my sex life is satisfactory" may have a substantially different meaning when asked of a 13-year-old in contrast to a 30-year-old. Further, awkwardly worded items, a source of concern in terms of administration of the MMPI to adults, had been a major problem in the assessment of adolescents. Finally, the MMPI item pool, although quite extensive, historically lacked items of specific relevance to adolescent experiences, including problem areas that typically emerge during the teenage years such as drug use, eating disorders, and school-related problems. In addition to modifications at the item level, the creation of MMPI items related to adolescence provided an opportunity to develop scale measures of specific relevance to adolescent development and psychopathology. Although several special MMPI scales, developed for adults, had been applied to adolescents (e.g., Welsh Anxiety and Repression scales, the MacAndrew Alcoholism scale), these scales were not specifically developed for this population.

On July 1, 1989, the MMPI Adolescent Project Committee, consisting of James N. Butcher, Auke Tellegen, and Robert P. Archer, was appointed by Beverly Kaemmer of the University of Minnesota Press to consider the advisability of creating an adolescent form of the MMPI, and the features such a form should incorporate if development was undertaken.

Goals of the MMPI-A Project

A number of goals were envisioned in the creation of the MMPI-A. Some of these goals were in conflict and required varying degrees of compromise for work to move forward on the adolescent form. It was clear that adult norms would not be applicable to an adolescent form (Archer, 1984, 1987b, 1990; Williams, Graham, & Butcher, 1986) and that a national normative sample representative of the general population of U.S. teenagers would be required for the MMPI-A. An emphasis was also placed on shortening the length of the MMPI while maintaining continuity between the original MMPI and the MMPI-A, including the preservation of the standard or basic MMPI Validity and Clinical scales. Within this context, however, opportunities were taken to modify and improve MMPI scales *F*, *Mf*, and *Si*, based on observations concerning adolescent response characteristics on these measures in the MMPI-A normative sample. If a form was to be developed for adolescent assessment, it was also deemed desirable to include items and scales directly relevant to adolescent development and expression of psychopathology. Finally, it was anticipated that the release of an adolescent form of the MMPI would help to standardize assessment practices with adolescents. As noted by Archer (1984, 1987b), there was considerable controversy and confusion regarding the optimal approach to interpreting adolescents' MMPI profiles. Questions concerning the most appropriate administration criteria, norm sets, special scales, and clinical correlates had been the subject of substantial debate, without clear and consistent resolution. The development and release of the MMPI-A, and the manual for this instrument (Butcher et al. 1992), served to standardize and improve assessment practices for both clinician and researcher.

The Experimental Booklet (Form TX)

The development of the MMPI-A was initiated with the creation of an experimental test booklet for adolescents, identified as MMPI Form TX. This experimental test booklet contained 704 items to be used in normative data collection efforts and in preliminary analyses to determine the feasibility of creating an adolescent form. The first section of this booklet contained 550 items from the traditional MMPI form, followed by the presentation of a new experimental item pool for which scale membership and clinical correlates had not yet been established. The 154 items included in the latter part of the test booklet involved content areas including negative peer group influence, alcohol and drug abuse, family relationship difficulties, school and achievement problems, eating disorders, and identity problems. Of the original 550 items, approximately 13% had been reworded to increase content clarity or quality. The 16 repeated items found on the traditional MMPI form were eliminated from MMPI Form TX.

In addition to MMPI Form TX, adolescents in the normative samples were administered a 16-item Biographical Information Form and a 74-item Life Events Form. The biographical questionnaire obtained data on a number of variables including age, ethnic background, family structure, parental education and occupation, and academic performance. The life events questionnaire requested information on the occurrence and effect of life events including major illnesses, loss of family members, and parental separation or divorce.

The MMPI-A Normative Sample

The collection of adolescent normative data was undertaken in eight states, seven of which also served as primary sites for adult normative data collection for the MMPI-2. Adolescent normative subjects were generally solicited by mail from the rosters of junior and senior high schools in predetermined areas, and subjects were tested in group sessions generally conducted within school settings. Adolescents who participated in the MMPI-A normative data collection were paid for their voluntary participation. A total of approximately 2,500 adolescents were evaluated with the MMPI Form TX in data collection procedures. Various exclusion criteria were applied to these data including the following: (a) subjects with incomplete data; (b) Carelessness scale values >35; (c) original F scale value >25; and (d) subject age <14 or >18. Employing these exclusion criteria resulted in the creation of a final adolescent normative sample that included 805 males and 815 females. The geographic distribution of this adolescent sample was as follows: Minnesota (n = 501), New York (n = 168), North Carolina (n = 203), Ohio (n = 210), California (n = 226), Virginia (n = 209), Pennsylvania (n = 89), and the State of Washington (n = 14). Approximately two-thirds of the adolescents in the MMPI-A normative sample reported that they lived with both parents, approximately 26% reported that they lived with their biological mother only, approximately 3.8% reported living with their biological father, and approximately 3.9% reported living in other home settings.

Table 2.3 provides age distribution data. The mean age of boys in the MMPI-A normative sample was 15.5 years (SD = 1.17 years) and the mean age for girls was 15.6 years (SD = 1.18 years). In the MMPI-A-RF normative sample, which is based on the MMPI-A normative sample with the random deletion of data from 10 girls, the mean age for girls was 15.6 years (SD = 1.18 years) and was identical to the MMPI-A values for boys.

Table 2.4 provides information concerning the ethnic origins of adolescents in the MMPI-A normative sample. The ethnic distribution of the MMPI-A normative sample represents a reasonable match against U.S. Census figures, with approximately 76% of data derived from Whites, 12% from Black adolescents, and the remaining 12% of data coming from other ethnic groups.

Tables 2.5 and 2.6 provide data on fathers' and mothers' educational levels, respectively, for adolescents in the MMPI-A normative sample. In general, these data show that the parents of adolescents used in the MMPI-A normative sample are well educated, and over-represent higher educational levels in comparison to the 1980 U.S. Census data. Specifically, roughly 49.9% of the fathers and 40.9% of the mothers of children in the MMPI-A normative sample reported an educational level of a bachelor's degree or higher. This may be compared with 20% of males and 13% of females in the 1980 U.S. Census data who reported comparable educational levels. This degree of over-representation of better educated individuals is very similar to that found in the MMPI-2 adult normative sample (Archer, 1997a). This phenomenon is probably related to the use of volunteer subjects in normative data collection procedures, in which better educated and higher socioeconomic status subjects are differentially more likely to participate. Black (1994) criticized specifically this aspect of

TABLE 2.3 Age Distribution of Adolescents in the MMPI-A and MMPI-A-RF Normative Samples

Age	MMPI-A and MMPI-A-RF[a] Boys (N = 805)		MMPI-A Girls (N = 815)		MMPI-A-RF Girls (N = 805)	
	Frequency	%	Frequency	%	Frequency	%
14	193	24.0	174	21.3	173	21.5
15	207	25.7	231	28.3	231	28.7
16	228	28.3	202	24.8	199	24.7
17	135	16.8	163	20.0	157	19.5
18	42	5.2	45	5.5	45	5.6

Source: Multiphasic Personality Inventory-Adolescent (MMPI®-A) Manual for Administration, Scoring, and Interpretation by Butcher, et al. Copyright © 1992 by the Regents of the University of Minnesota. MMPI-A-RF Administration, Scoring, Interpretation and Technical Manual by Archer, et al. Copyright © 2016 by the Regents of the University of Minnesota. Reproduced with the permission of the University of Minnesota Press. All rights reserved. "Minnesota Multiphasic Personality Inventory" and "MMPI" are trademarks owned by the Regents of the University of Minnesota.

Note

a The MMPI-A and MMPI-A-RF normative samples are identical for boys. Minnesota.

TABLE 2.4 Ethnic Origin of Adolescents in the MMPI-A and MMPI-A-RF Normative Samples

Ethnicity	MMPI-A and MMPI-A-RF[a] Boys (N = 805)		MMPI-A Girls (N = 815)		MMPI-A-RF Girls (N = 805)	
	Frequency	%	Frequency	%	Frequency	%
White	616	76.5	619	75.9	613	76.1
Black	100	12.4	100	12.3	99	12.3
Asian	23	2.9	23	2.8	23	2.9
Native American	21	2.6	26	3.2	25	3.1
Hispanic	18	2.2	16	2.0	15	1.9
Other	20	2.5	21	2.6	21	2.6
None reported	7	0.9	10	1.2	9	1.1

Source: Multiphasic Personality Inventory-Adolescent (MMPI®-A) Manual for Administration, Scoring, and Interpretation by Butcher, et al. Copyright © 1992 by the Regents of the University of Minnesota. MMPI-A-RF Administration, Scoring, Interpretation and Technical Manual by Archer, et al. Copyright © 2016 by the Regents of the University of Minnesota. Reproduced with the permission of the University of Minnesota Press. All rights reserved. "Minnesota Multiphasic Personality Inventory" and "MMPI" are trademarks owned by the Regents of the University of Minnesota.

Note

a The MMPI-A and MMPI-A-RF normative samples are identical for boys. Minnesota.

the MMPI-A normative sample and concluded that "the socioeconomic skewing of the normative sample brings into question the interpretation of protocols of respondents from low socioeconomic status levels" (p. 11).

Among the data collected for the MMPI-A normative sample was information concerning whether the adolescent had been "referred to a counselor or therapist" within the six months immediately prior to test administration. Hand, Archer, Handel, and Forbey (2007) removed data from the 193 adolescents who reported referral for counseling from the normative sample and recalculated uniform T-score values for the Basic Clinical scales based on the remaining 1,427 adolescents. Results of the study indicated that elimination of adolescents referred for counseling had little or no effect on normative transformation T-score values. Further, removal of adolescents referred for counseling did not substantively improve the overall hit rate, positive predictive power, or sensitivity when the refined norms were used to attempt to identify adolescents from normative samples versus adolescents in clinical samples. The authors observed that substantial improvements in classification accuracy might require more fundamental changes in the test instrument, including the potential development of Restructured Clinical (RC) scales for the MMPI-A.

TABLE 2.5 Fathers' Educational Level for Adolescents in the MMPI-A and MMPI-A-RF Normative Samples

Educational Level	MMPI-A and MMPI-A-RF[a] Boys (N = 805)		MMPI-A Girls (N = 815)		MMPI-A-RF Girls (N = 805)	
	Frequency	%	Frequency	%	Frequency	%
Less than high school	17	2.1	15	1.8	12	1.5
Some high school	59	7.3	88	10.8	86	10.7
High school graduate	173	21.5	191	23.4	189	23.5
Some college	114	14.2	108	13.3	108	13.4
College graduate	272	33.8	262	32.1	259	32.2
Graduate school	152	18.9	122	15.0	122	15.2
None reported	18	2.2	29	3.6	29	3.6

Source: Multiphasic Personality Inventory-Adolescent (MMPI®-A) Manual for Administration, Scoring, and Interpretation by Butcher, et al. Copyright © 1992 by the Regents of the University of Minnesota. MMPI-A-RF Administration, Scoring, Interpretation and Technical Manual by Archer, et al. Copyright © 2016 by the Regents of the University of Minnesota. Reproduced with the permission of the University of Minnesota Press. All rights reserved. "Minnesota Multiphasic Personality Inventory" and "MMPI" are trademarks owned by the Regents of the University of Minnesota.

Note

a The MMPI-A and MMPI-A-RF normative samples are identical for boys. Minnesota.

TABLE 2.6 Mothers' Educational Level for Adolescents in the MMPI-A and MMPI-A-RF Normative Samples

Educational Level	MMPI-A and MMPI-A-RF[a] Boys (N = 805)		MMPI-A Girls (N = 815)		MMPI-A-RF Girls (N = 805)	
	Frequency	%	Frequency	%	Frequency	%
Less than high school	9	1.1	11	1.3	9	1.1
Some high school	38	4.7	54	6.6	54	6.7
High school graduate	250	31.1	230	28.2	226	28.1
Some college	145	18.0	183	22.5	180	22.4
College graduate	260	32.3	244	30.0	243	30.2
Graduate School	91	11.3	68	8.3	68	8.4
None reported	12	1.5	25	3.1	25	3.1

Source: Multiphasic Personality Inventory-Adolescent (MMPI®-A) Manual for Administration, Scoring, and Interpretation by Butcher, et al. Copyright © 1992 by the Regents of the University of Minnesota. MMPI-A-RF Administration, Scoring, Interpretation and Technical Manual by Archer, et al. Copyright © 2016 by the Regents of the University of Minnesota. Reproduced with the permission of the University of Minnesota Press. All rights reserved. "Minnesota Multiphasic Personality Inventory" and "MMPI" are trademarks owned by the Regents of the University of Minnesota.

Note
a The MMPI-A and MMPI-A-RF normative samples are identical for boys. Minnesota.

Structure of the MMPI-A

After examining the preliminary data, a decision was reached by the MMPI Adolescent Project Committee during January 1990 to recommend the creation of the MMPI-A instrument. The final version of the MMPI-A contains 478 items. Administration of the first 350 items of the MMPI-A booklet are sufficient to score validity scales L, F_1, and K, and the standard clinical scales. The remaining 128 items are necessary to score the remaining Validity scales and the Supplementary and Content scales. The standard MMPI Clinical scales were retained in the MMPI-A form. As shown in Table 2.7, fifty-eight standard scale items were deleted from the original scales, however, 88% of these item deletions occurred on scales F, Mf, or Si. Items deleted from the MMPI-A standard scales included the 13 items that were also deleted from the traditional MMPI in the creation of the MMPI-2. In general, items deleted from the MMPI-A dealt with religious attitudes and practices, sexual preferences, bowel and bladder functioning, or items deemed inappropriate in terms of adolescents' life experiences. A variety of empirical criteria were used to delete items from scales *F*, *Mf*, and *Si*. Specifically, items deleted from the *F* scale were endorsed with a frequency of 21% or greater for either boys or girls in the MMPI-A normative sample. Items were deleted from *Mf* or *Si* if the item loaded only on that particular scale (i.e., did not overlap on other standard measures) and did not demonstrate significant gender differences for the *Mf* scale or did not contribute to factor patterns established for the *Si* scale. Table 2.7 indicates the number of items deleted and retained for each of the standard MMPI-A Validity and Clinical scales, and Table 2.8 provides a listing of items deleted from the basic Validity and Clinical scales.

The final form of the MMPI-A at the time of publication in 1992 included the original 13 standard scales combined with 4 new validity scales, 15 Content scales, 6 Supplementary scales, and the 28 Harris–Lingoes and 3 *Si* subscales. In the supplement to the MMPI-A Manual (Ben-Porath, Graham, Archer, Tellegen, & Kaemmer, 2006), 31 Content Components scales and the Personality Psychopathology Five (PSY-5) scales were formally added to the test. Table 2.9 provides an overview of the current scale structure of the MMPI-A.

The new validity measures for the MMPI-A include the F_1 and F_2 subscales of the standard *F* scale, and the True Response Inconsistency scale (*TRIN*) and the Variable Response Inconsistency scale (*VRIN*) developed by Auke Tellegen. The Supplementary scales for the MMPI-A involve measures that were developed for the original MMPI, including the Anxiety (*A*) scale, the

TABLE 2.7 Item Changes in Original MMPI Basic Scales and Resulting Effects on the MMPI-A Basic Scales

MMPI-A Scale	Items Retained	Number of Items Deleted
L	14	1
F	66[a]	27
K	30	0
1 (*Hs*)	32	1
2 (*D*)	57	3
3 (*Hy*)	60	0
4 (*Pd*)	49	1
5 (*Mf*)	44	16
6 (*Pa*)	40	0
7 (*Pt*)	48	0
8 (*Sc*)	77	1
9 (*Ma*)	46	0
0 (*Si*)	62	8

Note

a 12 items were deleted from the MMPI-A *F* scale, but retained in the MMPI-A item pool, 12 items from original test that were not scored on the *F* scale were transferred to the MMPI-A scale *F*, and 17 new items were also added to the MMPI-A *F* scale.

TABLE 2.8 Item Deletions From the Original MMPI Basic Validity and Clinical Scales in the Corresponding MMPI-A Scales

Scale	MMPI Item Numbers
L	255
F	14, 20, 31[a], 40[a], 53, 85, 112[a], 115[a], 139, 146, 156[a], 164[a], 169, 197, 199, 206, 211, 215[a], 218, 227, 245[a], 246, 247[a], 256[a], 258, 269[a], 276[a]
1(Hs)	63
2(D)	58, 95, 98
4(Pd)	20
5(Mf)	4, 19, 25, 69, 70, 87, 126, 133, 198, 203, 204, 214, 229, 249, 261, 295
8(Sc)	20
0(Si)	25, 126, 229, 371, 427, 440, 455, 462

Source: Adapted from Butcher et al. (1992). Adapted from Minnesota Multiphasic Personality Inventory-Adolescent (MMPI®-A) Manual for Administration, Scoring, and Interpretation by Butcher, et al. Copyright © 1992 by the Regents of the University of Minnesota. Reproduced with the permission of the University of Minnesota Press. All rights reserved. "Minnesota Multiphasic Personality Inventory" and "MMPI" are trademarks owned by the Regents of the University of Minnesota.

Note
a Original MMPI *F* scale item not appearing on the MMPI-A *F* scale but appearing on other MMPI-A scales.

Repression (*R*) scale, and the MacAndrew Alcoholism scale (*MAC*). In addition, the supplementary scales include a variety of new measures developed for the MMPI-A, including the Immaturity (*IMM*) scale, the Alcohol/Drug Problem Acknowledgment (*ACK*) scale, and the Alcohol/Drug Problem Proneness (*PRO*) scale. Most of the 15 Content scales developed for the MMPI-A overlap with similar measures developed for the MMPI-2, but several of these scales were created specifically and uniquely for the adolescent form. The Content Component subscales are a set of 31 subscales that were developed by Sherwood, Ben-Porath, and Williams (1997) to identify meaningful item clusters within 13 of the 15 Content scales. The Harris–Lingoes content subscales developed for the original MMPI were carried over to the MMPI-A, with a few item deletions resulting from the deletion of items on the Basic scales. The *Si* subscales were directly carried over from their counterparts in the MMPI-2. The MMPI-A manual by Butcher et al. (1992) contains a listing of each MMPI-A item accompanied by data concerning endorsement frequencies and reading requirements. Further, Butcher et al. (1992) showed item number conversion information for the Group Form of the original MMPI and MMPI-A, and for conversions between items in the MMPI-2 and MMPI-A. Finally, the MMPI-A scale structure includes the Personality Psychopathology Five (PSY-5) scales developed by McNulty, Harkness, Ben-Porath, and Williams (1997) to assess key personality dimensions as identified by Harkness and McNulty (1994).

TABLE 2.9 Overview of the MMPI-A Scales and Subscales

Basic Profile Scales (17 scales)

Standard Scales (13)

        L through *Si*

Additional Validity Scales (4)

        F_1/F_2 (Subscales of *F* Scale)

        VRIN (Variable Response Inconsistency)

        TRIN (True Response Inconsistency)

Content and Supplementary Scales (21 scales)

Content Scales (15)

        A-anx (Anxiety)

        A-obs (Obsessiveness)

        A-dep (Depression)

        A-hea (Health Concerns)

        A-aln (Alienation)

        A-biz (Bizarre Mentation)

        A-ang (Anger)

        A-cyn (Cynicism)

        A-con (Conduct Problems)

        A-lse (Low Self-esteem)

        A-las (Low Aspirations)

        A-sod (Social Discomfort)

        A-fam (Family Problems)

        A-sch (School Problems)

        A-trt (Negative Treatment Indicators)

Supplementary Scales (6)

        MAC-R (MacAndrew Alcoholism-Revised)

        ACK (Alcohol/Drug Problem Acknowledgment)

        PRO (Alcohol/Drug Problem Proneness)

        IMM (Immaturity)

        A (Anxiety)

        R (Repression)

Harris-Lingoes and Si Subscales (31 scales)

Harris-Lingoes Subscales (28)

        D_1 (Subjective Depression)

        D_2 (Psychomotor Retardation)

        D_3 (Physical Malfunctioning)

        D_4 (Mental Dullness)

D_5　　(Brooding)
Hy_1　(Denial of Social Anxiety)
Hy_2　(Need for Affection)
Hy_3　(Lassitude–Malaise)
Hy_4　(Somatic Complaints)
Hy_5　(Inhibition of Aggression)
Pd_1　(Familial Discord)
Pd_2　(Authority Problems)
Pd_3　(Social Imperturbability)
Pd_4　(Social Alienation)
Pd_5　(Self-Alienation)
Pa_1　(Persecutory Ideas)
Pa_2　(Poignancy)
Pa_3　(Naïveté)
Sc_1　(Social Alienation)
Sc_2　(Emotional Alienation)
Sc_3　(Lack of Ego Mastery, Cognitive)
Sc_4　(Lack of Ego Mastery, Conative)
Sc_5　(Lack of Ego Mastery, Defective Inhibition)
Sc_6　(Bizarre Sensory Experiences)
Ma_1　(Amorality)
Ma_2　(Psychomotor Acceleration)
Ma_3　(Imperturbability)
Ma_4　(Ego Inflation)

Si Subscales (3)

Si_1　(Shyness/Self-Consciousness)
Si_2　(Social Avoidance)
Si_3　(Alienation-Self and Others)

Content Component Scales (31)

$A\text{-}dep_1$　(Dysphoria)
$A\text{-}dep_2$　(Self-Depreciation)
$A\text{-}dep_3$　(Lack of Drive)
$A\text{-}dep_4$　(Suicidal Ideation)
$A\text{-}hea_1$　(Gastrointestinal Complaints)
$A\text{-}hea_2$　(Neurological Symptoms)
$A\text{-}hea_3$　(General Health Concerns)
$A\text{-}aln_1$　(Misunderstood)

(continued)

TABLE 2.9 *(continued)*

$A\text{-}aln_2$	(Social Isolation)
$A\text{-}aln_3$	(Interpersonal Skepticism)
$A\text{-}biz_1$	(Psychotic Symptomatology)
$A\text{-}biz_2$	(Paranoid Ideation)
$A\text{-}ang_1$	(Explosive Behavior)
$A\text{-}ang_2$	(Irritability)
$A\text{-}cyn_1$	(Misanthropic Beliefs)
$A\text{-}cyn_2$	(Interpersonal Suspiciousness)
$A\text{-}con_1$	(Acting-Out Behaviors)
$A\text{-}con_2$	(Antisocial Attitudes)
$A\text{-}con_3$	(Negative Peer Group Influences)
$A\text{-}lse_1$	(Self-Doubt)
$A\text{-}lse_2$	(Interpersonal Submissiveness)
$A\text{-}las_1$	(Low Achievement Orientation)
$A\text{-}las_2$	(Lack of Initiative)
$A\text{-}sod_1$	(Introversion)
$A\text{-}sod_2$	(Shyness)
$A\text{-}fam_1$	(Familial Discord)
$A\text{-}fam_2$	(Familial Alienation)
$A\text{-}sch_1$	(School Conduct Problems)
$A\text{-}sch_2$	(Negative Attitudes)
$A\text{-}trt_1$	(Low Motivation)
$A\text{-}trt_2$	(Inability to Disclose)

Personality Psychopathology Five (PSY-5) Scales (5)

AGGR	(Aggressiveness)
PSYC	(Psychoticism)
DISC	(Disconstraint)
NEGE	(Negative Emotionality/Neuroticism)
INTR	(Introversion/Low Positive Emotionality)

MMPI-A Normative Sample: Comparisons With Earlier Normative Groups

Newsom, Archer, Trumbetta, and Gottesman (2003) examined the changes in adolescent self-presentation on the MMPI and MMPI-A over a 40-year period. The primary samples used by these researchers for comparison included 1,235 adolescents between the ages of 14 and 16, inclusive, in the MMPI-A normative sample collected in 1989 and 10,514 adolescents between the ages of 14 and 16 collected between 1948 and 1954 in the Hathaway and Monachesi (1963) study of adolescent personality and behavior. MMPI basic scale and item-level data were also included for 817 adolescents, ages 14 through 16, collected by Colligan and Offord (1992) in their 1985 study of the original form of the MMPI. Overall, the result of these evaluations revealed that adolescents from the MMPI-A normative sample scored significantly higher across the Basic Clinical scales, and lower on validity scales *L* and *K*, than did adolescents from the Hathaway and Monachesi (1963) sample. The MMPI Basic Scale mean data reported by Colligan and Offord typically fell at a mid-range between these two. Results were interpreted as reflecting moderate to large changes in response frequencies between eras of data collection, with evidence of a relatively higher frequency of item endorsements by contemporary adolescents in the clinical direction on most MMPI Basic Clinical scales, particularly scales *Ma*, *Sc*, and *Hs*. Thus, contemporary normal adolescents not only endorse more psychopathological symptoms than do adults, but also endorse more pathology than did adolescents evaluated 40 years ago in the Monachesi and Hathaway sample. As we will explore in more detail later in this text, these response patterns may indicate that normal adolescents experience substantial psychological turmoil and distress which renders accurate discrimination between normal and abnormal functioning particularly difficult during this developmental age. Further, Archer, Handel, and Lynch (2001) demonstrated that many MMPI-A items, perhaps approaching nearly 50% of the Basic Scale item pool, did not show significantly higher rates of endorsement frequency among adolescent inpatients in contrast to adolescents from the normative sample. The implications of these findings led, in part, to the recent decision to modify the clinical elevation cutoff on the MMPI-A-RF to T ≥ 60.

MMPI-A Normative Sample: Comparisons With Later Non-Clinical Samples of Adolescents

As noted in the MMPI-A-RF Manual (Archer, Handel, Ben-Porath, & Tellegen, 2016a), eleven studies have been conducted between 1995 and 2012 in which the authors reported, at a minimum, mean and standard deviation data for the MMPI-A Validity and Clinical scales for boys and girls in non-clinical samples. Four of these studies also provided additional MMPI-A scale data, and two of these investigations (Carlson, 2001; Newton, 2008) included mean and standard deviation data for all of the 69 MMPI-A scales. Collectively, these studies include data from 1,899 adolescents evaluated following the release of the MMPI-A in 1992 and are relevant to the issue of the adequacy of the MMPI-A norms in providing an accurate reference point for the evaluation of contemporary adolescents.

The eleven studies were conducted for a variety of investigative purposes. Several of these studies, for example, focused on the detection of response sets such as random responding and overreporting by administering the MMPI-A to nine adolescent samples under standard instructions, and under instructions directing participants to simulate one or more response styles (Baer, Ballenger, Berry, & Wetter, 1997; Bagdade, 2004; Conkey, 2000; Stein, Graham, & Williams, 1995). Under standard instructions, these non-clinical samples of adolescents consistently produced mean T-score values on the Validity and Clinical scales generally within five T-score points of a mean value of 50. Additionally, three studies reported MMPI-A scores for samples of academically gifted adolescents (Cross, Adams, Dixon, & Holland, 2004; Cross, Cassady, Dixon, & Adams, 2008; Newton, 2008). These studies consistently produced mean T-score values ranging from the mid-40s to the low 50s. Cross et al. (2004, p.174), for example, concluded based on their findings that "The data from this study supports the contention that academically gifted adolescents . . . were not different from their non-gifted counterparts relative to the numerous scales measured by the MMPI-A." Two studies used non-clinical samples to compare MMPI-A results obtained by computer administrations versus paper-and-pencil test administrations (Carlson, 2001; Hays, 2003). In addition to establishing that test results are essentially equivalent across administration modalities, the results of these studies also indicated that T-score values across MMPI-A scales generally ranged within a 2- to 3-point grouping of a T-score value of 50, and standard deviations typically averaged approximately 10 T-score points. A study by Henry (1999) examined MMPI-A results produced by a non-clinical sample of African–American adolescents and found T-score values consistent with normative expectations. Finally, Yavari (2012) reported T-score values of around 50, with standard deviation values of about 10, for MMPI-A clinical scales derived in a sample of high school students in an investigation of K scale correlates. Collectively, the results of these studies indicate that no major normative shifts or changes have occurred in adolescent response patterns since the publication of the MMPI-A norms in 1992. These findings are consistent with the continuation of the 1992 MMPI-A norms for contemporary samples of adolescents evaluated with the MMPI-A, and also laid the foundation for the decision to use a derivation of the MMPI-A normative sample in the creation of the MMPI-A-RF non-gendered norms. This latter topic will be discussed in more detail in Chapter 7, which describes the MMPI-A-RF.

Clinical Popularity of the MMPI-A

As previously noted, Archer, Maruish, et al. (1991) presented survey findings on the popularity of the MMPI among psychologists who performed psychological assessments with adolescent clients. Archer and Newsom (2000) designed an investigation to update these results by examining the test use practices reported by 346 psychologists who worked with adolescents in a variety of clinical and academic settings. These respondents represented an adjusted survey return rate of 36%, and predominantly consisted of doctoral prepared psychologists (95%) in private practice settings (51%). The survey respondents had a mean of 13.6 years of post-degree clinical experience, and spent an average of 45% of their clinical time working with adolescents. Table 2.10 presents the usage rating totals, arranged in order of decreasing weighted scores, for the ten most frequently reported instruments in the Archer and Newsom survey.

The ten most frequently used instruments shown in Table 2.10 consisted of the Wechsler Intelligence Scales, several projectives, one objective self-report measure (MMPI-A), and Parent and Teacher Behavioral Rating Forms. The MMPI-A was ranked fifth in both total mentions by respondents in the survey, and by a score weighted by frequency of use. Further, the MMPI-A was the only self-report objective personality assessment instrument included in these top ten ranked instruments. In general, there is a considerable degree of similarity between survey findings in the 1991 survey by Archer et al. and in the Archer and Newsom (2000) results. For example, the Wechsler Intelligence Scales, the Rorschach, the TAT, and the MMPI remain among the most widely used tests with adolescents. In addition to questions related to test utilization,

TABLE 2.10   Test Usage Ratings for Ten Most Widely Used Assessment Instruments
           With Adolescents

Instrument	Usage Rating Totals							
	a	*b*	*c*	*d*	*e*	*f*	*TM*	*WS*
Wechsler Intelligence Scales	82	23	37	27	63	101	251	935
Rorschach Inkblot Technique	108	46	48	22	38	71	225	715
Sentence Completion Tasks (any form)	109	31	57	32	49	55	224	712
Thematic Apperception Test	114	46	55	38	33	47	219	637
MMPI-A	128	45	55	25	39	41	205	591
Child Behavior Checklist, Parent Report Form	133	62	50	18	30	41	201	541
The House-Tree-Person Technique	139	52	63	18	23	38	194	514
Wide Range Achievement Test (any format)	154	44	50	26	31	28	179	486
Child Behavior Checklist, Teacher's Report Form	138	54	65	25	29	22	195	485
Conners Rating Scales—Revised	135	46	82	27	31	12	198	475

Source: Adapted from Archer and Newsom (2000). Copyright © 2000 by Sage Publications. Reproduced with permission.

Note
a = Never; b = Infrequently; c = Occasionally; d = About 50% of the time; e = Frequently; f = Almost always. TM = Total mentions; WS = Weighted score (sum of n x numerical weight of ratings; a = 0, b = 1, c = 2, d = 3, e = 4, f = 5.

Archer and Newsom requested respondents to indicate the primary strengths associated with the use of the MMPI-A. The responses were, in order, the MMPI-A's ability to provide a comprehensive clinical picture, the availability of contemporary adolescent norms, ease of administration, and the psychometric soundness and comprehensive research base available for the instrument. The most frequently cited disadvantages reported by the respondents in connection with the MMPI-A included, in order, length of test instrument and associated demands for prolonged cooperation, a reading level that is too demanding or difficult for many adolescents, time requirements for scoring and interpretation, time requirements related to the administration of the test, and, finally, the expense associated with purchasing and using the test instrument in a managed care environment. Overall, Archer and Newsom observed that the MMPI-A has rapidly attained the status achieved by its predecessor as the most widely used objective personality assessment instrument with adolescents.

Research Popularity of the MMPI-A

In 1987, Archer noted that there were roughly 100 studies reported on the original form of the MMPI in adolescent populations from its release in 1943 to the mid-1980s. In contrast, Baum, Archer, Forbey, and Handel (2009) reviewed the literature on the MMPI-A and identified 277 articles, books, chapters, dissertations and monographs on this instrument since its release in 1992 until 2007. As a point of further comparison, Baum and her colleagues also noted that the Millon Adolescent Clinical Inventory (MACI), the second most frequently investigated objective personality self-report measure for adolescents, had only 84 publications or dissertations across the same 15-year timeframe. Baum et al. observed that the content areas addressed in this developing MMPI-A literature have been fairly broad and she grouped these publications into several non-mutually exclusive categories. Restricting review to published material, these categories included the use of the MMPI-A as an external criterion in validation of other instruments (five studies), 28 studies in which the MMPI-A had been used to address forensic issues, 21 investigations in which the MMPI-A addressed cross-cultural or cross-national issues, 21 articles related to the use of the MMPI-A with specific populations such as academically gifted adolescents or eating disordered adolescents, 44 MMPI-A articles dealing with specific methodological issues, 25 test reviews, 11 studies of MMPI-A Validity scales, and seven investigations of the factor structure of the MMPI-A. Overall, Baum et al. concluded that research with the MMPI-A is progressing at a much faster pace than shown in research investigations of the original form of the MMPI with adolescents and that the MMPI-A was the most widely researched objective personality assessment instrument used with adolescents. In support of this latter observation, Archer, Buffington-Vollum, Stredny, and Handel (2006) surveyed a group of 152 forensic psychologists concerning their utilization of a wide variety of test instruments and evaluations of both adults and children. Results of the survey indicated that the MMPI-A was the most widely used self-report instrument in evaluating adolescent's functioning in forensic settings.

Development of the MMPI-A-RF

As previously noted, the MMPI-A was developed to maintain continuity with the Validity and Clinical scales of the original MMPI, and was therefore subject to the same limitations inherent in the criteria-keying methodology used by Hathaway and McKinley in their development of these scales. These limitations included scale multidimensionality and content heterogeneity, as well as excessive item overlap between scales. These characteristics resulted in well documented high levels of intercorrelations between the MMPI-2 Basic scales as well as the MMPI-A Basic scales, and substantive limitations in the discriminant validity of these scales, the latter reflected in higher than expected correlations between specific scales and external criteria believed to be unrelated to the basic constructs assessed by these scales. A secondary issue concerned the 478-item length of the MMPI-A item tool, which had been identified by many as a significant disadvantage in comparison to shorter test instruments available for adolescents. Therefore, the target length of the MMPI-A-RF was set at 250 items or less by the test developers.

Table 2.11 provides a summary of the factors that contributed to the decision to develop the MMPI-A-RF. The MMPI-A-RF development project began in late 2007 with the goal of exploring the potential for developing an adolescent instrument modeled after the approach used in developing the MMPI-2-RF. Committee members included Robert Archer and Richard Handel at the Eastern Virginia Medical School, Yossi Ben-Porath at Kent State University, and Auke Tellegen of the University of Minnesota. The initial responsibility of the committee was to advise the University of Minnesota Press concerning the feasibility of creating an adolescent form of the MMPI-2-RF, using the MMPI-2-RF as the template to inform the development of the adolescent instrument.

TABLE 2.11 Factors Contributing to the Development of the MMPI-A-RF

I	Need to reduce the high degree of MMPI-A scale intercorrelation
	A. Reduce redundant influence of demoralization factor across scales
	B. Reduce item overlap between scales
	C. Reduce scale content multidimensionality
II	Develop a test based on roughly 250 items
	A. Test length of MMPI-A viewed by some as a significant disadvantage
	B. Develop an adolescent self-report measure comparable to the MMPI-2-RF but adapted to include measures uniquely related to adolescent psychopathology

Accordingly, the first step in developing the MMPI-A-RF was to identify a measure of demoralization, a major factor contributing to the high intercorrelation between the MMPI-A Basic Clinical scales. The second step was to identify major distinctive components for each of the MMPI-A Basic Clinical scales which could be differentiated from the demoralization factor through the use of factor analyses. This process essentially led to the development of Restructured Clinical (RC) scales for the MMPI-A-RF. The third step was to develop additional substantive scales to cover other content areas available in the MMPI-A item pool that were not directly addressed by the RC scales. The MMPI-2-RF Specific Problem scales served as the initial template for scale development, but were also augmented by scales uniquely developed for the MMPI-A-RF to address adolescent problem areas. In developing the MMPI-A-RF Specific Problems scales, procedures similar to those used to develop the MMPI-A-RF RC scales were followed by the test developers. Specifically, each of the MMPI-2-RF Specific Problem scales was examined to evaluate the extent to which corresponding MMPI-A items were available within the MMPI-A item pool. There was also a group of 58 items unique to the MMPI-A item pool which are not found on the MMPI-2-RF, for example those items uniquely found in the MMPI-A Content scales. After deriving a preliminary set of Specific Problem scales for the MMPI-RF, each scale was subjected to factor analysis to reduce the extent to which Specific Problem scales were strongly associated with the demoralization factor dimension. The remaining seed or core scales were further refined by dropping candidate items that appeared to be too highly correlated with other Specific Problem (SP) scales. Finally, we correlated each of the candidate SP scales with all remaining items from the 478-item pool of the MMPI-A. In this final stage, items with relevant content were added to a scale if they sufficiently correlated with that scale and showed a pattern of lower correlations with other SP scales.

As with the MMPI-2-RF, the process of deriving a final set of SP scales included numerous analyses of different subsets of items conducted in various age and gender subsamples. The development samples used for the construction of the MMPI-A-RF scales were initially based on a sample of 11,093 boys and 7,238 girls from a variety of settings including inpatient and outpatient psychiatric settings, correctional, drug and alcohol treatment, general medical, and school settings. Because of the relatively small number of participants in the drug/alcohol treatment and general medical settings, these latter samples were removed from any further analyses. Additionally, a variety of exclusion criteria were applied which included the following:

1. Age restricted to adolescents between 14 through 18, inclusive;
2. MMPI-A Cannot Say scores less than 30;
3. MMPI-A *VRIN*, *TRIN*, *L*, and *K* scale scores less than 80;
4. MMPI-A *F* scale score less than 90.

After applying these inclusion criteria, the final developmental sample consisted of 15,128 adolescents including 9,286 boys and 5,842 girls. The mean age for these samples which were derived from outpatient, inpatient, correctional and school settings was 15.61. In order to evaluate the influence of age and gender on scale construction, samples were further subdivided by age and gender, creating four developmental samples used in scale development. These four samples were: (1) younger boys (14 to 15); (2) older boys (16 to 18); (3) younger girls (14 to 15), and (4) older girls (16 to 18).

Finally, a revised set of Personality Psychopathology Five (PSY-5) scales was developed for the MMPI-A-RF by John McNulty and Alan Harkness based on their five-factor personality model. Harkness, McNulty, and Ben–Porath (1995) originally created a set of PSY-5 scales for the MMPI-2, and McNulty, Harkness, Ben-Porath, and Williams (1997) developed PSY-5 scales for the MMPI-A. McNulty and Harkness developed the MMPI-A-RF PSY-5 scales using a similar methodology to that employed for the MMPI-2 and MMPI-A. Items were selected on a rational basis, and internal consistency and external criteria analyses were conducted based on samples divided into developmental and validation studies. A cycle of internal analyses was conducted in four large databases, separately by gender.

The development process used to create the MMPI-A-RF resulted in 48 scales (six validity scales and 42 substantive scales). Table 2.12 provides brief descriptions of these 48 scales. The 48 MMPI-A-RF scales, similar to the MMPI-2-RF, have a three-tiered hierarchical structure that includes three Higher–Order broad-base scales at the top of the hierarchy, nine Restructured Clinical (RC) scales at the mid-level, and 25 SP scales at the lowest level as well as five PSY-5 scales. While the Higher-Order scales, RC scales, and many of the SP scales are identical in name to their counterparts on the MMPI-2-RF, it is important to note that the item composition of these scales differs, often significantly, from their MMPI-2-RF counterparts. The Validity scales shown in Table 2.12 include a non-content-based Validity scale which is not found in the MMPI-2-RF, the Combined Response Inconsistency (*CRIN*) scale. It should also be noted that the Infrequent Responses (*F-r*) scale shown in Table 2.12 is based on infrequent responses as defined by response frequencies obtained in both the normative and clinical samples, and therefore the *F-r* scale combines aspects of both the *F* and *Fp* scales on the MMPI-2-RF.

The MMPI-A-RF SP scales are organized into five Somatic/Cognitive scales, related to elevations on *RC1*, and nine Internalizing scales measuring aspects or facets of demoralization (*RCd*) and Dysfunctional Negative Emotions (*RC7*). There are also six Externalizing scales which measure facets of Antisocial Behavior (*RC4*) and Hypomanic Activation (*RC9*). It should be noted that three of the six Externalizing scales (Negative School Attitudes, Conduct Problems, and Negative Peer Influences) are unique to the MMPI-A-RF and do not have a counterpart on the MMPI-2-RF. The MMPI-A-RF also contains five

TABLE 2.12 MMPI-A-RF Scale and Descriptions

The MMPI-A-RF Scales

Validity Scales

 VRIN-r (Variable Response Inconsistency) Random responding

 TRIN-r (True Response Inconsistency) Fixed responding

 CRIN (Combined Response Inconsistency)—Combination of fixed and random inconsistent responding

 F-r (Infrequent Responses) Responses infrequent in the general population

 L-r (Uncommon Virtues) Rarely claimed moral attributes or activities

 K-r (Adjustment Validity) Uncommonly high level of psychological adjustments

Higher-Order (H-O) Scales

 EID (Emotional/Internalizing Dysfunction) Problems associated with mood and affect

 THD (Thought Dysfunction) Problems associated with disordered thinking

 BXD (Behavioral/Externalizing Dysfunction) Problems associated with under-controlled behavior

Restructured Clinical (RC) Scales

 RCd (Demoralization) General unhappiness and dissatisfaction

 RC1 (Somatic Complaints) Diffuse physical health complaints

 RC2 (Low Positive Emotions) A distinctive, core vulnerability factor in depression

 RC3 (Cynicism) Non-self-referential beliefs that others are bad and not to be trusted

 RC4 (Antisocial Behavior) Rule-breaking and irresponsible behavior

 RC6 (Ideas of Persecution) Self-referential beliefs that others pose a threat

 RC7 (Dysfunctional Negative Emotions) Maladaptive anxiety, anger, and irritability

 RC8 (Aberrant Experiences) Unusual perceptions or thoughts associated with psychosis

 RC9 (Hypomanic Activation) Over-activation, aggression, impulsivity, and grandiosity

Specific Problems (SP) Scales

 Somatic/Cognitive Scales

  MLS (Malaise) Overall sense of physical debilitation, poor health

  GIC (Gastrointestinal Complaints) Nausea, recurring upset stomach, and poor appetite

  HPC (Head Pain Complaints) Head and neck pain

  NUC (Neurological Complaints) Dizziness, weakness, paralysis, and loss of balance

  COG (Cognitive Complaints) Memory problems, difficulties concentrating

 Internalizing Scales

  HLP (Helplessness/Hopelessness) Belief that goals cannot be reached or problems solved

  SFD (Self-Doubt) Lack of self-confidence, feelings of uselessness

  NFC (Inefficacy) Belief that one is indecisive and inefficacious)

  OCS (Obsessions/Compulsions) Varied obsessional and compulsive behaviors

  STW (Stress/Worry) Preoccupation with disappointments, difficulty with time pressure

AXY (Anxiety) Pervasive anxiety, frights, frequent nightmares

ANP (Anger Proneness) Easily angered, impatient with others

BRF (Behavior-Restricting Fears) Fears that significantly inhibit normal behavior

SPF (Specific Fears) Multiple specific fears

Externalizing Scales

NSA (Negative School Attitudes) Negative attitudes and beliefs about school

ASA (Antisocial Attitudes) Various antisocial beliefs and attitudes

CNP (Conduct Problems) Difficulties at school and at home, stealing

SUB (Substance Abuse) Current and past misuse of alcohol and drugs

NPI (Negative Peer Influence) Affiliation with negative peer group

AGG (Aggression) Physically aggressive, violent behavior

Interpersonal Scales

FML (Family Problems) Conflictual family relationships

IPP (Interpersonal Passivity) Being unassertive and submissive

SAV (Social Avoidance) Avoiding or not enjoying social events

SHY (Shyness) Feeling uncomfortable and anxious around others

DSF (Disaffiliativeness) Disliking people and being around them

Personality Psychopathology Five (PSY-5) Scales

AGGR-r (Aggressiveness-Revised) Instrumental, goal-directed aggression

PSYC-r (Psychoticism-Revised) Disconnection from reality

DISC-r (Disconstraint-Revised) Under-controlled behavior

NEGE-r (Negative Emotionality/Neuroticism-Revised) Anxiety, insecurity, worry and fear

INTR-r (Introversion/Low Positive Emotionality-Revised) Social disengagement and anhedonia

---

Interpersonal scales, three of which (Family Problems, Social Avoidance, and Shyness) are interpretable in terms of both high and low scores. Finally, the Personality Psychopathology Five (PSY-5) scales are based on the revision undertaken by McNulty and Harkness to accommodate the 241 items of the MMPI-A-RF.

The MMPI-A-RF was released in 2016. Test materials released at that time included the *MMPI-A-RF manual for administration, scoring, interpretation, and technical manual* (Archer et al. 2016a) and scoring and automated interpretation systems available through Pearson Assessment. The MMPI-A-RF norms are derived from the normative sample for the MMPI-A, and focus on the assessment of adolescents ages 14 through 18, inclusive. A more comprehensive discussion of the MMPI-A-RF, including the development and interpretation of the Validity scales, Higher-Order scales, RC scales, and SP scales, is provided in Chapter 7.

TABLE 2.13 Comparison of the MMPI, MMPI-A, and MMPI-A-RF

Variable	MMPI	MMPI-A	MMPI-A-RF
Year of Publication	1942	1992	2016
Number of Items	566	478	241
Items required for abbreviated administration	400	370	Not available
Normative group size	1,766 (Marks & Briggs, 1972)	1620	1610
Administrative age range	12 and up	14–18 (possible with selected 12- and 13-year-olds)	14–18 (possible with selected 12- and 13-year-olds)
Validity Scales	L, F, K	VRIN, TRIN, L, F_1, F, L, and K	VRIN-r, TRIN-r, CRIN, F-r, L-r, and K-r
Critical Items	Multiple sets of critical items developed for adults	Forbey and Ben-Porath Critical Items List	Forbey and Ben-Porath Revised Critical Item List

As shown in Table 2.13, various forms of the MMPI have been used to evaluate adolescent psychopathology for over seven decades. The original form of the MMPI, while primarily developed for use with adults, was also widely used with adolescents from its original publication in 1942 until the publication of the MMPI-A in 1992. The MMPI-A is an instrument which is heavily interrelated to both the original form of the MMPI, as well as to the MMPI-2. The MMPI-A rapidly became the most widely used objective personality assessment instrument with adolescents, in both research and clinical settings. The development of the MMPI-A represented the first time in the history of this instrument that a specialized set of adolescent norms were created, and that a specific test form was developed by the test publisher for the assessment of adolescents. The MMPI-A-RF was heavily influenced by the theoretical underpinnings and methodological approach used in developing the MMPI-2-RF. The MMPI-A-RF is a 241-item self-report instrument which was derived from the 478 items of the MMPI-A. As we will discuss later in this text, the MMPI-A-RF is not simply a revision of the MMPI-A, and is most productively viewed as a new and innovative instrument that shares many of the features of the MMPI-A, but represents a new test instrument.

3

ADMINISTRATION AND SCORING ISSUES

Qualification and Background of Test Users

The use of the MMPI-A or MMPI-A-RF with adolescents requires specific training and experience in several areas. First, the clinician should be adequately trained in the essential features of test theory and test construction, as well as more specifically in the development and uses of these instruments. Therefore, the test user should have completed graduate-level courses in psychological testing and reviewed introductory or basic texts, such as those by Archer and Krishnamurthy (2002) and by Williams & Butcher (2011). Those seeking greater familiarity with the development of the MMPI-2 including the composition of the basic validity and clinical scales, or basic interpretive strategies, should also refer to the general guides provided by Friedman, Bolinskey, Levak, and Nichols (2015), Graham (2012), and Greene (2011), and to Ben-Porath (2012) for comparable information on the MMPI-2-RF. Archer (1987b), Hathaway and Monachesi (1963), and Marks et al. (1974) provided reference works concerning the use of the original MMPI form in the assessment of adolescents. Before administering the MMPI-A or MMPI-A-RF, the clinician should also thoroughly review the MMPI-A manual (Butcher et al., 1992), or the MMPI-A-RF manual (Archer et al., 2016a), which provide summaries of the development, administration, scoring, and interpretation of these instruments.

In addition to background and training in psychological assessment issues, individuals who apply the MMPI-A or MMPI-A-RF with adolescents should also have additional preparation in the areas of adolescent development, personality, psychopathology, and psychodiagnosis.

Administration Personnel

Because the actual administration of the MMPI-A or MMPI-A-RF appears deceptively simple, this task is frequently entrusted to individuals operating under the supervision of a psychologist. If these individuals are carefully trained, closely supervised, and well informed concerning appropriate test procedures, such a test administration procedure should not negatively affect test validity. Unfortunately, there are instances of invalid MMPI findings that are related to incorrect administration procedures used by untrained or unsupervised clerks or secretaries. Greene (2011) noted that although a clinician may delegate the task of MMPI administration to an assistant, a clinician cannot delegate the responsibility for proper administration. Responsibility for appropriate administration remains with the clinician utilizing and interpreting test findings. Because testing conditions, test instructions, and responses to clients' questions concerning test materials or purposes can all profoundly affect test results, the clinician must ensure that these areas meet the accepted standards for administration procedures.

Purpose of MMPI-A and MMPI-A-RF Administration

The MMPI-A and MMPI-A-RF are designed to assess psychopathology for adolescents ages 14 through 18, inclusive, and may be selectively used with 12- and 13-year-old adolescents under certain circumstances, which are discussed later. As noted in the MMPI-A and MMPI-A-RF manuals, 18-year-olds may be evaluated with this instrument if they are living with their parents in a dependent environment, but should be assessed with an adult form of the MMPI, that is, the MMPI-2 or MMPI-2-RF, if living independently. The MMPI-A and MMPI-A-RF are appropriate for evaluating adolescents who are experiencing, or suspected of experiencing, some form or type of psychopathology. The MMPI-A and MMPI-A-RF have two major functions in the assessment of adolescent psychopathology. First, these instruments provide the ability to objectively evaluate and describe an adolescent's level of functioning in relation to selected standardized dimensions of psychopathology. We may examine MMPI-A or MMPI-A-RF test findings, for example, in order to assess the degree to which an adolescent's psychological functioning deviates from that typically reported by normal adolescents. For these purposes, we compare an adolescent's test scores against those obtained by the test's normative sample. If an adolescent produces clinical levels of psychopathology on the MMPI-A or MMPI-A-RF, we may also consult the clinical literatures on these tests to find the most appropriate descriptors for that adolescent. These descriptors are established based on research with adolescents who have produced similar MMPI-A or MMPI-A-RF patterns. Second, the repeated administration of the MMPI-A or MMPI-A-RF can provide the clinician with a means of assessing changes in psychopathology across time. The ability to assess temporal changes is particularly important in dealing with adolescents, because this developmental stage is defined by rapid changes in personality and psychopathology. When the MMPI-A or MMPI-A-RF is administered at various stages in the treatment process, test results may also provide the clinician with a sensitive index of therapeutic change. Because the MMPI-A and MMPI-A-RF were developed as a means of describing psychopathology, the tests were not intended to serve as a primary measure for describing normal-range personality traits or functioning.

Administration Issues

A number of administration guidelines or criteria may be offered for using the MMPI-A or MMPI-A-RF with adolescents. Table 3.1 provides an overview of these criteria, with suggested responses that may be utilized by the clinician in dealing with specific administration issues and problems.

Age Criteria

Since the item pool and norms for the MMPI-A-RF are subsets of those for the MMPI-A, similar administration recommendations apply to both instruments. Guidelines for the administration of the MMPI-A have been provided

TABLE 3.1 Administration Guidelines for Adolescents Using the MMPI-A and MMPI-A-RF

Criteria	Possible Responses
1. Adolescent should be 14 to 18 years old.	A. 12- and 13-year-old adolescents may be evaluated with the MMPI-A or MMPI-A-RF if they meet all other criteria.
	B. Above 18, administer the MMPI-2 or the MMPI-2-RF
	C. Under age 12, do not administer MMPI (any form).
2. Adolescent must be able to read and understand item pool.	A. Evaluate reading ability on standardized measure of reading comprehension.
	B. If below sixth-grade reading level, administer by CD audio presentation.
	C. If IQ is below 70 or reading level below third grade, do not administer MMPI (any form).
3. Adolescent must have appropriate supervised environment.	A. Provide continuous supervision by trained personnel in appropriate setting.
	B. Do not attempt MMPI-A or MMPI-A-RF testing in non-supervised environments.
4. Adolescent must be willing to tolerate testing with lengthy instrument.	A. Establish rapport with subject prior to testing.
	B. Discuss the importance of MMPI-A testing.
	C. Clearly explain to adolescents that they will receive test feedback.
	D. Consider dividing testing session into two or more segments.

by Archer and Krishnamurthy (2002) and by Williams and Butcher (2011), and are provided in Archer et al. (2016a) for the MMPI-A-RF. The MMPI-A test manual observes that the test can be administered to "bright immature adolescents" as young as age 12, and this guidance is also applicable to the MMPI-A-RF. In recognition of the difficulty that many 12- and 13-year-old adolescents encounter in attempting to respond to the MMPI-A or MMPI-A-RF, the normative samples for these tests were restricted to 14- through 18-year-old adolescents. If a 12- or 13-year-old adolescent meets all administration criteria, however, including adequate reading ability and cognitive and social maturity, it is possible to administer the MMPI-A or the MMPI-A-RF to these adolescents. A set of MMPI-A adolescent norms for 13-year-old boys and girls, based on linear T-score conversions and using the same exclusion criteria employed for the 14- through 18-year-old MMPI norms (e.g., original F scale raw score >25) is included in the Archer (1992) text.

A study by Janus, de Grott, and Toepfer (1998) examined two questions concerning the use of the MMPI-A with 13-year-old inpatients. These questions involved the extent to which the profiles of 13-year-old inpatients differed substantively from those produced by 14-year-olds, and the effects of scoring 13-year-olds using the standard MMPI-A norms versus the MMPI-A norms for 13-year-olds reported by Archer (1992). Janus and his colleagues analyzed the protocols from 56 13-year-olds and 85 14-year-old psychiatric inpatients. They reported no significant differences by age in mean T-scores, and no clear pattern of age differences were found in the percentage of elevated profiles. A strong multivariate effect was found, however, for the use of the Archer (1992) MMPI-A norms for 13-year-olds, resulting in lower T-score values in contrast to the use of the standard MMPI-A adolescent norms. However, pervasive univariate differences based on the use of 13-year-old versus standard adolescent norms were not found, and statistically significant differences occurred for only two of 38 scales for boys and seven of 38 scales for girls. In general, the results of this study suggest that 13- and 14-year-old adolescents respond in similar ways, and that the use of a separate set of 13-year-old norms may not result in any tangible improvements in MMPI-A interpretation for this age group.

It is cautioned, however, that 13-year-old adolescents typically represent a difficult age group to evaluate with the MMPI-A or MMPI-A-RF. All criteria for administration must be carefully assessed to determine if these younger adolescents are capable of producing valid responses. Younger adolescents may not have a wide enough range of life experiences, including exposure to cultural and educational opportunities commonly encountered in the U.S. society, to render the item content psychologically and semantically meaningful. Limitations in developmental opportunities, as well as reading abilities, clearly contraindicate the administration of the MMPI or MMPI-A-RF to younger adolescents.

At the other end of the adolescent age range, the adult and adolescent forms of the MMPI normative samples overlap at age 18, and it is possible that an

18-year-old respondent could be evaluated with either the adult or adolescent instrument. The MMPI-A manual contains the following recommendations concerning the evaluation of 18-year-olds:

> The clinician should make a case-by-case judgment about whether to use the MMPI-A or the MMPI-2 with 18-year-olds because the normative and clinical samples for both tests include 18-year-olds. A suggested guideline would be to use the MMPI-A for those 18-year-olds who are in high school and the MMPI-2 for those who are in college, working, or otherwise living an independent adult lifestyle.
>
> (Butcher et al., 1992, p. 23)

However, in the application of these guidelines, it is quite possible to encounter an occasional adolescent for whom the selection of the most appropriate form would be a difficult or ambiguous decision. For example, an 18-year-old single mother with a 6-month-old infant who is in her senior year in high school but living at home with her parents presents a considerable challenge in terms of identifying the most appropriate MMPI form for use with this individual. In these difficult cases, an important question arises concerning what effects, if any, the selection of the adolescent versus the adult form of the MMPI might have on the resulting profile in terms of T-score elevation and configuration. Shaevel and Archer (1996) examined the effects of scoring 18-year-old respondents on the MMPI-2 and MMPI-A and found that substantial differences can occur in T-score elevations as a function of this decision. Specifically, these authors reported that 18-year-olds scored on MMPI-2 norms generally produced lower validity scale values and higher clinical scale values than the same adolescents scored on MMPI-A norms. These differences ranged as high as 15 T-score points and resulted in different single-scale and two-point profile configurations in 34% of the cases examined in this study. Shaevel and Archer concluded that for those relatively rare assessment cases in which the selection of the MMPI-A versus the selection of the MMPI-2 is a difficult decision for the 18-year-old respondent, a reasonable practice would be to score that individual on both MMPI-A and MMPI-2 norms in order to permit the clinician to assess the relative effects of instrument selection on profile characteristics.

Two additional studies have examined the effects of scoring 18-year-olds on MMPI-A versus MMPI-2 norms. Gumbiner (1997) compared the MMPI-2 versus MMPI-A profiles of a group of 18-year-old male and female college students. In general, the resulting MMPI profiles were often dissimilar in terms of codetype classifications, with a marked tendency for MMPI-2 profiles to produce greater T-score elevations. Osberg and Poland (2002) also administered both the MMPI-2 and the MMPI-A to 18-year-old male and female college students. In addition, the Global Severity Index (GSI) of the SCL-90-R was used to classify participants as either psychopathology present or psychopathology absent to permit an assessment of the degree of usefulness between

MMPI-A and MMPI-2 scores in detecting the presence of psychopathology. Consistent with prior findings, the MMPI-A and MMPI-2 produced profiles in this study that were often inconsistent in terms of clinical elevation status (46% of respondents produced incongruent findings). All of the 70 participants in this study who produced incongruent MMPI-2 versus MMPI-A profiles had the same overall pattern, i.e., clinically elevated MMPI-2 T-scores and normal-range MMPI-A T-scores. Further, analysis of incongruent profiles by Osberg and Poland, in comparison with subject classification as psychopathology present or absent based on SCL-90-R scores, indicated that 18-year-olds were over-pathologized based on scores from the MMPI-2 and, in contrast, MMPI-A scores tended to under-pathologize respondents.

Reading Requirements

Reading level is obviously a crucial factor in determining whether an adolescent can complete the MMPI-A. Inadequate reading ability may serve as one of the major causes of invalid test protocols for adolescents. Ball and Carroll (1960) found that adolescents with lower IQs and below average academic records tended to produce higher Cannot Say scores, suggesting that the failure to respond to MMPI items often reflects problems in item comprehension. A modest inverse relationship ($r = -.10$, $p < .05$) between reading grade level and raw score values on the Cannot Say scale was also found by Archer and Gordon (1991a). This study was based on a sample of 495 normal adolescents who completed the MMPI-A and the Ohio Literacy Test, a measure of reading comprehension. Thus, adolescents who have difficulty reading MMPI or MMPI-A items tend to omit items at a higher frequency than other adolescents. Unfortunately, many adolescents also attempt to respond to items that they cannot adequately read or comprehend, often resulting in invalid test protocols.

For many years a sixth-grade reading level was generally accepted as a requirement for MMPI evaluation. Johnson and Bond (1950), for example, assessed the readability of MMPI items using the Flesch Reading Ease Formula (Flesch, 1948) and derived an overall estimate of sixth-grade reading difficulty for a sample of MMPI items. The sixth-grade reading level estimate was used in most standard texts on the MMPI. Ward and Ward (1980), however, reevaluated the MMPI items using the Flesch readability measure and reported that MMPI items on the Basic scales have an average reading difficulty level at the 6.7 grade level. Individual scale readability levels ranged from a 6.4 grade level on the *Mf* scale to a 7.2 grade level for the *K* scale. Their findings resulted in the recommendation of a seventh-grade reading level for individuals taking the MMPI. Further increasing reading ability requirements, Butcher et al. (1989) recommended that clients have at least an eighth-grade reading level in order to ensure adequate comprehension of the MMPI-2 item pool. This recommendation was based on the analysis of MMPI-2 items using item difficulty ratings referred to as *Lexile* ratings in the MMPI-2 manual. Paolo, Ryan, and Smith (1991) also examined the Lexile values for the 567 items of the MMPI-2 and for each of the scales and subscales associated with this measure. Paolo and his colleagues reported that approximately 90% of MMPI-2 items require less than a ninth-grade reading level, and that the mean for all items corresponded roughly to the fifth-grade reading level. In addition, the authors identified a number of scales or subscales in which at least 25% of the total number of scale items required more than an eighth-grade reading level. When the MMPI-2 item pool is evaluated using other standardized measures of reading difficulty such as the Flesch Reading Ease Formula (Flesch, 1948), however, there are indications that the Lexile ratings may have produced an overestimate of reading requirements.

Part of the complexity in attempting to evaluate the reading requirements of the MMPI involves the differences in standardized methods of estimating the reading difficulty of individual items. Additionally, lack of agreement on the number or percentage of items that must be successfully read and comprehended before an individual is deemed suitable to take the inventory has added to variations in estimates. Unfortunately, reading ability is frequently discussed in a dichotomous manner; that is, the subject either does or does not have the reading ability to take the MMPI. Many subjects, however, can successfully comprehend some, but not all, of the MMPI item pool. The central question concerns the number of items that must be successfully read in order to ensure the overall validity of the test findings.

The MMPI-A (Butcher et al., 1992) and MMPI-A-RF (Archer et al. 2016a) manuals provide analyses of the reading difficulty for each of the test items using standardized measures of reading difficulty. The measures include the Flesch–Kincaid method, which has been used in previous studies of the MMPI and other assessment instruments. Based on the Flesch–Kincaid, the MMPI-A and MMPI-A-RF item pools vary in reading difficulty from the 1st-grade to the 16th-grade level. Employing a criterion that at least 70% of the MMPI-A item pool should be accurately read and comprehended in order to ensure valid test findings, a seventh-grade reading level would be required for the MMPI-A and MMPI-A-RF, based on the Flesch–Kincaid reading comprehension standard.

Dahlstrom, Archer, Hopkins, Jackson, and Dahlstrom (1994) evaluated the reading difficulty of the MMPI, MMPI-2, and MMPI-A using various indices of reading difficulty including the Flesch Reading Ease and the Lexile Index. One important finding derived from this study was that the instructions provided in the MMPI test booklets tended to be more difficult to read than the typical item contained within the inventories. Therefore, clinicians should ensure that the instructions are fully understood by respondents and it is often appropriate to ask the test taker to read the instructions aloud, and to explain the meaning of the instructions, in order to ensure adequate comprehension. The average difficulty level for all three forms of the MMPI was approximately the sixth-grade level. The MMPI-A test instructions and items were slightly easier to read than the MMPI-2 or the original form of the MMPI; however, the total differences tended to be relatively small. If the most difficult 10% of items were excluded, the remaining 90% of items on all three versions of the MMPI had an average difficulty level of the fifth grade. On average, the most difficult items appeared on Scale 9, whereas the easiest items tended to be presented within the item pool of Scale 5. The authors also reported, based on the Reading Ease Index, that approximately 6% of the MMPI-A items required a 10th-grade reading level or better. Dahlstrom et al. noted that the number of years of education completed by a subject is often an unreliable index of the individual's reading competence.

As noted in the MMPI-A-RF manual (Archer et al., 2016a), some test developers have based estimates of required reading levels for self-report instruments on applying item difficulty measures to the entire item pool of the test, i.e., treating the entire item pool as a continuous text. Applying this approach to the MMPI-A-RF item pool produces a Flesch–Kincaid index at the 4.5 grade level. This appears to be an unrealistically low estimate of the required reading level for the MMPI-A-RF, however, given that 141 of the 241 MMPI-A-RF items produce a Flesch–Kincaid value of 5th grade or higher. Further, 98 MMPI-A-RF items produce a Flesch–Kincaid reading level of sixth grade or higher, and 65 test items show a reading level of 7th grade or higher.

Based on the numerous studies that have been conducted on the reading requirements of the MMPI-A, and the preliminary evaluation of the MMPI-A-RF, it would appear that the mean grade level of items on both tests is between fifth and sixth grade, depending on the method used to evaluate reading difficulty, and that the substantive majority of test items require a sixth-grade reading level or less. Therefore, the reading requirements for both the MMPI-A and the MMPI-A-RF can be reasonably estimated to be at the sixth-grade level.

Adolescents' reading abilities may be evaluated by the use of any of a number of reading comprehension instruments, including the Gray Oral Reading Test (GORT-5; Wiederholt & Bryant, 2012), the Peabody Individual Achievement Test – Revised (PIAT-R; Markwardt, 1989), or the reading component of the Wide Range Achievement Test – Fourth Edition (WRAT-4, Wilkinson and Robertson, 2006). Results of analyses by Dahlstrom et al. (1994) indicated that both the GORT and the Wechsler Individual Achievement Test showed a relatively smooth progression of scores in relation to student grade levels, and both measures were recommended if a reading test was employed for evaluating individual's competence to deal with the item difficulty of any MMPI form. A reasonably accurate reading screen can also be accomplished, however, by requesting the adolescent to read aloud and explain several MMPI-A items. The items that appear to be the most useful markers in this regard are items that have a sixth-grade reading level difficulty rating. Among the abbreviated MMPI-A and MMPI-A-RF test statements, sixth-grade level items include those shown in Table 3.2.

TABLE 3.2 Examples of MMPI-A/MMPI-A-RF Items Requiring a 6th Grade as Determined by the Flesch-Kincaid Grade Level Formula

	MMPI-A Item	MMPI-A-RF Item
Retaliate when wronged	24	233
Rarely quarrel with family	79	201
People honest because they don't want to be caught	100	24
I vomit to lose weight	108	205
Seldom notice heart pounding or shortness of breath	196	78

An adolescent may have difficulty in responding to the MMPI-A or MMPI-A-RF because of specific reading ability deficits rather than limitations in overall intellectual cognitive functioning. Under these circumstances, test administration may still be undertaken using the standardized audio versions of this instrument available through Pearson Assessments. Generally, procedures in which an examiner reads test items to the adolescent are not recommended because of the degree of intrusion on the response process associated with this method. Research by Newmark (1971), for example, indicated that MMPI profiles produced by adolescents for whom items were read aloud by an examiner resulted in higher K scale scores than results obtained with traditional administration methods. In contrast, Brauer (1992) showed that there is no significant effect found for the signer when selected MMPI items were translated into American Sign Language and recorded on videotape for use with hearing-impaired or deaf individuals. If an adolescent scores below 70 on the standardized IQ assessment measure or has less than a fourth-grade reading level, administration of the MMPI-A or MMPI-A-RF should not be attempted through any format.

When questions are asked by adolescents concerning the specific meaning of an MMPI-A statement or word, the examiner should attempt to provide useful but neutral information. For example, dictionary definitions can be given to commonly misunderstood words (e.g., *constipation, nausea,* or *brood*). However, the frequency with which adolescents encounter unfamiliar or awkwardly worded items is lower on the MMPI-A and MMPI-A-RF in comparison with the original test instrument, because 69 of the original items have been reworded or modified in order to improve the item readability or relevance to contemporary adolescents' life experiences. Research by Archer and Gordon (1994) and by Williams, Ben-Porath, and Hevern (1994) indicate that these revised items may be considered to be psychometrically equivalent to the original items in terms of response characteristics. When questions are raised by the adolescent concerning items that he or she clearly understands and comprehends, however, the examiner must always be careful to remind the subject to respond to the item as it applies to him or her, based on the adolescent's own judgments and opinions.

Despite reasonable efforts to evaluate reading ability, the clinician is likely to encounter adolescents who have responded to the MMPI-A or MMPI-A-RF item pools without reading and/or understanding many items. These problems may occur because of reading deficits, motivational issues, or a combination of these factors. A simple method of checking for most types of random response patterns involves recording the total MMPI-A/MMPI-A-RF administration time. Total administration time provides one useful index for aiding in the identification of random response sets among adolescents, particularly for adolescents who provide unusually brief administration times of less than 40 minutes for the full-length MMPI-A or 20 minutes for the MMPI-A-RF. Unless test administration time is recorded, however, this valuable information source is lost. Other methods of detecting potential problems in reading ability, based on MMPI-A scales including *TRIN* and *VRIN*, and MMPI-A-RF scales *TRIN-r, VRIN-r* and *CRIN*, are discussed in later chapters.

MMPI-A Translations

The original form of the MMPI was associated with a wide range of foreign language translations and an impressive amount of research on the cross-cultural applications of this test instrument. The MMPI-2 is currently available in a wide array of translations including Bulgarian, Croatian, Chinese, Czech, Danish, Dutch/Flemish, French, French-Canadian, German, Greek, Hebrew, Hmong, Hungarian, Italian, Korean, Norwegian, Polish, Romanian, and Swedish, and three Spanish language translations for use in the United States and in Central and South America. The MMPI-A is following in the same tradition of the MMPI and MMPI-2 in terms of foreign language translations, currently having a Spanish version available for use in the United States from Pearson Assessment and Spanish translations for Mexico and Central and South America (University of Minnesota Test Division, 2014). Translations of the MMPI-A have also been developed in Bulgarian, Croatian, Dutch/Flemish, French, Hungarian, Italian, and Korean. Butcher, Cabiya, Lucio, and Garrido (2007) have provided an interpretive guide for the MMPI-2 and MMPI-A with Hispanic clients.

Supervision Requirements

It is important that the adolescent is provided with an appropriate testing environment in which to complete the MMPI-A or MMPI-A-RF. This environment should include adequate privacy and supervision. The testing environment should be as comfortable as possible, minimizing the presence of extraneous noise or other distracting influences. It is inappropriate to allow an adolescent to complete the MMPI-A or MMI-A-RF in any unsupervised setting, or in settings in which privacy cannot be assured, such as at home. Unsupervised test administration does not provide adequate data for valid test interpretation, and is subject to successful legal challenge if such findings are presented in a courtroom setting. Adequate test supervision means that a proctor or examiner is available to continuously monitor the test-taking process, and to provide appropriate assistance when necessary. Adequate proctoring does not require, however, that the proctor monitor each individual response by the subject, or otherwise become overly intrusive in the testing process.

Increasing Adolescents' Cooperation With Testing Procedures

A final criterion in the evaluation of adolescents involves their willingness to answer the lengthy 478-item pool of the MMPI-A, or the more modest attention and time demands of the 241-item MMPI-A-RF. For the angry and oppositional adolescent, the MMPI-A or MMPI-A-RF may present a welcome opportunity to exhibit hostility and resistance by refusing to respond to items, or responding in an inappropriate or random manner (e.g., Newmark & Thibodeau, 1979). Once the adolescent has entered into an "anal-retentive" struggle with the examiner over test completion, there is often little the examiner can do that will effectively decrease the conflict. Prior to the administration of the MMPI-A or MMPI-A-RF, however, several steps may be taken to increase the motivation of most adolescents. These procedures include the following: (a) establishing adequate rapport with the adolescent prior to testing, (b) providing clear and concise instructions concerning the purposes of testing, and (c) providing the adolescent with an opportunity to receive testing feedback.

Clear and concise instructions should be given to the adolescent that provide them with a general understanding of the purposes of test administration. When clear instructions are not provided, many adolescents will project their own meaning onto the testing in a manner that may serve to render test results invalid. For example, an adolescent may erroneously believe that test results are being utilized to determine whether a psychiatric hospitalization is indicated, or are being used by the therapist to attribute blame or punishment for family conflict or family dysfunction. Poorly worded instructions may also negatively influence a subject's test-taking attitude and cooperation with testing procedures. The instructions, therefore, should be carefully presented in the standardized manner. The adolescent should read the instructions provided in the test booklet and also receive a verbal summary, which might, for example, include the following: "Read each statement and decide whether it is true as applied to you or false as applied to you. Remember to give your own opinion of yourself. There are no right or wrong answers. Your test results will help us to understand you."

In addition to these introductory instructions, adolescents frequently ask questions concerning various aspects of testing, which often reflects their anxiety concerning the evaluation process. The following are frequently encountered questions, with suggested responses, as adapted from the Caldwell Report (Caldwell, 1977a) and from Friedman et al. (2001).

1. Q. How long will this take?
   A. About an hour to an hour and a half, usually (or 45 minutes for the MMPI-A-RF). Some teenagers take longer, whereas other teenagers finish in less time.
2. Q. Will it make any difference if I skip some questions and come back to them?
   A. If you do it carefully, skipping some questions and returning to them probably will not make any difference. But it is easy to get mixed up in marking your answers, and that will make a difference, so it is better to do them in order, if possible.
3. Q. Suppose I cannot answer all the questions?
   A. Try to answer all of them. If you omit a few items, it will not matter, but try to do them all. When you are finished, take a few minutes to check your answer sheet for any missing answers, incomplete erasures, or double-answered questions.
4. Q. What is the MMPI-A (or MMPI-A-RF)?
   A. It is a widely used test to help understand the kinds of problems that happen to teenagers.
5. Q. How do I try to answer these questions?
   A. Answer the questions as you currently feel. Work quickly, and do not spend time worrying over your answers.
6. Q. What if I don't agree with the results from the test or the test results are wrong?
   A. That is something that you and I will get a chance to discuss during the feedback process. Teenagers often learn some things about themselves that they did not know, and the therapist often learns which parts of the testing were more accurate than others. It is hoped we will *both* learn something from the feedback process.

It is important to present the MMPI-A or MMPI-A-RF to adolescents in a careful and serious manner that underscores the importance of the testing process. Attempts to assist the adolescent in feeling more comfortable by minimizing the importance of the MMPI-A evaluation are usually counterproductive. A "casual" presentation of the MMPI-A may actually result in a reduction in the adolescent's cooperation and motivation to complete testing because his or her doubts concerning the importance of test findings will appear to have been validated.

Test Administration Procedures to Increase Cooperation

Several additional steps may be taken in order to increase adolescents' willingness to cooperate with testing procedures. For example, it is often feasible to divide the administration of the MMPI-A or MMPI-A-RF across several sessions, when the total test administration can be accomplished over a few days.

If administration is attempted in one session, particularly for the MMPI-A, it is advisable to provide rest periods if an adolescent is becoming fatigued during the testing process. Placement of the MMPI-A or MMPI-A-RF at the earlier stages of an extensive test battery decreases the probability that an adolescent may employ a random response set in order to finish the testing session as quickly as possible. Finally, a clinician may elect to administer only the first 350 items in the MMPI-A form as an abbreviated administration of the test. If the motivation or cooperation of an adolescent would be increased significantly by an abbreviated administration format, or if time restrictions impose such limitations, this option allows the clinician to fully score and interpret the standard Clinical Scales, three of the Validity scales (L, F_1, and K) and the Harris–Lingoes and Si subscales. Abbreviated administrations of the MMPI-A do not, however, provide scores concerning the Content scales, the Supplementary scales, Validity scales $VRIN$, $TRIN$, F, and F_2. Another alternative to the full administration of the MMPI-A under time limited situations is the MMPI-A-RF, which is roughly half the item length of the MMPI-A and 109 items shorter than the abbreviated form of the MMPI-A, the Content Component scales, or the PSY-5 scales.

Short Form Issues Related to the MMPI-A

Ball, Archer, and Imhof (1994) reported findings from a national survey of practitioners related to the time requirements associated with the administration, scoring, and interpretation of 24 commonly used psychological test instruments. Findings derived for the MMPI indicated a mean administration time of 66.16 minutes, and a modal value of 90 minutes. This modal time estimate was exceeded only by the time requirements associated with administration of the Halstead–Reitan neuropsychological test battery. In response to the problems created by the lengthy MMPI item pool, Newmark and Thibodeau (1979) recommended the development and use of short forms of the MMPI in the assessment of adolescents. As defined by Butcher and Hostetler (1990), the term *short form* is

> used to describe sets of scales that have been decreased in length from the standard MMPI form. An MMPI short form is a group of items that is thought to be a valid substitute for the full scale score even though it might contain only 4 or 5 items from the original full scale.
>
> (p. 12)

The MMPI-168 was developed by utilizing the first 168 items to appear in the group booklet form of the MMPI (Overall & Gomez-Mont, 1974). The 71-item Mini-Mult was devised by Kincannon (1968) based on factor analyses used to identify item cluster groups. Investigations of MMPI-168 characteristics in adolescent samples were provided by MacBeth and Cadow (1984) and Rathus (1978). In addition, Mlott (1973) reported Mini-Mult findings for adolescent inpatients. Vondell and Cyr (1991) evaluated the influence of gender on eight MMPI short forms, including the Mini-Mult and the MMPI-168, in a sample of 318 male and 248 female adolescent psychiatric inpatients. The authors concluded that gender differences occur on all of these short forms in adolescent populations, a result that parallels similar findings obtained in short form investigations of adult samples.

Butcher (1985) and Butcher and Hostetler (1990) noted a series of potential problems with the use of MMPI short forms. The reduced number of items within MMPI scales entailed in short form versions reduces the overall reliability of the measurement of scale constructs. The shortened versions of the MMPI have also not been sufficiently validated against external criteria. Additionally, the short form profiles and codetypes are frequently different from results that would have been achieved for an individual based on the administration of the full MMPI item pool. Research by Hoffmann and Butcher (1975), for example, showed that the Mini-Mult and administration of the standard MMPI tend to produce the same MMPI codetypes in only 33% of cases, and that the full MMPI and the MMPI-168 produce similar codetypes in only 40% of adult cases. Consistent with these findings, Lueger (1983) reported that two-point codetypes derived from standard and MMPI-168 forms were different in over 50% of their sample of male adolescents. Greene (1982) suggested that short forms of the MMPI may constitute new test measures that require additional validation to identify external correlates. In addition to issues related to scale reliability and codetype congruence, Butcher and Hostetler (1990) questioned the ability of the MMPI short forms to accurately determine profile validity.

The problems with MMPI short forms, as identified in studies with adult populations, appear to have important implications for clinical and/or research uses of the MMPI-A. In particular, there is a significant loss of valuable clinical information when short forms are used in place of the full MMPI. The use of a short form procedure, although it saves administration time with adolescent respondents, appears likely to introduce more than an acceptable range of confusion and "noise" into the interpretation process for adolescent profiles. In recognition of these problems, no efforts were made by the MMPI-2 or MMPI-A advisory committees to preserve any of the currently existing MMPI short forms. Consequently, as noted by Butcher and Hostetler (1990), "Some of the items constituting previously developed MMPI short forms may have been deleted from the MMPI in the revision process" (p. 18).

Archer, Tirrell, and Elkins (2001) reported psychometric properties related to a short form of the MMPI-A based on the administration of the first 150 items of this test instrument. Results were based on analysis of the MMPI-A normative sample of 1620 adolescents and a clinical sample of 565 adolescents in a variety of treatment settings. Correlational analysis showed short form to full administration Basic Scale score correlations in the range of .71 for the *Mf* scale to a high of .95 for the *L* scale when computed for all the MMPI-A Basic Validity and Clinical scales. In addition to the correlational analyses, these authors also examined the degree of differences found in mean T-score values produced for the MMPI-A Basic scales by the full administration of the test instrument and when T-score values were pro-rated from MMPI-A short form results. Although comparisons for several of the Basic Validity and Clinical scales reached significance, at least partially because a relatively large sample size was utilized in these analyses, the mean T-score differences between the actual and pro-rated values exceeded two T-score points only for scales 4 and 9 in the clinical sample. While these analyses showed relatively high scale correlations and mean profile similarities, relatively lower rates of congruence in profile configural patterns were produced in this study. Specifically, only 30.6% of the normative sample and 32.2% of the clinical sample produced Basic scale profiles that were congruent in terms of identical two-point elevations produced by short form and full-length administrations. The potential advantages of this MMPI-A 150 included the reduction of the total item pool by nearly 70% and the reduction in typical administration time from 60 to 20 minutes. This item and time savings, however, are more than offset by the limitations in profile congruency illustrated in this study, and in all prior research findings related to MMPI short forms.

The use of MMPI-A short forms, particularly in light of the 241-item length of the MMPI-A-RF, is not recommended in the assessment of adolescents. As previously noted, however, the abbreviated form of the MMPI-A, or the administration of the MMPI-A-RF, may serve as a reasonable resource in coping with poorly motivated or resistant adolescents. Additionally, several approaches to abbreviating the administration of the MMPI-2 item pool by adapting the presentation of MMPI-2 items to computer administration have been developed and evaluated (e.g., Ben-Porath, Slutske, & Butcher, 1989; Roper, Ben-Porath, & Butcher, 1991, 1995). Computer-adapted administration approaches are strategies of presenting only those items that add to clinically relevant information about the patient, given the patient's prior MMPI-2 responses. Several approaches have been developed for this purpose, including strategies based on Item Response Theory (IRT) and the "countdown method," the latter approach terminating item administration for a given scale once sufficient information for that scale has been obtained from the respondent. Butcher and Hostetler (1990) noted that at that time although none of these approaches had proved practical, it was likely that effective, adaptive programs will be developed in the future for automated administration of the MMPI-2 and MMPI-A. In this regard, Forbey, Handel, and Ben-Porath (2000) evaluated a real data simulation of a computerized adaptive administration of the MMPI-A conducted using the item responses from three groups of participants. The first group included 196 adolescents (ages 14 through 18) tested at a midwestern residential treatment facility for adolescents. The second group consisted of the MMPI-A normative sample, and the third group was the clinical sample reported in the MMPI-A test manual (Butcher et al., 1992). The MMPI-A data for each group was run through a modified version of the MMPI-2 adaptive testing computer program to determine the amount of item savings produced by simulations based on three different orderings of MMPI-A items. These orderings included the presentation of items from least to most frequently endorsed in the critical or key direction, from the least to the most frequently endorsed in the keyed direction for the first 120 items arranged in the test booklet, or for all items administered in the test booklet. The mean number of items administered for each group were computed for each administration using T-score cutoffs of 60 and 65 to define clinical range elevations. Substantial item administration savings were achieved for the groups, and the mean number of items saved ranged from 50 items to 123 items, (in contrast to the 478 item total item pool), depending on the T-score cutoff classification method. This study shows promise in terms of the potential item saving ability that could be associated with the development of a computerized adaptive administration format for the MMPI-A.

Test Materials

Original MMPI Forms

Several forms of the original MMPI were developed, including the MMPI Group Form, which was a reusable group booklet form, and MMPI Form R, which was a hardcover, spiral-bound test booklet. Of these two forms, the Group Form was more widely used. Furthermore, as Greene (1980) noted, most of the MMPI research literature has been based on data derived from the Group Form. The Form R booklet had been particularly useful, however, when a subject does not have a hard surface on which to enter responses to the test items. The Form R answer sheet is inserted over two pegs in the back of the test booklet. Form R pages follow a step-down format in which the turning of each consecutive page reveals another column of answer spaces matched with the booklet column of the corresponding questions. The step-down procedure reveals only one column of questions and answers at a time, thereby reducing the possibility of misplacing a response to a specific question.

The numbering system for items in the group booklet form and Form R of the original MMPI were identical for the first 366 items, but diverged for the latter parts of the item pool. This discrepancy created substantial confusion for both researchers and clinicians. Dahlstrom et al. (1972), however, provided item conversion tables between the Group Form and Form R formats. Administration of the first 399 items on Form R allowed for an abbreviated testing, permitting the scoring of all basic standard and validity scales. Unfortunately, there was not a straightforward method of providing an abbreviated administration for the Group Form booklet.

On September 1, 1999, the University of Minnesota Press and the test distributor (Pearson Assessments) discontinued publication of the original form of the MMPI. The original form of the MMPI was discontinued because the material surrounding its use had become considerably dated, and the MMPI-2 and MMPI-A had largely replaced the original MMPI in clinical and research uses. The University of Minnesota Press also noted that the concurrent use of the original form of the MMPI with the revised forms of the MMPI had become a source of potential confusion for many test users, particularly those in forensic settings. Further, the MMPI-2 and MMPI-A had the benefit of containing a more appropriate and contemporary item pool as well as more contemporary and nationally representative normative samples.

MMPI-A and MMPI-A-RF Test Materials

Testing materials related to the use of the MMPI-A and MMPI-A-RF are available from Pearson Assessments. The order of the item presentation is identical across paper-and-pencil, computer, and audio versions of the MMPI-A and the 241 items of the MMPI-A-RF are also presented in the same order across formats. The CD versions of the MMPI-A and MMPI-A-RF are useful for the visually impaired, as well as for adolescents with significant reading-related disabilities that make the standard form administration impractical. This method of administration requires approximately one hour and 40 minutes (Archer & Krishnamurthy, 2002) for the MMPI-A and is estimated to require roughly 50 minutes for the MMPI-A-RF. Computerized administrations of MMPI-A and MMPI-A-RF items are also available through the purchase of software from Pearson Assessments.

Different answer sheets are available for the MMPI-A and MMPI-A-RF. Further, depending on whether the examiner intends to score the test by the use of hand-scoring keys or by computer scoring, different answer sheets are provided within each of these tests. Therefore, the examiner should consider the scoring mechanism that will be utilized before selecting the answer sheet to be used for the MMPI-A or MMPI-A-RF.

Scoring the MMPI-A and the MMPI-A-RF

The examiner should take substantial care to eliminate the common sources of error that occur in scoring and profiling MMPI-A or MMPI-A-RF responses. This process should start with a careful examination of the adolescent's answer sheet to ensure that items were not left unanswered, or endorsed in both the true and false directions. Additionally, answer sheets should be examined for evidence of response patterns indicative of random markings, or all-true or all-false response sets.

Obtaining the raw scores for all of the MMPI-A or MMPI-A-RF scales may be accomplished by computer or hand-scoring keys. If hand-scoring is used, conversion of raw scores to T-score values should be done using MMPI-A profile sheets based on the gender-specific adolescent norms for the MMPI-A or the non-gendered norms developed for the MMPI-A-RF. Adolescent profile sheets for the MMPI-A and MMPI-A-RF are available through Pearson Assessments, which utilize the normative values for the MMPI-A described and presented in Appendix A of the MMPI-A manual (Butcher et al., 1992) and in Appendix A of the MMPI-A-RF manual (Archer et al. 2016a). It is important to clarify that the raw score K-correction procedure is *not* used in deriving or profiling T-scores for adolescents with either the MMPI-A or MMPI-A-RF. As previously noted, Marks et al. (1974) reported several reasons why the K-correction procedure was not developed for adolescent norms, including their preliminary evidence that adolescent MMPI profiles achieve greater discrimination between adolescent subgroups without the addition of a K-correction factor. As is presented in more detail later, an investigation by Alperin, Archer, and Coates (1996) examined the effectiveness of a K-correction factor for the MMPI-A, and concluded that the adoption of a K-correction procedure would not result in systematic improvement in test accuracy for this instrument.

As reviewed by Archer (1989) and by Archer and Krishnamurthy (2002), the procedures for scoring and profiling adolescent responses on the MMPI-A (and by extension the MMPI-A-RF) may be summarized as follows. First, carefully examine the answer sheet for evidence of deviant response sets, unanswered items, or double-marked items. Second, obtain the raw score value for each scale, utilizing the computer scoring reports available from Pearson Assessments or the hand-scoring keys. Third, convert the non-K-corrected raw scores to T-scores for each scale using the appropriate adolescent norm tables, with attention to the gender of the respondent for the MMPI-A. Fourth, plot T-score values on the appropriate MMPI-A or MMPI-A-RF profile sheet. The MMPI-A Profile for Basic Scales (Male Form) is shown in Figure 3.1 and the MMPI-A-RF Profile for RC scales (non-gendered) is shown in Figure 3.2.

Scoring of the MMPI-A or MMPI-A-RF may be accomplished through several different methods. A computer software program is available through Pearson Assessments that permits test users to administer and score all test scales using their personal computers. Specifically, the MMPI-A Basic Scale Profile Report provides raw and T-score values for four validity scales (L, F, F_1, K) and the ten Basic Clinical scales, and is suitable for scoring abbreviated administrations that are based on responses to the first 350 MMPI-A items. The MMPI-A and MMPI-A-RF Extended Score Reports include raw and T-scores for all test scales and subscales, including a list of items omitted by the adolescent. Examples of the output from the MMPI-A and MMPI-A-RF Extended Score Reports are included in Chapter 8. The tests may also be administered via the standard paper-pencil format, with the responses hand-scored or key-entered into the scoring package later by trained support staff. High-volume test users might wish

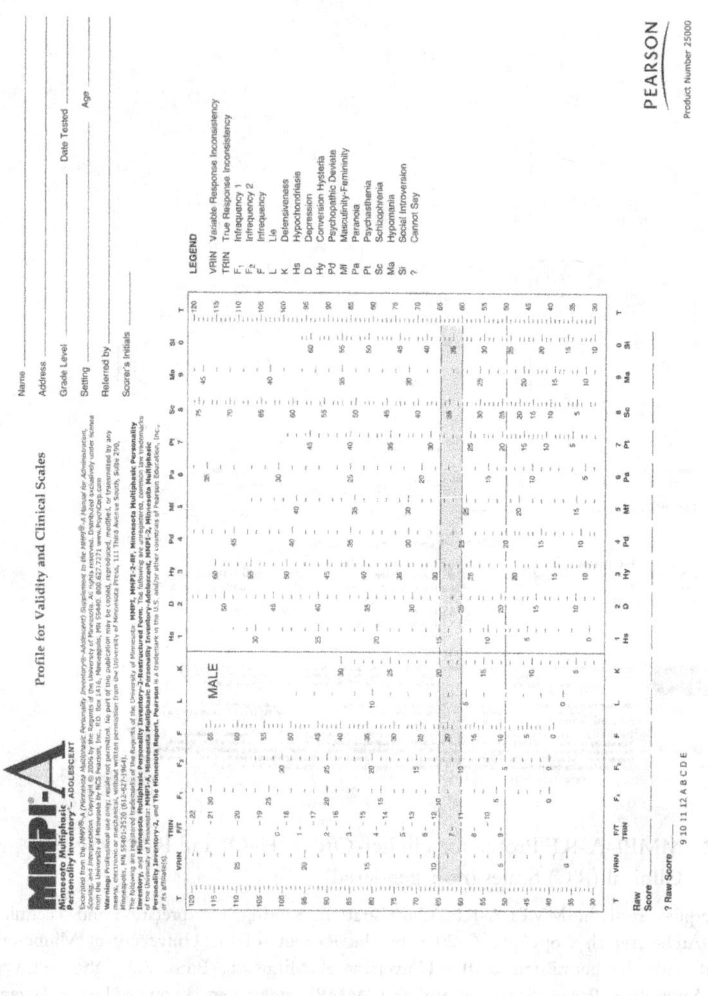

FIGURE 3.1   MMPI-A Profile for Basic Scales (male).

Source: Reproduced with the permission of the University of Minnesota Press. All rights reserved. "Minnesota Multiphasic Personality Inventory" and "MMPI" are trademarks owned by the Regents of the University of Minnesota.

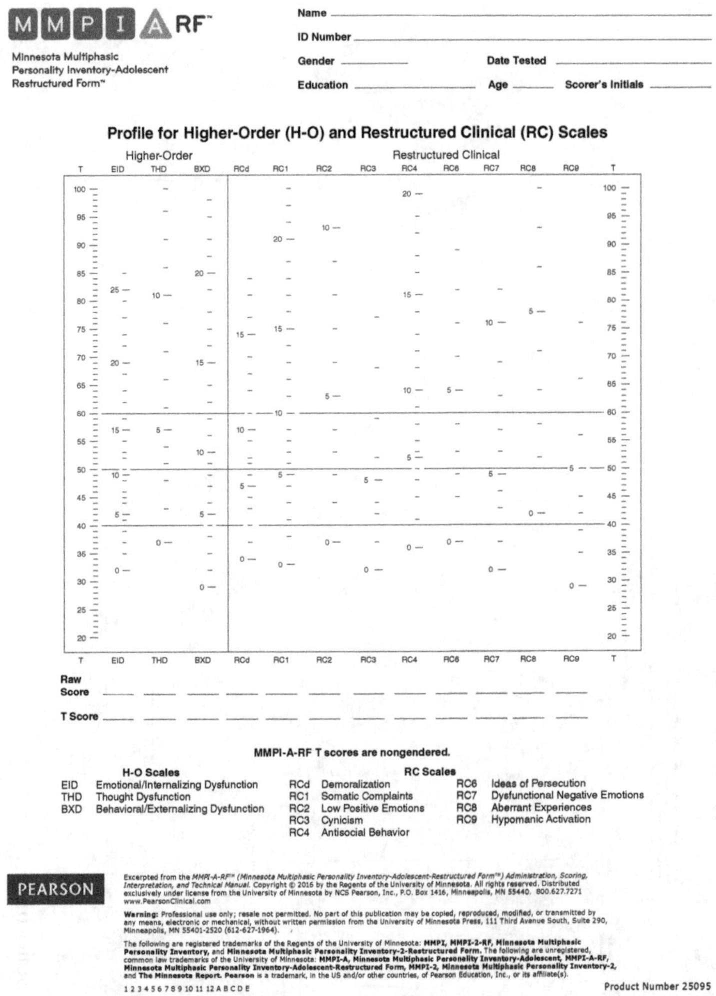

FIGURE 3.2 MMPI-A-RF Profile for Higher-Order (H-O) and Restructured Clinical (RC) Scales (non-gendered).

Source: Excerpted from the MMPI-A-RF Administration, Scoring, Interpretation and Technical Manual by Archer, et al. Copyright © 2016 by the Regents of the University of Minnesota. Reproduced with the permission of the University of Minnesota Press. All rights reserved. "Minnesota Multiphasic Personality Inventory" and "MMPI" are trademarks owned by the Regents of the University of Minnesota.

to consider the scanner option for their personal computer, in which answer sheets are scanned and responses tabulated by the scoring program. In addition, answer sheets may be mailed to Pearson Assessments in Minnesota, where test responses are scored and returned to the test user.

In addition to computerized scoring services, hand-scoring templates, for use with specialized answer sheets, are available for all MMPI-A and MMPI-A-RF scales and subscales, sold separately by test. Templates for each MMPI-A or MMPI-A-RF scale are placed over the answer sheet, and the number of darkened spaces is counted, representing the raw score for the scale being scored. Special care should be taken when scoring the MMPI-A scale 5 (Masculinity-Femininity) to use the scoring key designed for the adolescent's gender. Response Consistency scales are available on the MMPI-A and MMPI-A-RF. On the former test, these are the True Response Inconsistency (*TRIN*) scale and the Variable Response Inconsistency (*VRIN*) scale. On the MMPI-A-RF, the consistency scales are True Response Inconsistency (*TRIN-r*), Variable Response Inconsistency (*VRIN-r*), and Combined Response Inconsistency (*CRIN*). Given the complexity of scoring these consistency scales, special caution should also be used in applying the complex scoring grids for hand-scoring purposes with these scales. The scoring and interpretation of these consistency scales, a subset of the Validity scales, are described in more detail in later chapters.

Computer Administration and Scoring Issues

There are several special considerations that should be evaluated when using computer software for administering or scoring the MMPI-A or MMPI-A-RF. With online administration of these inventories, clear instructions for entering and changing responses should be provided to the respondent. The examiner should ensure that the respondent is instructed in how to accurately enter or change their responses. The respondents' entry of responses should be monitored to ensure that they have understood the instructions. Computer administration programs often have summary or editing screens that permit the monitoring of item omissions.

Several studies have examined the possibility that computer-administered MMPI scores may differ from values produced by administration using the standard paper-and-pencil test booklet. Watson, Thomas, and Anderson (1992) undertook a meta-analysis that compared the MMPI scaled scores produced by standard test-booklet and computer-administered MMPIs as reported in nine studies encompassing 967 respondents. The authors concluded that computer-administered MMPIs produced systematically lower scores than the standard test booklet administration, although these differences were small and typically accounted for less than 1.5 T-score points. Watson and his colleagues concluded that the computer-based underestimates, although small, appeared consistent enough to suggest the possibility that the development of separate norms and profile sheets might be useful for computer-administered protocols, particularly for MMPI-A Basic scales 3, 4, and 8. In contrast, Hays and McCallum (2005) administered the MMPI-A by computer and paper-and-pencil across a one-week interval in a counterbalanced design to 102 students between 14 and 18, inclusive. They reported no significant mean differences found for any of the Basic Validity or Clinical scales for administration method, and scale score distributions and relative score rankings were similar across administration methods. Taken together, the results of these two studies are consistent in reflecting little or no differences between test results obtained by paper-and-pencil versus computer administrations of the MMPI.

As previously noted, a mail-in scoring service from Pearson Assessment is available for the MMPI-A and MMPI-A-RF. When this option is utilized, the respondent enters his or her responses on the computer-scored answer sheet, which is sent to Pearson for scoring and reporting. As with the hand-scored versions, the computer-scored answer sheets should be checked by the examiner for item omissions, double-marking, and deviant response sets before the answer sheet is sent to Pearson Assessment for processing. The clinician should also eliminate any stray marks or incomplete erasures because these may be interpreted as valid responses in the computer scoring process. These same cautions apply to those examiners who use in-office scanning equipment for response entry. Although clinical lore has held that the degree of neatness or sloppiness displayed by the respondent in filling out an MMPI response sheet may be related to personality features, findings by Luty and Thackrey (1993) provided no evidence of a meaningful relationship between neatness and test scores. MMPI-A or MMPI-A-RF users who elect to employ a computer scoring method should be aware that the profiles will be printed only if the adolescent's age is entered within the 14 to 18 range, inclusive.

Selection of Appropriate Norms

The adolescent norms to be utilized with the MMPI-A are based on the 1,620 adolescents in the MMPI-A normative sample described in Chapter 2. As will be described in more detail in Chapter 7, the norms for the MMPI-A-RF are a subset of 1,610 adolescents from the MMPI-A normative sample and, unlike the MMPI-A, are based on non-gendered normative conversions. Archer et al. (2016a) noted that the use of gender-specific norms is based on the assumption that gender differences in raw scores are irrelevant to the constructs measured and therefore may be eliminated by use of gender-specific norms to transform scale raw scores to standard scores. When the MMPI-A was developed (Butcher et al., 1992), the use of gender-specific T-scores was standard practice. Ben-Porath and Forbey (2003) developed a set of non-gendered norms for all MMPI-2 scales because of the requirements of the 1991 Federal Civil Rights Act on the application of the MMPI-2 in pre-employment screening, and non-gendered norms were incorporated into the development of the MMPI-2-RF. Because gender differences cannot be dismissed as irrelevant on the MMPI-A-RF, non-gendered norms were also incorporated into this test.

Adolescent Norm Transformation Procedures

The adolescent norms developed by Marks and Briggs (1972) for the original form of the MMPI were based on linear transformation procedures that converted raw scores to T-score values. This is identical to the transformation procedures used in developing the adult norms for the original MMPI by Hathaway and McKinley (Dahlstrom et al., 1972). The MMPI-A retains the use of linear T-scores for the Validity scales (i.e., $VRIN$, $TRIN$, F_1, F_2, F, L, and K), for Basic scales 5 (Masculinity-Femininity) and 0 (Social Introversion), and for the Supplementary scales, including MacAndrew Alcoholism Scale – Revised (MAC-R), Alcohol/Drug Problem Acknowledgment (ACK), Alcohol/Drug Problem Proneness (PRO), Immaturity (IMM), Repression (R), and Anxiety (A). Eight of the clinical scales on the MMPI-A (1, 2, 3, 4, 6, 7, 8, and 9) and all of the 15 Content scales have T-score values derived from uniform T-score transformation procedures. The MMPI-A-RF used the traditional linear T-scores for Validity scales $VRIN$-r, $TRIN$-r, $CRIN$, F-r, L-r, and K-r.

Uniform transformation procedures were developed to address a problem that has been associated with the use of linear T-score values for the MMPI. This problem is that identical T-score values do not represent the same percentile equivalents across the standard MMPI scales when derived using linear procedures. This phenomenon occurs because MMPI scale raw score distributions are not normally distributed, and the degree to which they vary from the normal distribution fluctuates from scale to scale. Thus, using linear T-score conversion procedures, a T-score value of 70 on one scale does not represent an equivalent percentile value that may be represented by a T = 70 score on another MMPI clinical scale. This discrepancy resulted in difficulty when directly comparing T-score values across the MMPI scales. The problems related to use of linear T-score conversion procedures for the MMPI were first discussed in detail by Colligan et al. (1983).

In the development of the MMPI-2, uniform T-score transformation procedures were used in order to provide equivalent T-score values across the Clinical and Content scales (Tellegen & Ben-Porath, 1992). This same approach was taken in the development of the MMPI-A and in the development of the MMPI-A-RF substantive scales. For example, uniform T-score values were developed for the MMPI-A Clinical scales by examining the distributions for scales 1, 2, 3, 4, 6, 7, 8, and 9 for males and females separately. MMPI-A scales 5 and 0 were not included in the uniform T-score procedures because these scales were derived in a manner different than the other clinical scales, and the distribution of scores on scales 5 and 0 are less skewed; that is, more normally distributed. A composite or averaged distribution of raw scores was then created across the eight Basic scales for each gender, adjusting the distribution of each individual scale so that it would match the composite distribution. The purpose of developing a composite distribution was to allow for the assignment of T-score conversion values for each scale such that a given T-score value would convert to equivalent percentile values across each of these scales. Uniform T-score conversions were separately derived for the 15 Content scales based on the distribution of scores for this group of measures. Uniform T-scores were developed for all of the scales on the MMPI-A-RF with the exception of the MMPI-A-RF Validity scales.

Because uniform T-scores represent composite linear T-scores, this procedure serves to produce equivalent percentile values across a given group of scales for a given T-score. This procedure, however, also maintains the underlying positive skew in the distribution of scores from these measures. Thus, uniform T-scores are generally similar to values that would be obtained from linear T-scores (Edwards, Morrison, & Weissman, 1993b). Nevertheless, differences in T-score transformation procedures can produce different T-score values for a specific response pattern, particularly when combined with the effects of non-gendered norms on the MMPI-A-RF that generated uniform T-scores based on combined raw score distributions for boys and girls.

The Equivalency Issue

Honaker examined the issue of equivalency between the MMPI and MMPI-2 in the assessment of adults at a 1990 symposium. According to Honaker, the issue of psychometric equivalence between the MMPI and MMPI-2 was critically important because this factor determined, to a large extent, the degree to which the vast research literature on the original instrument could be generalized to the revised and restandardized form. Honaker noted that psychometric theory and standards require four conditions to be met in order to consider two forms equivalent or parallel. These conditions are as follows:

1. The forms should yield identical scores (e.g., equal mean scores, high-point codes, etc.).
2. The forms should yield the same distribution of scores.
3. Individual rank ordering produced by each form should be identical (e.g., individuals should be ranked on a given dimension in the same order based on test scores from each form).
4. Scores generated from each form should correlate equally well with independent external criteria.

In evaluating this issue, Honaker examined a sample of 101 adult psychiatric patients who had received both the MMPI and the MMPI-2 in a counterbalanced, repeated-measures design. Findings indicated that the MMPI and the MMPI-2 did produce parallel score dispersion and rank ordering of respondents, but did not yield equivalent mean scores. MMPI-2 scores were consistently lower for scales F, 2, 4, 8, 9, and 0. Further, the congruence of high-point codes between the MMPI and MMPI-2 was lower than that found for repeated administrations of the MMPI or the MMPI-2. These findings indicate that the MMPI and MMPI-2 are highly interrelated, but not equivalent, test forms. A similar conclusion was supported in research findings by Archer and Gordon (1991a) who administered the MMPI-A and the MMPI to a sample of normal high school students. Findings from this study indicated significant and pervasive elevation differences between T-scores produced by these two instruments, with MMPI-A scores significantly lower on most clinical scales.

While it is clear that the MMPI-A and MMPI are not psychometrically equivalent forms using the criteria offered by Honaker (1990), there is also substantial research literature that indicates that a high degree of congruence is found between adolescent profiles generated from the original MMPI and from the MMPI-A. As we shall see in later chapters, this issue is a central determinant of the conclusion that much of the research literature developed for adolescents using the original test form may be validly generalized to users of the MMPI-A.

It is important to note that the MMPI-A and MMPI-A-RF are not psychometrically equivalent forms of the same test, but rather reflect different test instruments that share items in common, and have heavily overlapping normative sets. Further, research findings from the MMPI-A are not generalizable to the MMPI-A-RF, and the MMPI-A-RF is most appropriately viewed as a new adolescent assessment instrument that will require its own research literature to evaluate the reliability and validity of MMPI-A-RF scale test scores.

Deriving the Welsh Code for the MMPI-A

Two major coding systems have been developed for MMPI profiles, the first by Stark Hathaway (1947), which in turn was modified and made more comprehensive in a revision by George Welsh (1948). Because the Welsh system is more widely used than the Hathaway code, and allows for a more precise classification of profile features, this system was recommended for classification of adolescents' MMPI-A responses in the MMPI-A manual (Butcher et al., 1992). A comprehensive description of both the Hathaway and Welsh systems, however, is contained in such texts as Dahlstrom et al. (1972) and Friedman et al. (2001). The use of a profile coding system was not developed for the MMPI-A-RF and therefore the following discussion applies only to the coding of scale scores for MMPI-A.

The general function of profile coding is to provide a quick notation that summarizes the most salient features of the profile. These features include the range of elevation of scales and the pattern of relationships between the scales when ordered from highest to lowest elevation. The code provides a quick and convenient way of summarizing the major features of the profile, without the loss of substantial information.

The Welsh Code requires that all standard clinical scales (designated by number) be arranged (left to right) in descending order of magnitude of T-score elevation. The traditional validity scales (*L*, *F*, and *K*) are then coded immediately to the right of the clinical scales, again arranged from most to least elevated. The relative degree of elevation for any scale within the code is denoted by the system of symbols (as modified for the MMPI-A and described in the test manual for this instrument) shown in Table 3.3.

In the Welsh Coding System, the relevant symbol is placed to the immediate right of the scale or scales related to that range of elevation. For example, if scale *2* has a T-score value of 98 and scale *4* has a T-score value of 92, the expression 24* would symbolically represent this occurrence. Further, if two or more scales are within 1 T-score point of each other, this occurrence is denoted by underlining all affected scales. For example, if scale *2* were elevated at 53 and scale *3* were elevated at 52, they would be denoted as follows: *23/*. The example shown in Table 3.4, adapted from Friedman et al. (2001), illustrates the Welsh Coding System for the MMPI-A.

Several features of this illustration may be noted. For example, scales *3* and *6* both produced an identical T-score value of 62, and therefore by convention the scale identified by the lowest numerical value (i.e., scale *3*) is presented first in the descending order. Additionally, scales *3*, *6*, and *8* vary by only one T-score value and therefore all three scales are underlined in the code. Finally, the " symbol is immediately adjacent to the * symbol that follows scale *2*. This indicates that no MMPI scale produced values in the T-score range of 80 to 89, illustrating the convention that although no value in this specific T-score range may occur, the appropriate symbol should nevertheless be recorded in the code. Typically, most clinicians apply the Welsh Code first to the standard

TABLE 3.3 Symbols Designating T-score Elevation Ranges

T-score Values	Symbol
120 and above	!
110–119	!!
100–109	**
90–99	*
80–89	"
70–79	'
65–69	+
60–64	−
50–59	/
40–49	:
30–39	#
29 and below	No symbol (scale is presented to the right of the # symbol)

TABLE 3.4 Sample Profile Used to Illustrate the Welsh Coding Method

Scales:	L	F	K	1	2	3	4	5	6	7	8	9	0
T-scores:	44	60	49	49	99	62	50	67	62	79	63	38	70
Welsh													
Code:	2*"70'5+<u>836</u>-4/1:9# F-/KL:												

clinical scales, and then repeat the coding exercise for the validity scales. An example of the use of Welsh coding for the MMPI-A is also provided in the manual for this test instrument (Butcher et al., 1992).

Providing Test Result Feedback

In addition to establishing rapport with the adolescent prior to testing, and providing clear and concise test instructions, it is very helpful to inform the adolescent that he or she will receive feedback on the test results. If an adolescent does not have the opportunity to learn from the testing experience, there is often little inherent motivation to cooperate with the demanding testing procedures. Finn and Tonsager (1992) reported data indicating that the provision of MMPI-2 feedback to college students awaiting psychotherapy was associated with a significant decline in subjects' psychological distress and a significant increase in their levels of self-esteem. The MMPI-2 test feedback process has served as a central focus in three texts entitled *MMPI-2 in psychological treatment* (Butcher, 1990), the *Therapist guide to the MMPI and MMPI-2: Providing feedback and treatment* (Lewak, Marks, & Nelson, 1990), and in the *Manual for using the MMPI-2 as a therapeutic intervention* (Finn, 1996). The text by Finn stresses the importance of involving the client in the assessment process by identifying what the client would like to learn from testing, and providing this information to them during feedback.

Archer and Krishnamurthy (2002) emphasized a method of providing feedback to the adolescent which encourages the adolescents' curiosity concerning the testing process and increases the personal relevance of test findings. Adapting the general guidance from Finn (1996), these authors recommend actively engaging the adolescent in constructing questions that can be answered from test findings prior to the administration of the MMPI. The ultimate goal is to encourage the adolescent to produce a manageable number of practical issues or questions that can be systematically addressed in test feedback. Archer and Krishnamurthy presented the following illustration of a typical discussion that might ensue in this collaborative process (2002, pp. 24–25):

Examiner: I understand that you are not sure about how this testing may be useful to you. Often, this type of testing helps teenagers to learn things about themselves that they hadn't been fully aware of, or actively thought about.

Adolescent: What kinds of things?

Examiner: For example, most people don't really think about how they come across to other people, or whether their ways of thinking and feeling are very different from those of others. The MMPI-A can shed light on these issues. Does that make sense to you?

Adolescent: I guess.

Examiner: The testing could also help you to better understand things that adolescents might already suspect about themselves. For example, a teenager might be aware that she often feels unhappy or grouchy but not have a clear idea about what's going on. The MMPI-A results may help her to realize that she is depressed, which may include being very sensitive to other's reactions, having negative thoughts about herself, and feeling that no one really understands her. Does this give you an idea of how this works?

Adolescent: Yes.

Examiner: Okay. Now all of this can be best done if you take a few moments to think about some questions you have about yourself that you would like answered by the testing.

Adolescent: Uh . . . about feeling depressed?

Examiner: The type of question varies from person to person and is up to you. What are some things that you have wondered about regarding yourself?

Adolescent: I don't know . . . Sometimes I feel that everyone in my class, and all my friends, are so sure of themselves and know what they want better than I do.

Examiner: That is a good place to start. It sounds like you feel uncertain about yourself and your goals, and don't feel like you have as much confidence as other teenagers. Is that correct?

Adolescent: Yes. Seems like I'm the only one who doesn't have a clue.

Examiner: The question for testing, then, can be, "Am I low in self-confidence and self-esteem compared to other teenagers?" How does that sound?

Adolescent: That sounds right.

Examiner: Good. The MMPI-A can certainly give us an answer to this question and help us see what kinds of things contribute to this feeling. Let's make a note of that question and then try another one.

Adolescent: Well, I also get mad at people who show off or are in my face. My parents make me mad too. I can really pitch a fit and it comes out of nowhere. I guess I wonder why I blow up so easily.

Examiner: That is an excellent issue for which we should get useful information from the MMPI-A. It sounds like there are two related questions here, one being, "Do I get angry more quickly than other people?" and the other one being, "Why do I get easily angered?"

Adolescent: That's exactly it.

Archer and Krishnamurthy (2002) note that this collaborative process involves the adolescent identifying issues of concern and the examiner helping to restate and clarify these issues. This pre-administration dialogue should be conducted in an unhurried pace until a satisfactory list of queries has been produced. Archer and Krishnamurthy note that modified versions of this procedure may be used in which the adolescent and his or her legal guardians are included in the process, or, alternatively, another referring professional who is involved in the adolescents' care may take the place of the adult party in the collaborative process.

Butcher (1990) has provided general guidelines for MMPI-2 feedback that are also applicable to the MMPI-A and MMPI-A-RF. Among Butcher's recommendations are suggestions that the test should be explained to the patient, including a brief description of the meaning of scales and T-scores, and that the therapist should then review the patient's scores in relation to test norms. Furthermore, responses are encouraged from the client during the feedback session in order to make feedback an interactive experience. Butcher also underscored the therapist's need to appraise the degree of acceptance of test feedback by asking the client to summarize their understanding of, and reaction to, major findings. Butcher cautioned that therapists should present feedback as "provisional" information, and that the therapist should gauge how much feedback the client can realistically absorb or incorporate without becoming overwhelmed or excessively defensive.

4

MMPI-A AND MMPI-A-RF VALIDITY SCALES AND VALIDITY INTERPRETATION

There are several methods of assessing the technical validity of adolescents' MMPI-A and MMPI-A-RF profiles. These methods involve the individual and configural interpretation of standard validity scale findings, and may extend to include an analysis of the overall profile configuration for evidence of atypical response set features. Because the majority of MMPI-A-RF validity scales represent shortened counterparts to corresponding MMPI-A validity scales, and because the validity scale interpretation process is similar for both instruments, this chapter will present the validity scales for both tests. On the MMPI-A, validity measures were developed which are the Variable Response Inconsistency ($VRIN$) and True Response Inconsistency ($TRIN$) scales, and the F_1 and F_2 subscales. The inclusion of these four new validity scales at the beginning of the MMPI-A Basic Scale profile (in conjunction with reordering L, F, and K to F, L, and K) is among the most readily apparent changes associated with this revision of the instrument.

For the MMPI-A-RF, revised $VRIN$ and $TRIN$ scales were developed, i.e., the $VRIN$-r and $TRIN$-r scales, as well as a new consistency scale which represents the sum of scores from the $VRIN$-r and $TRIN$-r scales, that is, the Combined Response Inconsistency ($CRIN$) scale. Further, the MMPI-A-RF contains a revision of the MMPI-A L scale entitled Uncommon Virtues (L-r) and a revised form of the K scale labeled Adjustment Validity (K-r). Finally, the MMPI-A-RF Validity scales include the Infrequent Responses (F-r) scale, which reflects a substantive modification of the MMPI-A F scale. In addition to these validity assessment tools, this chapter also reviews a conceptual model developed by Roger Greene (2000, 2011) for interpreting technical validity patterns. This model emphasizes the distinction between response consistency and response accuracy as components of technical validity and is applicable to

TABLE 4.1 MMPI-A and MMPI-A-RF Validity Scales

MMPI-A Scale	MMPI-A-RF Scale
Consistency Scales	
VRIN (Variable Response Inconsistency)	VRIN-r (Variable Response Inconsistency)
TRIN (True Response Inconsistency)	TRIN-r (True Response Inconsistency)
-----	CRIN (Combined Response Inconsistency)
Over-Reporting Scales	
F_1 (F subscale)	-----
F_2 (F subscale)	-----
F (Infrequency)	F-r (Infrequent Responses)
Under-Reporting Scales	
L (Lie)	L-r (Uncommon Virtues)
K (Defensiveness)	K-r (Adjustment Validity)

both the MMPI-A and the MMPI-A-RF. Table 4.1 presents the MMPI-A and MMPI-A-RF Validity scales.

MMPI-A and MMPI-A-RF Validity Scales

MMPI Validity Scales and Derivative Subscales

The traditional validity (F, L, and K) scales originally developed for the MMPI by Hathaway and McKinley were created to detect deviant test-taking attitudes and responses primarily among adult respondents. However, determining the technical validity of the adolescents' MMPI-A and MMPI-A-RF profiles is particularly important because invalid profiles probably occur with a higher frequency in adolescent samples, resulting from problems related to response consistency as well as response accuracy. Pogge, Stokes, Frank, Wong, and Harvey (1997), for example, observed that while the MMPI-A has scales specifically designed to evaluate the effects of response styles on adolescents' disclosure of psychopathology, many of the more commonly used self-report instruments with adolescents (e.g., the Symptom Checklist-90-Revised) do not contain validity scales. Further, these researchers noted that some clinicians prefer the use of observer ratings of adolescents, rather than self-report data, as a means of attempting to minimize the possible effects of response styles.

Pogge and his colleagues examined these issues in a study of self-report and therapist ratings of psychopathology for 235 adolescent psychiatric inpatients. All the participants in this study completed three self-report rating scales including the MMPI, the SCL-90-R, and the BDI. The results from this study demonstrated that the best prediction of self-reported and therapist ratings of adolescent symptomatology was based on a prediction model incorporating individual scores from clinical scales and from the validity scales *L, F,* and *K*. In fact, one-third of the adolescent patients utilized in this study manifested clinical range elevations on at least one of these three MMPI validity scales, underscoring the relatively high prevalence of validity scale issues for this population. Pogge et al. concluded that their findings strongly indicate that the use of validity scales is central in any effort to assess psychopathology among adolescents, and that the use of clinician ratings does not eliminate self-presentation biases and does not serve as an adequate substitute for the evaluation of self-reported psychopathology. As research has accumulated on the standard validity measures, however, Graham (2012) noted that we have come to view the traditional validity scales as additional sources of inferences about the respondents' extra-test behaviors. Thus, these validity scales provide data regarding not only the technical validity of the MMPI response pattern, but also valuable information concerning behavioral correlates or descriptors that are likely to apply to the respondent.

The Cannot Say Scale

The Cannot Say (*CNS*) scale consists of the total number of items that a respondent fails to answer, or answers in both the true and false directions. Thus, the *CNS* scale is not a formal scale because it does not have a consistent or fixed item pool. Profile sheets for the original MMPI have shown the *CNS* scale as the first in the series of standard validity scales on the profile grid. The MMPI-A and MMPI-A-RF profile sheets, although still providing a space to record the raw score for the *CNS* scale, have deemphasized its role as a "scale" by its new placement in the lower portion of the profile sheet.

Although several studies have examined the characteristics of *CNS* values in adult populations (as reviewed in Greene, 1980, 1989a, 1991, 2000, 2011), little research has been focused on this issue among adolescent respondents. Ball and Carroll (1960) examined correlates of the *CNS* scores among 262 ninth-grade public school students in Kentucky. They reported that male respondents had a higher mean number of *CNS* responses than females. The items omitted by these adolescents tended to fall into broad categories, including statements not applicable to adolescents, religious items, items related to sexuality and bodily functions, and items that require adolescents to make a decision concerning personal characteristics about which they are ambivalent. Similarly, Hathaway and Monachesi (1963) found 23 items that were left unanswered by at least 2% of the male or female respondents in their statewide Minnesota sample of normal adolescents. They reported that content related to religion and sex appeared to be the most frequently omitted items for both boys and girls. Additionally, girls tended to leave a significantly larger number of sex-related items unanswered.

In general, findings on the original MMPI by Ball and Carroll (1960) and on the MMPI-A by Archer and Gordon (1991a) indicated a relationship between intellectual functioning/reading ability and CNS scale scores. Ball and Carroll found no evidence of a relationship between CNS scores and delinquent behaviors in their sample, but did find higher CNS scale scores to be inversely associated with adolescents' scores on intelligence measures and their academic grades. Archer and Gordon (1991a) found a modest but significant relationship ($r = -.10, p < .05$) between the number of unanswered MMPI-A items and adolescents' reading abilities in a sample of 495 junior high and high school students. These findings suggest that adolescents' failure to complete items may at times be related to intellectual and reading limitations, rather than oppositional and defiant characteristics.

Table 4.2 provides information from Greene (1991) concerning the frequency of omitted items for the original MMPI in psychiatric samples of adults and adolescents. This table shows approximately equivalent rates of item omissions between these two age groups.

Gottesman et al. (1987) reported that the mean CNS scale value for normal adolescents in the Hathaway and Monachesi (1963) dataset was roughly three. Further, a raw score value of five to six converts to a T-score range of 70 to 80 in the Gottesman et al. adolescent norms. It should be noted, however, that the

TABLE 4.2 Frequency of Omitted Items on the MMPI in Adult and Adolescent Psychiatric Samples by Gender

Number of Omitted Items	Psychiatric patients (Hedlund & Won Cho, 1979)			
	Adults		Adolescents	
	Male (N = 8,646)	Female (N = 3,743)	Male (N = 693)	Female (N = 290)
0	29.8%	28.4%	28.0%	27.9%
1–5	32.3%	30.4%	31.0%	30.8%
Cumulative (0-5)	62.1%	58.8%	59.0%	58.7%
6–10	16.8%	17.2%	21.1%	21.7%
Cumulative (0-10)	78.9%	76.0%	80.1%	80.4%
11–30	14.7%	17.4%	14.6%	13.1%
Cumulative (0-30)	93.6%	93.4%	94.7%	93.5%
31+	6.4%	6.6%	5.3%	6.5%
M	8.7	9.3	7.7	8.4
SD	18.1	19.2	13.1	15.1

Source: Roger L. Greene. The MMPI-2/MMPI: An Interpretive Manual, 1st © 1991. Printed and electronically reproduced with the permission of Pearson Education, Inc., New York, NY.

Marks and Briggs (1972) adolescent norms for the traditional MMPI indicate that a *CNS* raw score value of 30 converts to a T-score value of 50 for both male and female adolescents. This T-score conversion appears to be a continuation of the arbitrary assignment of T-score values to *CNS* raw score values of 30 used by Hathaway and McKinley (1967) in the original adult MMPI norms. In both adolescent and adult samples, however, a raw score value of 30 on the *CNS* scale occurs *much* less frequently than is implied by the T = 50 value. The data from the MMPI-A normative samples, for example, indicate that the mean raw score value for the *CNS* scale is approximately 1 for both boys and girls.

Greene (1991) identified traditional MMPI items most frequently omitted in a sample of 983 adolescent psychiatric patients. Of these 17 items, 10 were deleted in the formation of the MMPI-A, and 3 additional items underwent revision. The very low *CNS* scale mean raw score values found for the MMPI-A normative sample suggest that the MMPI-A item revision process may have been successful in creating a test booklet of increased relevance to adolescents when contrasted with the original test form. It should be noted, however, that MMPI-A *CNS* scale mean values were affected by the elimination of adolescents from the normative sample with *CNS* scale raw score values ≥ 35. Tables 4.3 and 4.4 show the abbreviated items most frequently omitted by 805 boys and 815 girls, respectively, in the MMPI-A normative sample. These tables also show those items retained within the item pool of the MMPI-A-RF.

TABLE 4.3 Most Frequently Omitted Items for 805 Male Adolescents in the MMPI-A Normative Sample

MMPI-A Item No.	Item Content	Freq. of Omission	% of Sample
203	Ruminate a lot.	25	3.1
441	Not thought attractive.	13	1.6
16	Life unfair.	10	1.2
199	Lead life based on duty.	8	1.0
395	Have worked for people who take all the credit but blame others for any mistakes.*(31)	8	1.0
404	Sometimes feel I'm going to "fall apart."*(128)	8	1.0
177	Think about killing self.* (46)	7	.9
406	Many misbehave sexually.	7	.9
448	Thought to be dependable.	7	.9
467	Like marijuana.* (235)	7	.9

Note
Items with asterisks also appear in the MMPI-A-RF with the latter item number shown in parentheses.

TABLE 4.4 Most Frequently Omitted Items for 815 Male Adolescents in the MMPI-A
Normative Sample

MMPI-A Item No.	Item Content	Freq. of Omission	% of Sample
203	Ruminate a lot.	24	2.9
199	Lead life based on duty.	12	1.5
93	Head feels "full."* (227)	10	1.2
16	Life unfair.	8	1.0
31	No trouble because of sexual activities	7	.9
213	Fine for people to take all they can get.	7	.9
431	Talking about problems often more helpful than taking medicine	7	.9
196	Seldom notice heart pounding or shortness of breath.* (78)	6	.7
244	Very few fears.	6	.7
251	Bothered by sexual thoughts	6	.7
429	Harmful habits.	6	.7
432	Have faults I can't change.* (121)	6	.7
442	Follow beliefs no matter what.* (99)	6	.7

Source: MMPI-A abbreviated items reproduced with permission. MMPI®-A Booklet of Abbreviated Items. Copyright © 2005 by the Regents of the University of Minnesota. MMPI-A-RF Test Booklet. Copyright © 2016 by the Regents of the University of Minnesota. Reproduced with the permission of the University of Minnesota Press. All rights reserved. "Minnesota Multiphasic Personality Inventory" and "MMPI" are trademarks owned by the University of Minnesota.

Note
Items with asterisks also appear in the MMPI-A-RF with the latter item number shown in parentheses.

Table 4.5 provides interpretive guidelines for the MMPI-A *CNS* scores. As noted in this table, adolescents who omit more than 30 items should be requested to complete the unanswered items or retake the entire test. Research findings relating omissions to intelligence and reading ability, however, strongly indicate that the examiner should assess an adolescent's capacity to comprehend items before instructing the teenager to respond to unanswered MMPI-A statements. Clopton and Neuringer (1977) demonstrated that random omissions of 30 items or fewer from the traditional MMPI do not seriously distort MMPI profile features when scored on adult norms. As previously noted, a substantial majority of adolescents would be expected to omit fewer than 10 items on either the traditional MMPI or the MMPI-A. Raw score values of 11 to 30 on the *CNS* scale represent substantially more omissions than might typically be expected. This degree of item omission may be produced by adolescents who have impaired reading ability, or have limitations in their life experiences that render some items meaningless or unanswerable. It is unlikely, however, that this range of *CNS* scale values will result in profile configuration distortions unless omitted items are concentrated within a few scales.

TABLE 4.5 Interpretation Guidelines for MMPI-A Cannot Say (*CNS*) Scales

Raw Score	Interpretation
0–3	*Low.* These adolescents are willing and capable of responding to the item pool and were not evasive of item content.
4–10	*Moderate.* These adolescents have omitted a few items in a selective manner. Their omissions may be the result of limitations in life experiences that rendered some items unanswerable. There is little probability of profile distortions unless all omissions occurred from a single scale.
11–29	*Marked.* These adolescents are omitting more items than expected and may be very indecisive. Their omissions may have distorted their profile elevations. Check the scale membership of missing items to evaluate profile validity.
30 and above	*Invalid.* Adolescents in this range have left many items unanswered, possibly as a result of a defiant or uncooperative stance or serious reading difficulties. The profile is invalid. If possible, the adolescent should complete unanswered items or retake the entire test.

Source: Adapted from Archer (1987b). Copyright © 1987 by Lawrence Erlbaum Associates, Inc. Reprinted with permission.

The 241-item MMPI-A-RF is roughly one-half the length of the 478-item MMPI-A, and therefore new *CNS* score interpretation guidelines were developed for *CNS* scores on the former test. Table 4.6 provides interpretation guidelines for the *MMPI-A-RF CNS* scale. As noted in this table, conservative *CNS* score guidelines were developed for the MMPI-A-RF because of the potential impact of omitted items on many of the relatively short substantive scales of this test. Therefore, a *CNS* score of 10 or greater on the MMPI-A-RF raises significant concerns regarding protocol validity. For adolescents who produce *CNS* scores within the range of 1 to 9, inclusive, it is recommended that the percentage of omitted items on the briefer scales should be evaluated in order to determine the relative impact of omitted items on that scale. MMPI-A-RF scales which have less than 90% of items answered should not be interpreted because these results may produce serious underestimates of the problems associated with these scales.

The MMPI-A Infrequency (F) Scale and F$_1$ and F$_2$ Subscales

The original MMPI *F* scale consisted of 64 items selected using the criterion that no more than 10% of the Minnesota normative adult sample answered these items in the deviant direction. As a result of this development procedure, the *F* scale was often referred to as the Frequency or Infrequency scale. The *F* scale includes a variety of items related to strange or unusual experiences, thoughts, sensations, paranoid ideation, and antisocial attitudes and behaviors. The *F* scale on the original MMPI was also one of the most problematic scales when applied

TABLE 4.6 Interpretation Guidelines for MMPI-A-RF Cannot Say (*CNS*) Scores

Raw Score	Protocol Validity Concerns	Possible Reasons for Score	Interpretive Implications
≥ 10	Scores on some scales may be invalid.	Reading or language limitations Severe psychopathology Obsessiveness Lack of insight Lack of cooperation	Examine the content of unscorable items to detect possible themes. The impact is scale-dependent. For scales on which less than 90% of the items are scorable, the absence of elevation is uninterpretable. Elevated scores on these scales may underestimate the significance or severity of associated problems.
1–9	Scores on some of the shorter scales may be invalid.	Selective non-responsiveness	Examine the content of unscorable items to detect possible themes. The impact is scale-dependent. For scales on which less than 90% of the items are scorable, the absence of elevation is uninterpretable. Elevated scores on these scales may underestimate the significance or severity of associated problems.
0	None	The test taker provided scorable responses to all 241 items.	The test taker was cooperative insofar as his or her willingness to respond to the test items.

in adolescent populations, because adolescents typically produced much higher *F* scale raw scores than adults. Significant *F* scale mean raw score differences between adolescent and adult respondents were consistently reported in both normal and clinical samples (e.g., Archer, 1984, 1987b). Because of the high *F* scale values typically found for adolescents, the use of *F* scale validity criteria to assess the technical validity of teenagers' MMPI profiles was very complex and often ineffective. Interestingly, elevated *F* scale values have also been found in other populations or groups, including Chinese subjects from the People's Republic of China and Hong Kong when their responses are placed on standard norms developed in the United States (e.g., Cheung, Song, & Butcher, 1991). Cheung et al. (1991) attributed these *F* scale elevations produced by Chinese respondents to cultural differences in attitudes, practices, and beliefs.

Thus, *F* scale item endorsement patterns have been shown to be affected by both developmental and cultural factors.

In the development of the MMPI-A, it was apparent that adolescents produced marked elevations on the *F* scale because many of the *F* scale items did not function effectively for this age group. Specifically, 11 of the 60 *F* items that appear on the MMPI-2 form for adults produced item endorsement frequencies exceeding 20% in the MMPI-A normative sample. For example, roughly 26% of both male and female adolescents in the MMPI-A normative sample responded *true* to the traditional *F* scale item, "Sometimes I feel as if I must injure either myself or someone else," and roughly 36% of males and 45% of females answered *true* to the item, "Most any time I would rather sit and daydream than to do anything else." Table 4.7 provides the abbreviated item content and endorsement frequencies for the 11 *F* scale items most frequently endorsed by adolescents in the MMPI-A normative sample using the MMPI-TX experimental test form.

The traditional *F* scale also contains several items that might be deemed offensive because statement content was related to religious beliefs (e.g., "I believe there is a God"), or sexual attitudes and functioning (e.g., "Children should be taught all the main facts of sex"). Based on these observations, the *F* scale underwent a major revision in the development of the MMPI-A, leading to the creation of a new 66-item *F* scale, which is subdivided into the F_1 and F_2 subscales.

TABLE 4.7 MMPI-2 *F* Scale Items Producing Endorsement Frequencies Exceeding 20% in the MMPI-TX Normative Data Collection Sample

MMPI-2 Item No.	Item Content	Endorsement Frequency[a]
48	Like to daydream.	42.0%
288	Judged unfairly by family.	41.7%
12	Satisfactory sex life.	32.8%
174	Like to learn about things I'm working on.	32.3%
132	Believe in eternity.	31.2%
168	Sometimes do things and don't remember doing them.	29.8%
324	Like making people afraid of me.	28.2%
300	Jealous of some family members.	26.3%
150	Feel need to injure self or others.	26.3%
312	Like only the comic strips in newspapers.	25.8%
264	Used alcohol a lot.	22.6%

Source: MMPI-2 abbreviated items reproduced with permission. MMPI®-2 Booklet of Abbreviated Items. Copyright © 2005 by the Regents of the University of Minnesota. All rights reserved. Used by permission of the University of Minnesota Press. "MMPI" and "Minnesota Multiphasic Personality Inventory" are registered trademarks owned by the Regents of the University of Minnesota.

Note

a Analyses based on 1,435 adolescents sampled as part of the MMPI-A normative data collection.

The MMPI-A F scale was created by the selection of items endorsed in a deviant direction by no more than 20% of the 805 boys and 815 girls in the MMPI-A normative sample. In creating the MMPI-A F scale, 27 items were deleted from the original F scale because adolescents' endorsement of these items exceeded the 20% criterion for selection, or because the items contained content deemed inappropriate for inclusion in the MMPI-A. In addition, 12 items that appeared on the original form of the MMPI but were not tradition- ally scored on F were included on the MMPI-A F scale because these items met the 20% criterion rule. Finally, the MMPI-A F scale includes 17 new items that appear only on the MMPI-A.

Table 4.8 provides five levels of interpretive suggestions for the MMPI-A F scale. Adolescents who produce marked or extreme elevations on the MMPI-A F scale may be suffering from severe psychiatric illnesses, may be attempting to "fake-bad" or overreport symptomatology, or may be engaging in a random response pattern either through conscious intent or as a result of inadequate reading ability. For example, Krakauer (1991) investigated the relationship between MMPI-A F scale elevation and reading ability in a sample of 495 ado- lescents. She found that 11% of adolescents scored below a sixth-grade reading level in the total sample. In a subsample of 231 adolescents who produced F scale T-score values ≥ 65, however, the percentage of adolescents reading below the sixth-grade level increased to 18%. Similarly, the examination of 120 adolescents who produced an F scale T-score value of 80 or greater yielded a base rate of 24% for poor readers. This further increased to 29% when considering 68 adolescents who produced F scale T-score values of 90 or greater.

TABLE 4.8 Interpretation Guidelines for the MMPI-A F Scale

T-score	Interpretation
45 and below	*Low.* Scores in this range may reflect very conventional life experiences among normal adolescents, and possible "fake good" attempts among disturbed adolescents.
46–59	*Normal.* Adolescents in this range have endorsed unusual experiences to a degree that is common during adolescence.
60–65	*Moderate.* These adolescents are endorsing a range of F scores typically found among teenagers exhibiting some evidence of psychopathology.
66–89	*Marked.* Validity indicators should be checked carefully for adolescents in this range. Valid profiles most likely reflect significant psychopathology including symptoms typically exhibited by adolescents in inpatient settings.
90 and above	*Extreme.* Protocols with F scores in this range are likely to be invalid. If "fake-bad" and other response set issues are ruled out, may reflect severely disorganized or psychotic adolescents.

Source: Adapted from Archer (1987b). Copyright © 1987 by Lawrence Erlbaum Associates, Inc. Reprinted with permission.

The MMPI-A F_1 scale is a direct descendant of the original F scale and consists of 33 items, of which 24 appeared in the original. The remaining nine F_1 items are new items that did not appear on the original instrument. All of the F_1 items occur in the first 350 items of the MMPI-A booklet, and therefore may be used even when the MMPI-A is given in the abbreviated format. The F_2 scale also consists of 33 items, all of which occur after item 242, and 16 of which occur after item 350. The F_2 scale consists predominantly of items that appeared on the original MMPI, but only 12 of these items were scored on the F scale in the original instrument. Eight of the F_2 items are new items that did not appear on the original MMPI. Table 4.9 provides examples of MMPI-A F scale abbreviated items with the F_1 and F_2 membership indicated within the parentheses. All F_1 and F_2 items, as part of the MMPI-A F scale, were selected based on the criterion that fewer than 20% of normal adolescent subjects in the MMPI-A normative data collection endorsed the item in the scored or critical direction.

The F_1 and F_2 scales for the MMPI-A may be used in an interpretive strategy similar to that employed for the F and Fb scales found in the MMPI-2 (Butcher et al. 1989). Specifically, the F_1 scale provides information concerning the validity of the adolescent's responses to the Basic MMPI-A scales, whereas F_2 provides information concerning the adolescent's responses to the latter half of the MMPI-A test booklet, and data necessary to score the MMPI-A Content scales and Supplementary scales. If an adolescent's F_1 score is within acceptable ranges, but F_2 is extremely elevated (T $\geq$ 90), this pattern is indicative of the possible use of a random response pattern during the latter half of the MMPI-A test booklet. Under these conditions, it may be possible to interpret data from the standard scales, while treating Content scale and Supplementary scale findings as invalid. If F_1 scores exceed acceptable ranges, however, the entire protocol should be treated as invalid and further interpretation should not be undertaken regardless of the elevation on F_2.

TABLE 4.9 Sample Items From the MMPI-A F Scale With F_1 or F_2 Subscale Membership

---

Examples of items scored if true
    22.   Possessed by spirits. (F_1)
   250.   Spirit leaves body. (F_2)
Examples of items scored if false
    74.   Liked by most. (F_1)
   258.   Love[d] mother. (F_2)

The research data on the F_1 and F_2 scales is limited concerning the optimal cutoff score for identifying invalid records with these scales. Berry et al. (1991) demonstrated the usefulness of the MMPI-2 F and Fb scales in detecting random responding in a college student sample. However, Archer and Elkins (1999) reported that F, F_1 and F_2 were each useful when used individually to identify random MMPI-A profiles, but the T-score difference between F_1 and F_2 did not appear to be of practical usefulness in this task. Further, Archer, Handel, Lynch, and Elkins (2002) also found these F scales and subscales individually useful in detecting profiles with varying levels of random responding, but noted the $F_1 - F_2$ difference score was ineffective in this regard because, ". . . when the T-score difference cutoffs became large enough to generate acceptable levels of positive predictive power (probability an elevated score reflects a random protocol), so few random protocols were found above that criterion score that test sensitivity was markedly low" (p. 429). Archer et al. (2002) note that a partial explanation for the failure of the $F_1 - F_2$ index to produce useful results may lie in the tendency of the $F1$ subscale to produce higher T-score values than the F_2 subscale under standard administration conditions as well as in most random response conditions. As presented earlier, Table 4.8 provides some T-score interpretation guidelines for the MMPI-A F scale, and these T-score recommendations also appear to be applicable to the F_1 and F_2 subscales when interpreted as individual measures. Clinicians should be particularly cautious concerning validity inferences based on the observed T-score differences that occur between the F_1 and F_2 subscales, however, given the limited usefulness of this index found in the research conducted thus far on this issue.

The MMPI-A-RF Infrequent Responses (F-r) Scale

The MMPI-A-RF includes one measure of overreporting, the Infrequent Responses (*F-r*) scale. This scale differs from its counterpart on the MMPI-A, in that items were selected on the basis of infrequent endorsement in both the MMPI-A-RF normative sample and in the combined developmental samples of adolescents collected in clinical settings including outpatient, inpatient, correctional, and school samples. Items were initially selected for the *F-r* scale based on the criteria that the item was endorsed with a frequency below 15% in the normative sample, and below 20% in the clinical samples used for MMPI-A-RF scale development. After removing five items to reduce over-representation or redundancy of content areas within the preliminary *F-r* scale, the final version of the *F-r* scale includes 23 items. Table 4.10 provides interpretive guidelines for the MMPI-A-RF *F-r* scale. The levels of interpretation range from T-scores of 70 to 79, indicative of possible overreporting, to T-scores >89, strongly suggestive of an invalid protocol as a result of excessive response inconsistency or overreporting of symptomatology. As reported in the MMPI-A-RF Manual

(Archer et al., 2016a), none of the adolescents in the MMPI-A-RF normative sample produced *F-r* scale T-scores ≥ 90, while 65% of adolescents instructed to simulate psychopathology or "fake-bad" produced elevations in this range. As noted in Table 4.10, scores from the *VRIN-r*, *TRIN-r*, and *CRIN* scales may be useful in ruling out that elevations on the *F-r* scale were the result of inconsistent responding.

The MMPI-A Lie (L) Scale

The Lie scale in the original MMPI consisted of 15 items that were selected to identify individuals deliberately attempting to lie, or to avoid answering the item pool in an open and honest manner. The Lie scale was keyed in the false direction for all items, and was created based on a rational/intuitive identification of items. The MMPI-A Lie scale retained all but one item from the original measure, resulting in a 14-item scale. The traditional Lie scale item deleted in the creation of the MMPI-A *L* scale was, "Sometimes in elections I vote for men about whom I know very little," based on the limited relevance of this item for many adolescents. Table 4.11 presents examples of the abbreviated items contained in the MMPI-A *L* scale.

The MMPI-A Lie scale covers a variety of content areas, including the denial of aggressive or hostile impulses that constitute areas of common human failings for the majority of individuals. Higher range *L* scale values have been related to longer treatment duration for hospitalized adolescents (Archer, White, & Orvin, 1979). In general, the clinical correlates of Lie scale elevations for adolescents appear to be similar to the meaning of these elevations in adult populations. Thus, moderate elevations in the range of T-score values of 60 to 65 are related to an emphasis on conformity and the use of denial among adolescent respondents. Marked elevations in excess of T-score values of 65 raise questions concerning the possible use of a "nay-saying" response set or an unsophisticated attempt by a respondent to present personal characteristics in a favorable light and in a "saintly" manner. Stein and Graham (2005) investigated the ability of MMPI-A substance abuse and validity scales to detect attempts to fake-good in a sample that included substance abusing and non-substance abusing incarcerated adolescents. Adolescents were administered the MMPI-A twice; once under standard test instructions and once under instructions to fake-good. The *L* scale was able to detect accurately more than 75% of fake-good profiles and 77% of standard instruction profiles when an *L* ≥ 56 T criterion score was employed to predict group membership.

Because all *L* scale items are keyed in the false direction, scores on this measure (in conjunction with the *TRIN* scale discussed later in this chapter) serve as a valuable index in detecting all-true and all-false response patterns. Table 4.12 presents a variety of interpretive suggestions for four levels of *L* scale elevations on the MMPI-A.

TABLE 4.10 Interpretation Guidelines for the MMPI-A-RF Infrequent Responses (*F-r*) Scale

T-Score	Protocol Validity Concerns	Possible Reasons for Score	Interpretive Implications
≥ 90	The protocol is invalid. Over-reporting is indicated by assertion of a considerably larger than average number of symptoms rarely described by adolescents with genuine, severe psychopathology.	Inconsistent responding Over-reporting	Inconsistent responding should be considered by examining the *VRIN-r*, *TRIN-r* and *CRIN* scores. If it is ruled out, note that this level of infrequent responding is very uncommon even in individuals with genuine, severe psychopathology or emotional distress who report credible symptoms. Scores on the Substantive Scales should not be interpreted.
80–89	Possible over-reporting is indicated by assertion of a much later-than-average number of symptoms rarely described by adolescents with genuine, severe psychopathology.	Inconsistent responding Severe psychopathology Severe emotional distress Over-reporting	Inconsistent responding should be considered by examining the *VRIN-r*, *TRIN-r* and *CRIN* scores. If it is ruled out, note that this level of infrequent responding may occur in individuals with genuine, severe psychopathology or emotional distress who report credible symptoms, but it can also reflect exaggeration. For individuals with no history or current corroborating evidence of psychopathology, it very likely indicates over-reporting.
70–79	Possible over-reporting is indicated by assertion of a larger than average number of symptoms rarely described by adolescents with genuine, severe psychopathology.	Inconsistent responding Significant psychopathology Significant emotional distress Over-reporting	Inconsistent responding should be considered by examining the *VRIN-r*, *TRIN-r* and *CRIN* scores. If it is ruled out, note that this level of infrequent responding may occur in individuals with genuine, significant psychopathology or emotional distress who report credible symptoms. However, for individuals with no history or current corroborating evidence of psychopathology, it likely indicates over-reporting.

The MMPI-A-RF Uncommon Virtues (L-r) Scale

One of the most marked limitations of the MMPI-A Lie scale was the misleading label used to identify this scale. The term "lie" connotes a conscious effort at deception or distortion, a characteristic which is inaccurate for many of the adolescents who produce elevated scores on this measure. The MMPI-A-RF counterpart of the MMPI-A *L* scale was renamed the Uncommon Virtues (*L-r*) scale. This relabeling more accurately reflects the fact that many individuals who produce elevated scores on this scale employ a relatively unsophisticated defense mechanism of denial and repression, but are not engaged in a conscious effort to deceive or mislead the examiner.

The MMPI-A-RF *L-r* scale consists of 11 items that reflect common human shortcomings or faults that are reported by most adolescents. Three of these 11 items are scored if endorsed in the true directions, and the eight remaining items are scored if endorsed in the false direction. While an effort was made to achieve a better balance in items keyed in the false and true direction on the MMPI-A-RF *L-r* scale, it still remains important to rule out an excessive nay-saying or all-false response style before interpreting this scale. Table 4.13 provides interpretive guidance for four levels of elevation on the *L-r* scale. As shown in this table, protocols producing T-score values > 79 on the *L-r* scale are likely to be invalid and reflect an adolescent who presents himself or herself in the most positive light by denying common human failings. Non-elevated scores on the Clinical scales of the MMPI-A-RF are unlikely to be interpretable when *L-r* T-scores show this marked level of elevation.

The MMPI Defensiveness (K) Scale

In contrast to the extensive changes to the *F* scale, the *K* scale did not undergo any item deletions in the development of the MMPI-A, and only two items were modified in terms of wording. Thus, the MMPI-A *K* scale consists of 30 items that were empirically selected to identify individuals who display significant degrees of psychopathology but produced profiles that were within normal

TABLE 4.11 Sample Items From the MMPI-A *L* Scale (14 Items)

Items scored if true
None
Examples of items scored if false
26.   Sometimes want to swear.
38.   Sometimes don't tell truth.

Source: MMPI-A abbreviated items reproduced with permission. MMPI®-A Booklet of Abbreviated Items. Copyright © 2005 by the Regents of the University of Minnesota. Reproduced with the permission of the University of Minnesota Press. All rights reserved. "Minnesota Multiphasic Personality Inventory" and "MMPI" are trademarks owned by the University of Minnesota.

TABLE 4.12 Interpretation Guidelines for the MMPI-A *L* Scale

T-score	*Interpretation*
45 and below	*Low.* May reflect an open, confident stance among normal adolescents. "All-true" or "fake-bad" response sets are possible in this range.
46–55	*Normal.* Scores in this range reflect an appropriate balance between the admission and denial of common social faults. These adolescents tend to be flexible and non-rigid.
56–65	*Moderate.* May reflect an emphasis on conformity and conventional behaviors among adolescents. Scores in this range for adolescents in psychiatric settings may reflect the use of denial as a central defense mechanism.
66 and above	*Marked.* Scores in this range reflect extreme use of denial, poor insight, and lack of sophistication. Treatment efforts are likely to be longer and associated with guarded prognosis. An "all-false" or "fake-good" response set may have occurred.

Source: Adapted from Archer (1987b). Copyright © 1987 by Lawrence Erlbaum Associates, Inc. Reprinted with permission.

limits (Meehl & Hathaway, 1946). Only one of these items is scored in the true direction. Table 4.14 provides examples of abbreviated items from the MMPI-A *K* scale.

Item content on the *K* scale is quite diverse and covers issues ranging from self-control to family and interpersonal relationships (Greene, 2011). Although the *K*-correction procedure for Basic scales *1, 4, 7, 8,* and *9* has become standard practice with adult respondents, *K*-correction was *not* used with adolescent profiles on the original MMPI, and is *not* used with the MMPI-A or MMPI-A-RF. Marks et al. (1974) presented three reasons why *K*-correction procedures should not be employed with adolescents. First, they noted that *K*-correction was originally developed on a small sample of adult patients and "hence its applicability to adolescents is at best questionable" (p. 134). Second, they noted that Dahlstrom et al. (1972), as well as other authorities, have repeatedly cautioned against the use of *K*-weights with samples that differ significantly from those employed by Meehl in the development of the original *K*-correction weights. Finally, Marks et al. cited previous research using adolescent samples that indicated that adolescents' MMPI scores produced a stronger relationship to external criteria without use of the *K*-correction procedure. This pattern was also reported by Weed, Ben-Porath, and Butcher (1990) in MMPI data collected in adult samples, and by Archer, Fontaine, and McCrae (1998) in MMPI-2 results for adult psychiatric inpatients. These findings raise questions concerning the usefulness of *K*-correction even in interpretation of adult profiles.

Alperin et al. (1996) derived experimental *K*-weights for the MMPI-A to determine the degree to which the use of this correction procedure could improve test accuracy when weighting was based on results obtained in

TABLE 4.13 Interpretation Guidelines for the MMPI-A-RF *L-r* Scale

T-Score	Protocol/Concerns	Possible Reasons	Interpretive Implications
≥ 80	The protocol is likely invalid. Under-reporting is indicated by the test taker presenting himself or herself in an extremely positive light by denying many minor faults and shortcomings that most people acknowledge.	Inconsistent responding Under-reporting	Inconsistent responding should be considered by examining the *VRIN-r*, *TRIN-r* and *CRIN* scores. If it is ruled out, note that this level of virtuous self-presentation is very uncommon even in individuals with a background stressing traditional values. Any absence of elevation on the Substantive Scales is uninterpretable. Elevated scores on the Substantive Scales may underestimate the problems assessed by those scales.
70–79	Possible under-reporting is indicated by the test taker presenting himself or herself in a very positive light by denying several minor faults and shortcomings that most people acknowledge.	Inconsistent responding Under-reporting	Inconsistent responding should be considered by examining the *VRIN-r*, *TRIN-r* and *CRIN* scores. If it is ruled out, note that this level of virtuous self-presentation is uncommon, but it may to some extent reflect a background stressing traditional values. Any absence of elevation on the Substantive Scales should be interpreted with caution. Elevated scores on the Substantive Scales may underestimate the problems assessed by those scales.
65–69	Possible under-reporting is indicated by the test taker presenting himself or herself in a positive light by denying some minor faults and shortcomings that most people acknowledge.	Inconsistent responding Under-reporting	Inconsistent responding should be considered by examining the *VRIN-r*, *TRIN-r* and *CRIN* scores. Any absence of elevation on the Substantive Scales should be interpreted with caution. Elevated scores on the Substantive Scales may underestimate the problems assessed by those scales.
< 65	There is no evidence of under-reporting.		The protocol is interpretable.

TABLE 4.14 Sample Items From the MMPI-A *K* Scale

Item scored if true (one only)
   79. Rarely quarrel with family.
Items scored if false
   34. Sometimes feel like destroying things.
   72. Hard to convince people of truth.

Source: MMPI-A abbreviated items reproduced with the permission. MMPI®-A Booklet of Abbreviated Items. Copyright © 2005 by the Regents of the University of Minnesota. Reproduced with the permission of the University of Minnesota Press. All rights reserved. "Minnesota Multiphasic Personality Inventory" and "MMPI" are trademarks owned by the University of Minnesota.

adolescent samples. Empirically determined *K*-weights were systematically added to raw score values from the eight Basic scales (excluding *Mf* and *Si*) to optimally predict adolescents' membership in the MMPI-A normative sample of 1,620 adolescents versus a clinical sample of 122 adolescent psychiatric inpatients. Hit rate analyses were utilized to assess the degree to which the *K*-corrected uniform T-scores resulted in improved classification accuracy in contrast to the standard MMPI-A non-*K*-corrected adolescent norms. Results indicated that the use of a *K*-correction procedure for the MMPI-A did not result in any systematic improvement in test accuracy in the classification task used in this study. The authors concluded that their findings did not support the clinical application of a *K*-correction procedure with the MMPI-A.

    In general, the *K* scale is unique (relative to the basic clinical scales) in that *K* scale mean raw score values for adolescents tend to be *lower* than that found for adult samples. For example, the *K* scale mean raw score values for males and females in the MMPI-2 adult normative sample were 15.30 and 15.03, respectively (Butcher et al., 1989), whereas the normative values for males and females in the MMPI-A normative sample were 12.7 for males and 11.5 for females (Butcher et al., 1992). Although little research has been devoted to this issue, the available data indicate that *K* scale elevations in adolescents may be related to the same clinical correlate patterns that have been established for adult respondents. Thus, markedly low elevations on the *K* scale tend to be produced by adolescents who may be consciously or unconsciously exaggerating their degree of symptomatology in an attempt to fake-bad, or as a "cry for help" in response to acute distress. Conversely, elevations on the *K* scale are often produced by adolescents who are defensive and who underreport psychological problems and symptoms. Further, these adolescents often fail to perceive a need for psychological treatment and attempt to deny psychological problems. They often hide behind a facade of adequate coping and adjustment. In both the adolescent and adult MMPI literatures, high *K* scale profiles have been linked to a poor prognosis for positive response to psychological intervention because of the respondent's inability or refusal to cooperate with treatment efforts (Archer et al., 1979). Table 4.15 offers interpretive guides for four elevation levels on the MMPI-A *K* scale.

TABLE 4.15 Interpretation Guidelines for the MMPI-A *K* Scale

T-score	*Interpretation*
40 and below	*Low.* These adolescents may have poor self-concepts and limited resources for coping with stress. Scores in this range may be related to "fake-bad" attempts among normals, or acute distress for adolescents in psychiatric settings.
41–55	*Normal.* Scores in this range reflect an appropriate balance between self-disclosure and guardedness. Prognosis for psychotherapy is often good.
56–65	*Moderate.* Scores in this range among normal adolescents may reflect a self-reliant stance and reluctance to seek help from others. For adolescents in psychiatric settings, this level of *K* is related to an unwillingness to admit psychological problems and a denial of the need for treatment or psychiatric help.
66 and above	*Marked.* Scores in this range reflect extreme defensiveness often related to poor treatment prognosis and longer treatment duration. The possibility of a "fake-good" response set should be considered.

Source: Adapted from Archer (1987b). Copyright © 1987 by Lawrence Erlbaum Associates, Inc. Reprinted with permission.

The MMPI-A-RF Adjustment Validity (K-r) Scale

The Adjustment Validity (*K-r*) scale on the MMPI-A-RF consists of 12 items, two of which are scored if endorsed true, and the remaining items scored if endorsed in the false direction. Items on the *K-r* scale were primarily selected from the MMPI-A *K* scale, and reflect adolescents who present themselves as well-adjusted, self-reliant, and free from psychological symptoms. Table 4.16 presents four levels of interpretation guidance for the MMPI-A-RF *K-r* scale. As shown in this table, interpretation ranges from scores below 60, reflecting no evidence of underreporting, to T-scores > 74, indicating a level of psychological adjustment which is rare among adolescents and likely to represent an invalid protocol. *K-r* scale T-score values greater than 74 are also likely to render uninterpretable scores on the MMPI-A-RF substantive scales that occur within a normal range.

Validity Scales for Assessing Response Consistency on the MMPI-A and MMPI-A-RF

The MMPI-A Variable Response Inconsistency (VRIN) and True Response Inconsistency (TRIN) Scales

A Variable Response Inconsistency (*VRIN*) scale and a True Response Inconsistency (*TRIN*) scale were originally developed for the MMPI-2, and served as models for their counterparts in the MMPI-A instrument. Both *VRIN*

TABLE 4.16 Interpretation Guidelines for the MMPI-A-RF K-r Scale

T-Score	Validity Concerns	Possible Reasons	Interpretive Implications
≥ 75	The protocol is likely invalid. Under-reporting is indicated by the test taker presenting himself or herself as remarkably well-adjusted.	Inconsistent responding Under-reporting	Inconsistent responding should be considered by examining the VRIN-r, TRIN-r and CRIN scores. If it is ruled out, note that this level of psychological adjustment is rare among adolescents. The absence of elevation on the Substantive Scales is not interpretable. Elevated scores on the Substantive Scales may underestimate the problems assessed by those scales.
66–74	Possible under-reporting is indicated by the test taker presenting himself or herself as very well adjusted.	Inconsistent responding Very good psychological adjustment Under-reporting	Inconsistent responding should be considered by examining the VRIN-r, TRIN-r and CRIN scores. If it is ruled out, note that this level of psychological adjustment is relatively rare among adolescents. For individuals who are not especially well adjusted, any absence of elevation on the Substantive Scales should be interpreted with caution. Elevated scores on the Substantive Scales may underestimate the problems assessed by those scales.
60–65	Possible under-reporting is indicated by the test taker presenting himself or herself as well adjusted.	Inconsistent responding Good psychological adjustment Under-reporting	Inconsistent responding should be considered by examining the VRIN-r, TRIN-r and CRIN scores. If it is ruled out, for individuals who are not well adjusted, any absence of elevation on the Substantive Scales should be interpreted with caution. Elevated scores on the Substantive Scales may underestimate the problems assessed by those scales.
< 60	There is no evidence of under-reporting.		The protocol is interpretable.

and *TRIN* provide data concerning an individual's tendency to respond to MMPI-A items in a consistent manner. The *VRIN* scale consists of 50 pairs of items with either similar or opposite content. Each time an adolescent answers an item pair inconsistently, one raw score point is added to the *VRIN* scale score. Table 4.17 provides illustrations of *VRIN* scale items.

As shown in this table, the content of the item pairs determines the response combination that would result in a point added to the *VRIN* total. For some item pairs, two true responses are scored, for other combinations two false responses are scored, and for others a combination of true and false responses produces an inconsistent response pattern resulting in a point added to the raw score value. The *VRIN* findings can serve as a warning that an adolescent has responded to the MMPI-A in an indiscriminate and random manner. For example, Berry et al. (1992) and Berry et al. (1991) demonstrated the sensitivity of the MMPI-2 *VRIN* scale to the presence of random responding in college student samples. Elevated *VRIN* scale values can also be used to support the inference that an elevation on the *F* scale is likely to reflect carelessness or a random response pattern. Illustrating this point, Wetter, Baer, Berry, Smith, and Larsen (1992) demonstrated that both random and malingered responses produced elevations on the MMPI-2 *F* scale in a college student sample, whereas elevated *VRIN* scale scores result solely from random response patterns. Thus, a high *VRIN* score combined with a high *F* scale score strongly suggests the possibility of a random response pattern. It should be noted, however, that *VRIN* T-score values within acceptable ranges do not necessarily imply that an MMPI-A profile is subject to valid interpretation. Although *VRIN* scale values are related to inferences concerning the consistency of an adolescent's response pattern, findings from this scale do not permit judgments concerning the accuracy of the subjects' responses. The distinction between accuracy and consistency as subcomponents of validity assessment are discussed later in this chapter.

TABLE 4.17 Examples of Variable Response Inconsistency (*VRIN*) Scale Items

---

Sample VRIN pair that adds one point when both marked true
   70. Not self-confident.
      223. Wholly self-confident.
Sample VRIN pair that adds one point when both marked false
304. Try to avoid crowds.
      335. Like excitement of a crowd.
Sample VRIN pair scored when marked differently (T-F or F-T)
   6. Father a good man.
      86. Love (d) father.

The effectiveness of the MMPI-A *VRIN* scale in adolescent populations has been the focus of several studies. Baer, Ballenger, Berry, and Wetter (1997), for example, examined random responding on the MMPI-A in a sample of 106 normal adolescents. Participants were asked to report on the frequency, location, and reason for any random responses that occurred during the standard administration of the MMPI-A, and relationships between self-reported random responding and validity scale scores were examined including the F, F_1, F_2, and *VRIN* scales. In addition, participants were assigned to groups that varied in the extent of random responding (0%, 25%, 50%, 75%, or 100% random). Findings indicated that most adolescents acknowledged one or more random responses during the standard administration process, and the number of self-reported random responses were significantly correlated with the F scale. Further, scores on the F and *VRIN* scale were effective in discriminating standard protocols from protocols with various levels of randomness. The authors concluded that their study provided strong support for the utility of the *VRIN* scale because this scale is designed to be sensitive to random responding but, unlike the F scale, does not typically elevate under conditions of symptom overreporting. Archer and Elkins (1999) followed up this line of research by evaluating the utility of MMPI-A validity scales in detecting differences in response patterns between protocols produced by 354 adolescents in clinical settings and a group of 354 randomly produced MMPI-A protocols. Results indicated that the MMPI-A Validity scales F, F_1, F_2, and *VRIN* all appeared to be useful in correctly identifying protocols from actual clinical participants versus randomly generated response patterns. Further, it was noted that the optimal MMPI-A scale cutoffs for these validity scales were largely consistent with the interpretive recommendations provided in the MMPI-A test manual (Butcher et al., 1992), that is, $T \geq 80$ on *VRIN* and $T \geq 90$ on F, F_1, and F_2. Archer, Handel, Lynch, and Elkins (2002) extended this methodology by examining the ability of the MMPI-A Validity scales to detect varying degrees of protocol randomness. Samples were 100 adolescent inpatients administered the MMPI-A under standard conditions and samples of 100 protocols containing varying degrees of computer-generated random responses. In general, the overall classification accuracy reported by Archer et al. (2002) was highly consistent with overall classification accuracy reported by Archer and Elkins (1999) and by Baer et al. (1997). T-score values for the *VRIN* scale consistently climbed as increasing levels of randomness was introduced into protocols, with a T-score value ≥ 80 on the *VRIN* scale generally functioning as a useful cutoff across varying levels of random responding. However, the *VRIN* scale was more effective in distinguishing standardly administered protocols from protocols that contained larger proportions of random responding. No MMPI-A validity scale was particularly effective in detecting partially random responding that involves less than half of the items in the second half of the test booklet.

Pinsoneault (2005) evaluated the ability of the MMPI-A Validity scales to detect varying levels of random protocols. The author reported that the VRIN scale was the most effective scale in detecting all-random protocols with an optimal T-score cutoff of 75 or greater to identify all-random response patterns. More recently, Pinsoneault (2014) explored the ability of the MMPI-A to accurately detect half-random and all-random protocols from non-random protocols produced by adolescents referred for forensic evaluations by Juvenile and Domestic Relations Courts. In this study, the MMPI-A was administered in the short form 350-item format, resulting in truncated versions of the VRIN scale because approximately one-third of the item pairs in the VRIN scale are included after item 350 in the test booklet. As noted in prior studies, the effectiveness of the VRIN scale was related to the degree of randomness, with the truncated form of the VRIN scale most effective in detecting all-random protocols. In general, the MMPI-A *VRIN* scale has demonstrated sufficient effectiveness to serve as a model for similar attempts to detect random responding on other test instruments. For example, a variable response inconsistency scale has been developed for the Jesness Inventory, a self-report instrument designed for use with delinquent boys and girls aged 8 through 18 (Pinsoneault, 1997, 1999) and for the MMPI-A-RF (Archer et al., 2016a).

The True Response Inconsistency (*TRIN*) scale for the MMPI-A, like its counterpart on the MMPI-2, was developed to detect an individual's tendency to indiscriminately respond to items as either *true* (acquiescence response set), or *false* (nay-saying), regardless of item content. This MMPI-A scale consists of 24 pairs of items that are negatively correlated and semantically opposite in content. The *TRIN* scale was developed in such a manner that raw score values must convert to T-scores that are $\geq$50 (i.e., raw scores cannot convert to T-score values below 50). *TRIN* T-scores >50 may represent deviations from the mean in either the acquiescent or nay-saying direction. In the computer scoring of the MMPI-A provided by Pearson Assessments, the direction of deviation is indicated by a "T" or "F" that follows the T-score assigned to the *TRIN* scale. For example, 80 T would indicate inconsistency in the true-response direction, whereas 80 F would represent an equal magnitude of inconsistency in the direction of false responding.

Table 4.18 provides examples of *TRIN* items. As shown in the table, *true* responses to some item pairs, and *false* responses to other item pairs, result in scores on the *TRIN* scale. *TRIN* scores may be used to provide data concerning the degree to which an adolescent has tended to employ an acquiescent or nay-saying response style. As noted by Greene (2011), however, scores on the *TRIN* scale should not be used to determine whether an adolescent has endorsed MMPI-A items in a random manner. As shown later in this chapter in the example of a random profile, the *TRIN* scale may often produce acceptable T-score values under a random response set condition. The specific formula for *TRIN* scoring, as provided in the MMPI-A manual (Butcher et al., 1992, 2001), is as follows:

TABLE 4.18 Examples of True Response Inconsistency (*TRIN*) Scale Items

---

Sample TRIN pairs that add one point when both marked true
14. Work atmosphere tense.
    424. Don't have much stress.
Sample TRIN pairs that subtract one point when both marked false
46. Am friendly.
    475. Quiet around others.

Source: MMPI-A abbreviated items reproduced with permission. MMPI®-A Booklet of Abbreviated Items. Copyright © 2005 by the Regents of the University of Minnesota. Reproduced with permission of the University of Minnesota Press. All rights reserved. "Minnesota Multiphasic Personality Inventory" and "MMPI" are trademarks owned by the University of Minnesota.

1. For each of the following response pairs *add* one point:

14 T – 424 T	119 T – 184 T
37 T – 168 T	146 T – 167 T
60 T – 121 T	242 T – 260 T
62 T – 360 T	264 T – 331 T
63 T – 120 T	304 T – 335 T
70 T – 223 T	355 T – 367 T
71 T – 283 T	463 T – 476 T
95 T – 294 T	

2. For each of the following response pairs *subtract* one point:

46 F – 475 F	128 F – 465 F
53 F – 91 F	158 F – 288 F
63 F – 120 F	245 F – 257 F
71 F – 283 F	304 F – 335 F
82 F – 316 F	

3. Then *add* 9 points to the total raw score.

Limited information is currently available concerning the characteristics of the MMPI-A *TRIN* scale in adolescent samples. Handel, Arnau, Archer, and Dandy (2006) examined the MMPI-A and MMPI-2 *TRIN* scales as measures of acquiescence and non-acquiescence among the standard scales of these instruments. The study objective was to evaluate the effectiveness of the *TRIN* scale in discriminating respondents in one-half of the MMPI-A normative sample from adolescents in the remaining portion of the normative sample with varying degrees of inserted true or false responses in the latter group. For the MMPI-A, *TRIN* positive predictive power was relatively modest at the recommended T-score cutoff of T ≥ 75 until the true response insertion percentage reached 30% or greater. The authors concluded that their findings supported the *TRIN* cutoff score (i.e., T ≥ 80) recommended in the MMPI-A manual.

Because both scales include items beyond item 350, the full MMPI-A must be administered to score *TRIN* or *VRIN*. The following guidelines in interpreting these scales are recommended:

- *VRIN* T-scores of 70–79 indicate marginal levels of response inconsistency.
- *VRIN* T-scores ≥ 80 indicate unacceptable levels of response inconsistency.
- *TRIN* T-scores of 70–79 indicate marginal levels of response inconsistency.
- *TRIN* T-scores ≥ 80 indicate unacceptable levels of response inconsistency.

Inconsistent item endorsement patterns for adolescents may be related to inadequate reading ability, limited intellectual ability, active noncompliance or test resistance, or thought disorganization related to substance abuse-induced toxicity or active psychosis.

The MMPI-A-RF VRIN-r and TRIN-r Scales

The MMPI-2 and MMPI-A *VRIN* and *TRIN* scales served as the models for the development of similar scales on the MMPI-A-RF. The MMPI-A-RF Variable Response Inconsistency (*VRIN-r*) scale is based on 27 item pairs that are similar in content, so that the total number of true-false and false-true responses to item pairs equals the total score on the *VRIN* scale. The MMPI-A-RF True Response Inconsistency (*TRIN-r*) scale is based on the adolescent's responses to 13 pairs of items containing content which is contradictory. Eight of these *TRIN-r* scale item pairs are scored when answered in the true direction, and five of the pairs are scored when answered in a false-false direction. Similar to the scoring procedure for the MMPI-A *TRIN* scale, MMPI-A-RF *TRIN-r* raw scores are computed by summing the number of true-true responses and subtracting the number of false-false responses with a constant of 5 added to avoid the production of negative values. Consistent with the MMPI-A scoring for the *TRIN* scale, MMPI-A-RF *TRIN-r* T-scores below 50 are not possible. On the Pearson scoring program for the MMPI-A-RF, T-score values are followed by a "T" to reflect an acquiescence response set, or followed by an "F" to reflect a non-acquiescence or nay-saying response style. The following preliminary guidelines are offered for interpreting these scales:

- *VRIN-r* T-scores of 65 to 74 indicate marginal levels of response consistency.
- *VRIN-r* T-scores ≥ 75 indicate unacceptable levels of response inconsistency.
- *TRIN-r* T-scores of 65 to 74 indicate marginal levels of response inconsistency.
- *TRIN-r* T-scores ≥ 75 indicate unacceptable levels of response inconsistency.

The MMPI-A Combined Response Inconsistency (CRIN) scale

The Combined Response Inconsistency (*CRIN*) scale is a global measure of response inconsistency which does not have a counterpart on the MMPI-A. The *CRIN* scale includes item pairs from both the *VRIN-r* and *TRIN-r* scales scored by simply summing all items scored in an inconsistent direction, without subtraction of any constant value. The *CRIN* scale provides an additional scale beyond the *VRIN-r* and *TRIN-r* scales in identifying adolescents exhibiting an inconsistent response pattern. As noted in the MMPI-A-RF manual (Archer et al. 2016a), elevations on the *CRIN* scale may indicate protocol invalidity, even in the absence of comparable elevations on the *VRIN-r* or *TRIN-r* scales. The following are preliminary guidelines offered for the interpretation of the *CRIN* scale:

- *CRIN* T-score ≤ 65 indicates an acceptable protocol subject to valid interpretation.
- *CRIN* T-score of 65–74 indicates marginal levels of response consistency.
- *CRIN* T-score ≥ 75 indicates unacceptable levels of response consistency.

Effects of Response Sets on Standard Scales

Graham (2012) described the characteristics of MMPI-2 profiles that are generated by adults based on systematic response sets such as "all-true," "all-false," and random patterns, and Graham, Watts, and Timbrook (1991) described MMPI-2 fake-good and fake-bad profiles. Similar response set data for adolescents on the original test instrument was presented by Archer, Gordon, and Kirchner (1987) and summarized for the MMPI-A by Archer and Krishnamurthy (2002) and by Butcher and Williams (2000). Archer and Krishnamurthy (2002) noted that adolescents employing all-true and all-false response sets on the MMPI-A are easily detected, and the extreme validity scale profile features are similar to those produced by their adult counterparts. Additionally, the fake-bad or overreporting response set found for adolescents is relatively easy to identify based on the occurrence of an extremely elevated *F* scale combined with clinical range elevations on all clinical scales (excluding *Mf* and *Si*). In contrast, adolescents' production of random response sets, and particularly on fake-good or underreporting response sets, were more difficult to detect on the MMPI-A. The following section provides a summary of the effects of a variety of response sets on the MMPI-A and MMPI-A-RF.

All-True MMPI-A-Profiles

The MMPI-A all-true response pattern is indicated by extremely low scores on scales *L* and *K*, and markedly elevated scores (T > 90) on scales F, F_1, and F_2. The male and female all-true profile on MMPI-A norms is presented in Fig. 4.1. The raw score value for *TRIN* (raw score = 24) clearly indicates inconsistent responses, with *TRIN* indicative of an extreme "yea-saying" response style, whereas *VRIN* (raw score = 5) is within acceptable limits. In addition to the extreme "most open" validity scale pattern formed by scales F_1, F_2, F, L, and K, there is a very noticeable positive or psychotic slope to the profile, with elevations on scales 6, 7, 8, and 9. These characteristics are similar to those found for all-true response patterns among adolescents on the original form of the MMPI (Archer, 1989).

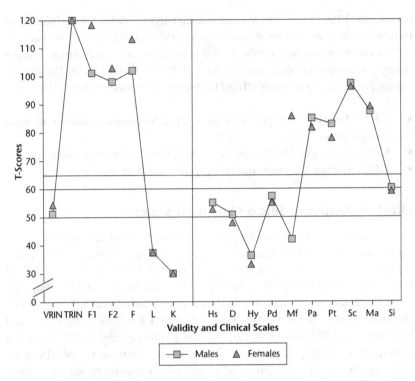

FIGURE 4.1 All-true MMPI-A response patterns for males and females (*TRIN* T-score = 120T for males and females).

Figure 4.2 provides the Content scale and Supplementary scale profile for the all-true response pattern. because the majority of items in the Content scales are keyed in the true direction, this profile exhibits very elevated T-score values for most Content scales.

All-True MMPI-A-RF Profiles

The all-true response pattern for the MMPI-A-RF Validity scales is shown in Figure 4.3. Figure 4.4 shows the all-true response pattern for the MMPI-A-RF Higher-Order (H-O) and Restructured Clinical (RC) scales. The all-true MMPI-A-RF Validity scale pattern is marked by extreme elevations on *TRIN-r* and *F-r*, while the H-O and RC profile exhibits extreme (T > 90) on *THD*, *RC8*, and *RC4*.

All-False MMPI-A Profiles

The profile shown in Fig. 4.5 will be produced if an adolescent responds *false* to all MMPI-A items. The *TRIN* raw score value is zero (T > 100) and the

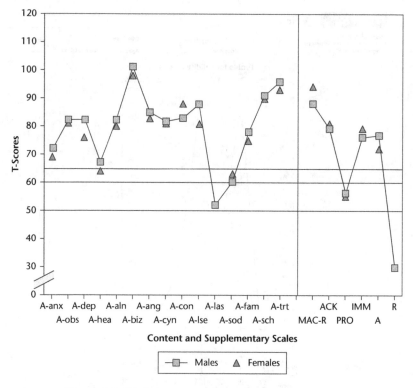

FIGURE 4.2 All-true MMPI-A Content and Supplementary scale patterns for males and females.

VRIN raw score value is 4. The *TRIN* value indicates response inconsistency, exhibiting an extreme nay-saying response style. In addition, F_1 values produce marginally elevated T-scores, whereas F_2 and F T-scores fall within normal limits. The all-false profile is characterized by extreme elevations on validity scales *L* and *K*, and on the first three clinical scales of the MMPI-A, which are frequently referred to as the *neurotic triad*. The clinical scale profile has a distinctive negative slope; that is, scale values greatly decrease as the scale's numerical designation increases. These findings are similar to the adolescent all-false profile for the original MMPI reported by Archer et al. (1987) and for adults on the MMPI-2 reported by Graham (2012). The characteristic profile features of both the all-true and the all-false patterns are easily discernible as invalid profiles. It should be clearly noted, however, that these deviant response sets should typically be detected by the inspection of the completed answer form prior to the profiling of response features.

Figure 4.6 shows the Content and Supplementary scale profile associated with an all-false pattern. Because all Content scales except Health Concerns (*A-hea*) and Low Aspirations (*A-las*) are composed of items predominantly keyed

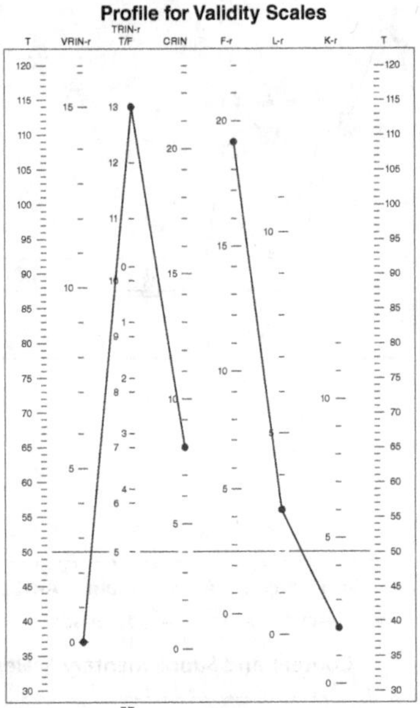

FIGURE 4.3 All-true MMPI-A-RF Validity scale response pattern.

Source: MMPI-A-RF Administration, Scoring, Interpretation and Technical Manual by Archer, et al. Copyright © 2016 by the Regents of the University of Minnesota. Reproduced with the permission of the University of Minnesota Press. All rights reserved. "Minnesota Multiphasic Personality Inventory" and "MMPI" are trademarks owned by the Regents of the University of Minnesota.

in the *true* direction, an all-false response set produces low T-scores for these scales. In contrast, the Repression (R) scale is composed of items exclusively keyed in the *false* direction and therefore produces a very elevated T-score value under this response set.

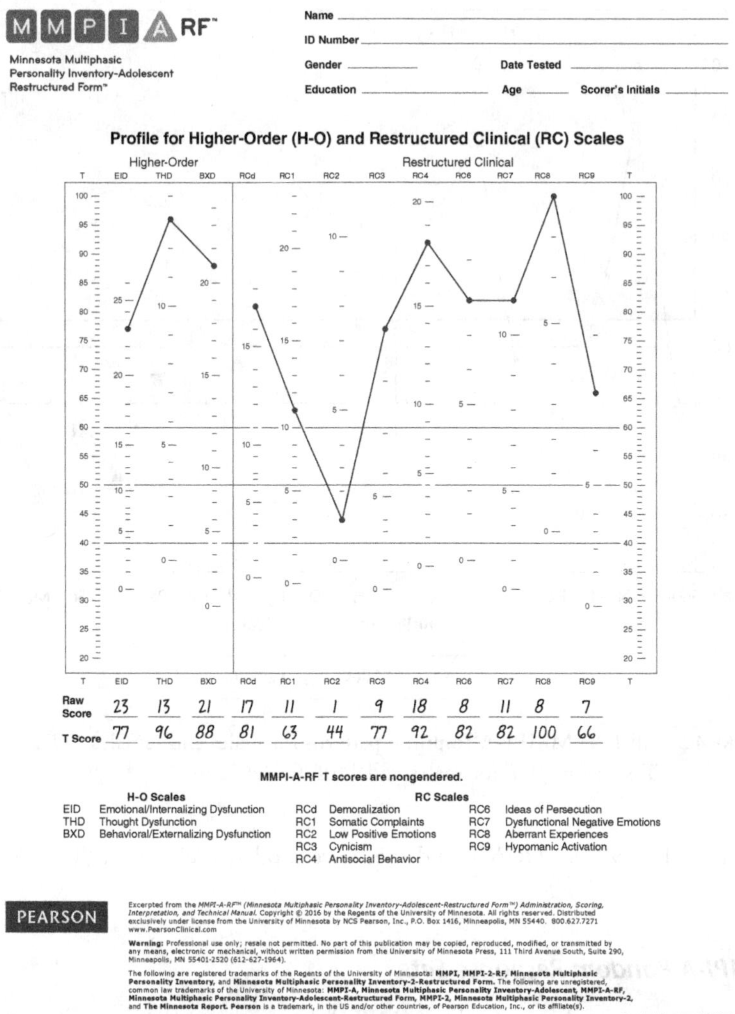

FIGURE 4.4 All-true MMPI-A-RF *H-O* and *RC* scale response pattern.

Source: MMPI-A-RF Administration, Scoring, Interpretation and Technical Manual by Archer, et al. Copyright © 2016 by the Regents of the University of Minnesota. Reproduced with the permission of the University of Minnesota Press. All rights reserved. "Minnesota Multiphasic Personality Inventory" and "MMPI" are trademarks owned by the Regents of the University of Minnesota.

All-False MMPI-A-RF Profiles

Figure 4.7 shows the MMPI-A-RF Validity scale profile associated with an all-false response pattern. Figure 4.8 shows the all-false pattern on MMPI-A-RF H-O and RC scales. The all-false Validity scale profile is notable for the extreme

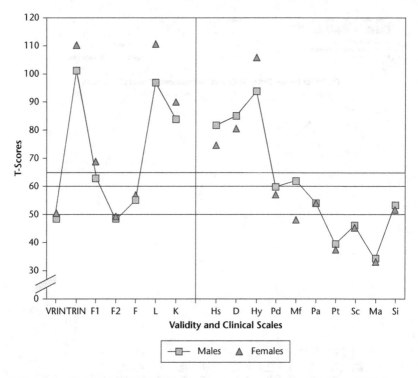

FIGURE 4.5 All-false MMPI-A response patterns for males and females (*TRIN* T-score = 101F for males and 110F for females).

elevation T > 90 on *TRIN-r,* and the more moderate elevation (T > 80) on *RC2.*

MMPI-A Random Response Sets

An adolescent may also respond to MMPI-A items in a random response pattern. The profile resulting from equal numbers of true and false item endorsements on each MMPI-A Basic scale (i.e., the effect of an infinite number of random sorts) is presented in Fig. 4.9.

Consistent with the findings for adolescents on the original test instrument (Archer et al., 1987), random MMPI-A profiles are more difficult to detect than other response sets. The MMPI-A *VRIN* scale is a useful indicator of random response sets in adolescents. The *TRIN* scale, however, may often produce acceptable T-score values under a random response set condition. The random profile is also characterized by a highly unusual validity scale configuration in which clinical range elevations on scales F, F_1, and F_2 are accompanied by a clinical range L scale elevation. The actual profile characteristics for a random response set will vary substantially, depending on the particular approach

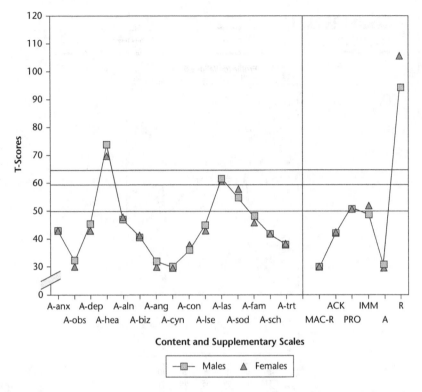

FIGURE 4.6 All-false MMPI-A Content and Supplementary scale patterns for males and females.

used to randomize the response pattern. The profile characteristics will also vary quite markedly depending on the degree or extent of randomness in the profile, and Archer et al. (2002) have demonstrated that "partially random" protocols may be difficult or impossible to detect through the examination of validity scale results. Random response patterns should always be considered when an adolescent completes the MMPI-A too quickly; that is, in less than 40 minutes.

Figure 4.10 shows the effects of a totally random response pattern on the MMPI-A Content and Supplementary scales. Similar to the corresponding Basic scale profile, even this profile is relatively difficult to detect based on shape and elevation features.

MMPI-A-RF Random Response Sets

Figure 4.11 shows the effects of a random response set on the MMPI-A-RF Validity scales, and Figure 4.12 shows the effects for the MMPI-A-RF H-O and RC scales. The MMPI-A-RF Validity scale profile for a random response

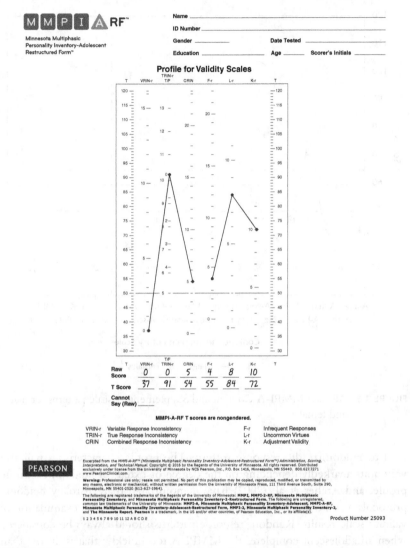

FIGURE 4.7   All-false MMPI-A-RF Validity scale pattern.

Source: MMPI-A-RF Administration, Scoring, Interpretation and Technical Manual by Archer, et al. Copyright © 2016 by the Regents of the University of Minnesota. Reproduced with the permission of the University of Minnesota Press. All rights reserved. "Minnesota Multiphasic Personality Inventory" and "MMPI" are trademarks owned by the Regents of the University of Minnesota.

pattern shows relatively moderate elevations on *CRIN* (T > 80). Similar to the effects of a random pattern on the MMPI-A Basic scales, a random response pattern on the H-O and RC scales of the MMPI-A-RF is more difficult

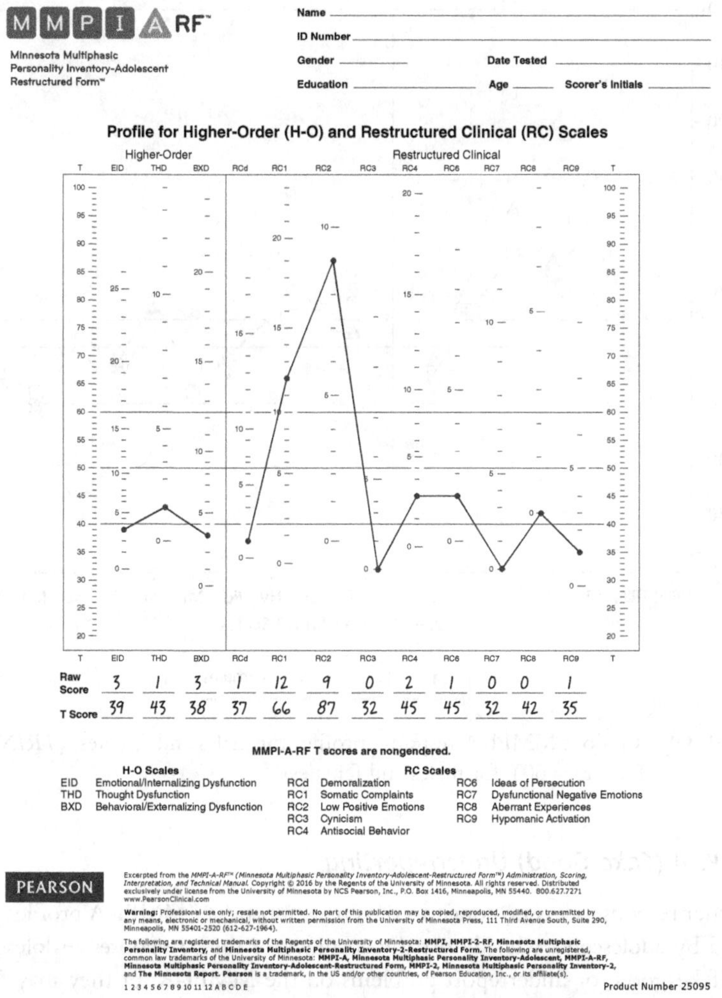

MMPI A RF™

Minnesota Multiphasic
Personality Inventory-Adolescent
Restructured Form™

Name _____

ID Number _____

Gender _____   Date Tested _____

Education _____   Age _____   Scorer's Initials _____

Profile for Higher-Order (H-O) and Restructured Clinical (RC) Scales

	EID	THD	BXD	RCd	RC1	RC2	RC3	RC4	RC6	RC7	RC8	RC9	
Raw Score	3	1	3	1	12	9	0	2	1	0	0	1	
T Score	39	43	38	37	66	87	32	45	45	32	42	35	

MMPI-A-RF T scores are nongendered.

H-O Scales
EID   Emotional/Internalizing Dysfunction
THD   Thought Dysfunction
BXD   Behavioral/Externalizing Dysfunction

RC Scales
RCd   Demoralization
RC1   Somatic Complaints
RC2   Low Positive Emotions
RC3   Cynicism
RC4   Antisocial Behavior
RC6   Ideas of Persecution
RC7   Dysfunctional Negative Emotions
RC8   Aberrant Experiences
RC9   Hypomanic Activation

FIGURE 4.8   All-false MMPI-A-RF *H-O* and *RC* scale pattern.

Source: MMPI-A-RF Administration, Scoring, Interpretation and Technical Manual by Archer, et al. Copyright © 2016 by the Regents of the University of Minnesota. Reproduced with the permission of the University of Minnesota Press. All rights reserved. "Minnesota Multiphasic Personality Inventory" and "MMPI" are trademarks owned by the Regents of the University of Minnesota.

to detect than other response styles, and may often produce an acceptable credible appearance. The effects of random responding on the MMPI-A-RF, therefore, are best detected by a reliance on the characteristic Validity scale configuration.

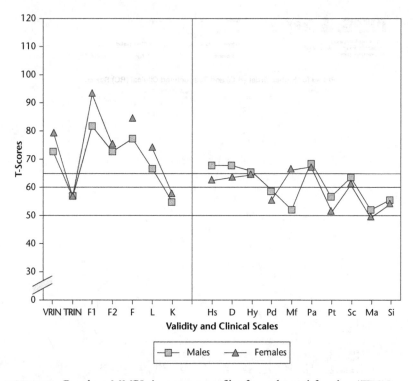

FIGURE 4.9 Random MMPI-A response profiles for males and females. (*TRIN* T–score = 60T for males and females).

MMPI-A (Fake-Good) Underreporting

Another response set issue concerns the characteristics of MMPI-A profiles produced by adolescents who distort the accuracy of their responses. Adolescents may fake-good, or underreport problems on the MMPI-A, or they may fake-bad, completing the MMPI-A in a manner that overreports symptomatology. Because these types of profiles may be produced by individuals who consciously or unconsciously distort their responses, Greene (2000) and Archer and Krishnamurthy (2002) emphasized the use of the terms *underreporting* and *overreporting*, respectively, to describe these response sets. Graham (2000) used the terms *positive self-presentation* and *negative self-presentation* to describe these distortions in the accuracy of a subject's test responses.

Studies with adult psychiatric patients have found that the ability to simulate a normal profile is significantly related to a favorable treatment outcome among schizophrenics (Newmark, Gentry, Whitt, McKee, & Wicker, 1983) and across psychiatric diagnoses (Grayson & Olinger, 1957). Additionally, Bonfilio and Lyman (1981) investigated the ability of college students to simulate the profile of "well-adjusted" peers. Results from this study indicated

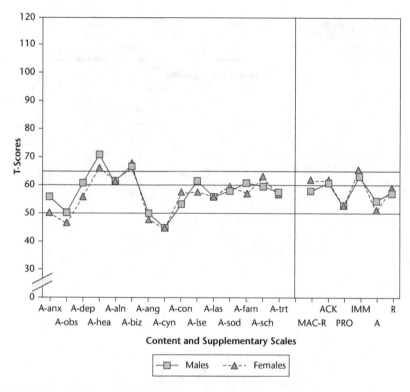

FIGURE 4.10   Random MMPI-A Content and Supplementary scale patterns for males and females.

that simulations produced by college students classified as *neurotic, normal,* and *psychopathic,* based on their actual MMPIs administered under normal instructions, were essentially within normal limits. Simulated profiles produced by psychotic or hypomanic college students, however, contained clearly pathological or clinical range features. Graham, Watts, and Timbrook (1991) provided MMPI-2 fake-good response features generated by college students who were administered the MMPI with instructions to respond as they would if they were applying for a highly valued job. The clearest indication of a fake-good profile in these data was the occurrence of a defensive validity scale configuration in which marked elevations occurred for scales *L* and *K,* particularly evident for scale *L.* Baer, Wetter, and Berry (1995) examined the effects of two levels of information about the MMPI-2 Validity scales on the ability of college students to underreport symptomatology. Findings indicated that the MMPI-2 standard Validity scales, including *L* and *K,* were effective in accurately identifying uncoached fakers. However, these scales were far less effective in discriminating standard subjects from coached subjects given either detailed or general information concerning the operation of the MMPI-2 Validity scales. These findings

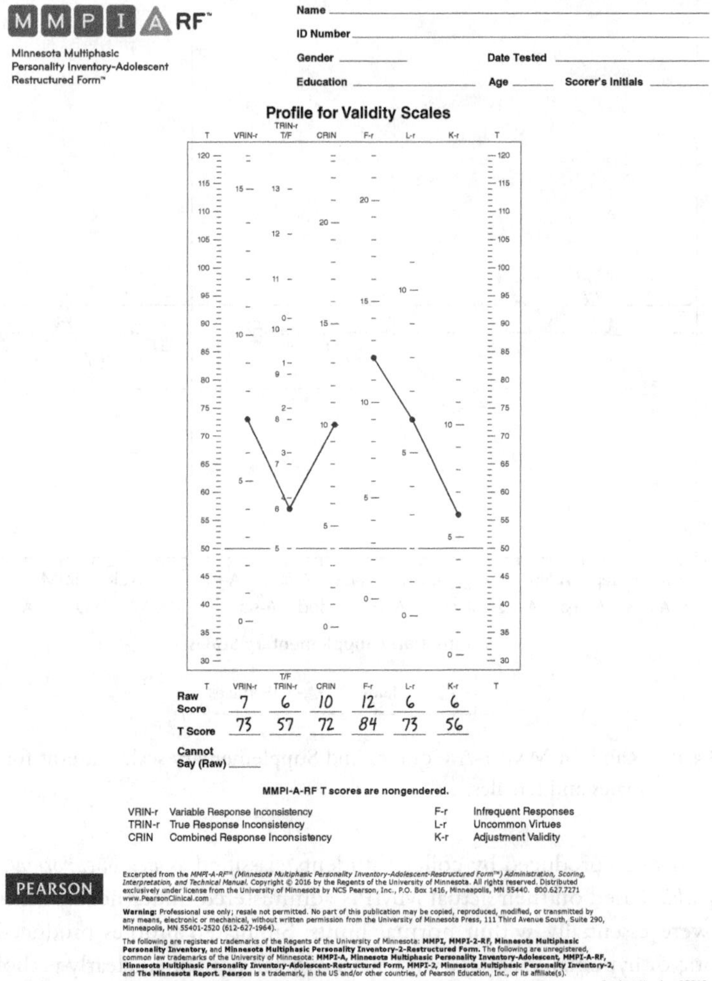

M M P I A RF™

Minnesota Multiphasic
Personality Inventory–Adolescent
Restructured Form™

Name _____

ID Number _____

Gender _____   Date Tested _____

Education _____   Age _____   Scorer's Initials _____

Profile for Validity Scales

	VRIN-r	TRIN-r T/F	CRIN	F-r	L-r	K-r	

Raw Score: VRIN-r 7, TRIN-r 6, CRIN 10, F-r 12, L-r 6, K-r 6

T Score: VRIN-r 73, TRIN-r 57, CRIN 72, F-r 84, L-r 73, K-r 56

Cannot Say (Raw) _____

MMPI-A-RF T scores are nongendered.

VRIN-r   Variable Response Inconsistency
TRIN-r   True Response Inconsistency
CRIN   Combined Response Inconsistency
F-r   Infrequent Responses
L-r   Uncommon Virtues
K-r   Adjustment Validity

FIGURE 4.11   Random MMPI-A-RF Validity scale pattern.

Source: MMPI-A-RF Administration, Scoring, Interpretation and Technical Manual by Archer, et al. Copyright © 2016 by the Regents of the University of Minnesota. Reproduced with the permission of the University of Minnesota Press. All rights reserved. "Minnesota Multiphasic Personality Inventory" and "MMPI" are trademarks owned by the Regents of the University of Minnesota.

suggest that providing information about the presence and functions of validity scales may enable some subjects to distort their response patterns to the MMPI-2 (and potentially the MMPI-A) in a way that effectively evades detection. Finally, Bagby, Rogers, and Buis (1994) examined the effectiveness of various

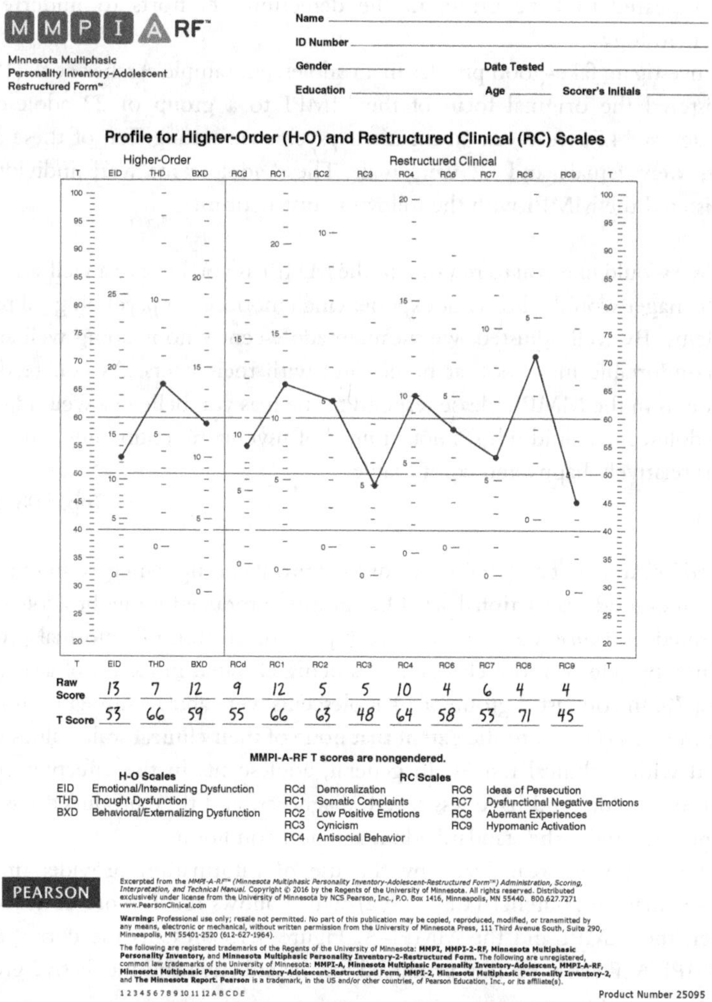

M M P I A RF™

Minnesota Multiphasic
Personality Inventory-Adolescent
Restructured Form™

Name _____

ID Number _____

Gender _____   Date Tested _____

Education _____   Age _____ Scorer's Initials _____

Profile for Higher-Order (H-O) and Restructured Clinical (RC) Scales

Higher-Order | Restructured Clinical

	EID	THD	BXD	RCd	RC1	RC2	RC3	RC4	RC6	RC7	RC8	RC9	
Raw Score	13	7	12	9	12	5	5	10	4	6	4	4	
T Score	53	66	59	55	66	63	48	64	58	53	71	45	

MMPI-A-RF T scores are nongendered.

H-O Scales
EID Emotional/Internalizing Dysfunction
THD Thought Dysfunction
BXD Behavioral/Externalizing Dysfunction

RC Scales
RCd Demoralization
RC1 Somatic Complaints
RC2 Low Positive Emotions
RC3 Cynicism
RC4 Antisocial Behavior
RC6 Ideas of Persecution
RC7 Dysfunctional Negative Emotions
RC8 Aberrant Experiences
RC9 Hypomanic Activation

PEARSON

FIGURE 4.12 Random MMPI-A-RF *H-O* and *RC* scale pattern.

Source: MMPI-A-RF Administration, Scoring, Interpretation and Technical Manual by Archer, et al. Copyright © 2016 by the Regents of the University of Minnesota. Reproduced with the permission of the University of Minnesota Press. All rights reserved. "Minnesota Multiphasic Personality Inventory" and "MMPI" are trademarks owned by the Regents of the University of Minnesota.

MMPI-2 validity scales and indices in the detection of malingering and faking-good in samples of 165 college students and 173 forensic inpatients. Although several validity indicators appear to be moderately effective at detecting fake-bad profiles, only the *F-K* index and the Subtle-Obvious index appeared to have utility in the detection of efforts to underreport symptomatology.

To investigate fake-good profiles in an adolescent sample, Archer et al. (1987) administered the original form of the MMPI to a group of 22 adolescents (mean age = 14.76 years) in an inpatient psychiatric setting. Ten of these adolescents were female and 12 were male. These adolescents were individually administered the MMPI with the following instructions:

> We would like you to respond to the MMPI as you believe a well-adjusted teenager would who is not experiencing emotional or psychological problems. By well-adjusted, we mean an adolescent who is doing well and is comfortable in school, at home, and with their peers. As you read the items in the MMPI, please respond to them as you believe a well-adjusted adolescent would who is not in need of psychiatric counseling, and who is relatively happy and comfortable.
>
> (pp. 508–509)

As noted by Archer et al. (1987), two distinct profile groups emerged in response to this fake-good instructional set. One profile, produced by eight adolescents and termed *ineffective*, consisted of a very poor simulation of a normal profile, as defined by one or more clinical scales being elevated in excess of a T-score value of 70. In contrast, a group of 14 adolescents were able to simulate a normal profile (termed *effective*) to the extent that none of their clinical scale values were elevated within clinical ranges. In general, adolescents in the effective group tended to be older and have less severe diagnoses, and they produced less elevated profiles under the standard administration conditions.

These data were reanalyzed by the use of information provided in the MMPI-A manual (Butcher et al., 1992) which allows for T-score conversions between the MMPI and the MMPI-A. Figure 4.13 presents the corresponding MMPI-A T-score profiles produced for the effective and ineffective groups under fake-good instructions.

These data indicate a validity scale configuration for the effective group characterized by elevations on scales *L*, *F*, and *K*, which are generally within acceptable ranges. Clinical scale values present a "hypernormal" configuration, with T-scores at or below 50 on most clinical scales. Therefore, the mean fake-good profile for the effective group would be difficult to distinguish from the responses of a somewhat guarded and defensive normal adolescent without significant psychiatric problems. The following guidelines, however, should serve to improve screening for adolescents who attempt to fake-good on the MMPI-A:

1. Elevations on validity scales *L* and $K \geq 65$.
2. All clinical scale T-score values are ≤ 60, but produced by an adolescent with known or established psychopathology.

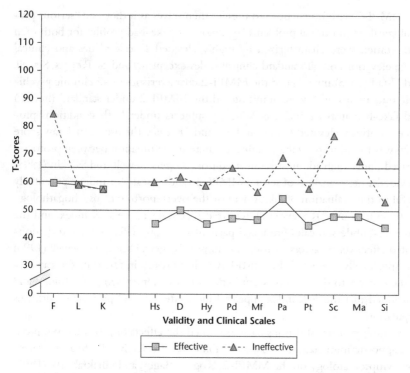

FIGURE 4.13 Fake-good MMPI-A Validity scale profile.

While the MMPI-A-RF research will be needed to reach firm recommendations, tentative guidelines for the MMPI-A-RF in detecting fake-good or
underreporting attempts are provided in the MMPI-A-RF Manual (Archer et al.,
2016a) are summarized as follows:

T-score elevations on Validity Scales L-r ≥ 80, or T-score elevations on
K-r ≥ 75.

Overreporting (Fake-Bad)

The ability of normal adults to simulate psychopathology (to fake-bad) has
been investigated by numerous researchers, including Anthony (1976), Exner,
McDowell, Pabst, Stackman, and Kirk (1963), Gough (1947, 1954), Lanyon
(1967), and Meehl and Hathaway (1946). Results have consistently shown that
adults fail to accurately simulate the types of symptomatology typically reported
by psychiatric patients. In general, normals tend to overreport psychopathology
on the MMPI in an exaggerated and non-specific manner that is easily detected
as a fake-bad attempt (Dahlstrom et al., 1975; Greene, 1980, 2000). Graham,
Watts, and Timbrook (1991) requested male and female college students to take

the MMPI-2 with instructions to present themselves as if they had "serious psychological or emotional problems" (p. 267). The fake-bad profiles for both men and women were characterized by highly elevated *F* scale values and clinical range elevations on all standard clinical scales except *Mf* and *Si*. Rogers, Sewell, and Ustad (1995) investigated the MMPI-2 characteristics of 42 chronic psychiatric outpatients who were administered the MMPI-2 under standard (honest) and fake-bad instructional sets. Whereas subjects under both conditions produced relatively elevated scores on the *F* and *Fb* scales, the use of an *F* raw score > 29 was found to produce a highly accurate discrimination between protocols derived under each administration condition. Rogers, Sewell, and Salekin (1994) provided a meta-analysis of several MMPI-2 validity scales or indices potentially useful in the evaluation of faking-bad or the overreporting of psychopathology. Of these measures, Rogers et al. reported that scale *F*, the *F-K* index, and the Obvious-Subtle subscales produced particularly strong effect sizes and demonstrated effectiveness across a variety of samples. Rogers, Hinds, and Sewell (1996) also specifically evaluated the MMPI-A validity scales in terms of the capacity of these scales to detect adolescents' efforts to overreport symptomatology and concluded that the *F-K* index appeared most effective and promising with this population.

A number of investigations have examined the effects of providing symptom or diagnostic information on subjects' ability to effectively fake-bad or overreport symptomatology on the MMPI-2. Rogers, Bagby, and Chakraborty (1993) compared the MMPI-2 profiles of subjects who had been provided information or coached on the symptoms of schizophrenia, coached on strategies used to detect faking-bad efforts on the MMPI-2, coached on both symptoms and detection strategies, or uncoached. These authors reported that knowledge concerning the operation and use of MMPI-2 scales and indices used to detect malingering was sufficient to allow approximately one-third of their sample to elude detection. In contrast, knowledge concerning schizophrenia appeared to be less useful to simulators attempting to feign a schizophrenic disorder "of sufficient severity as to warrant hospitalization" (p. 218). Wetter, Baer, Berry, Robison, and Sumpter (1993) provided two groups of normal adults with information concerning the symptoms of post-traumatic stress disorder and paranoid schizophrenia and instructed these subjects to simulate these disorders on the MMPI-2 with monetary rewards offered for successful simulations. Wetter and her colleagues concluded that providing symptom information about a psychological disorder did not enable fakers to avoid detection. Their fake-bad groups produced lower scores on *K*, and higher scores on *F* and the 10 clinical scales, than actual patient groups.

A variety of other investigations have examined the effects of providing symptom information on borderline personality disorder (Wetter, Baer, Berry, & Reynolds, 1994), somatoform disorder and paranoid psychosis (Sivec, Lynn, & Garske, 1994), and closed head injury (Lamb, Berry, Wetter, & Baer, 1994).

In general, the results of these investigations indicate that effects of symptom coaching are relatively limited and that the MMPI-2 validity scales are typically effective in accurately identifying malingered profiles. Illustrating this latter point, Bagby, et al. (1997) reported that psychiatric residents and clinical psychology graduate students, presumed to have considerable information about psychopathology and psychological testing, were easily detected when they attempted to feign schizophrenia on the MMPI-2. Further, Storm and Graham (1998) evaluated the scores of students who were instructed to simulate general psychopathology on the MMPI-2 after being provided with information concerning the validity scales in contrast to patients who took the MMPI-2 under standard instructions. Scores from the MMPI-2 F and $F(p)$ scales were effective in discriminating students simulating psychopathology from actual patients, and the $F(p)$ scale was found to be particularly effective in this regard. More recently, Veltri and Williams (2012) examined the effects of feigning specific psychiatric disorders (i.e., schizophrenia, post-traumatic stress disorder, or generalized anxiety disorder) among 265 college undergraduates who were either coached about validity scales and disorders or not provided with coaching. The study results indicated that the specific psychiatric disorder being feigned served to moderate the impact coaching had on the detection of overreporting on the MMPI-2 and on the PAI. For example, participants coached to feign PTSD or generalized anxiety disorder were more successful in avoiding detection than participants coached to feign schizophrenia. These results suggest that the usefulness of validity scales may vary as a function of the type of disorder an individual attempts to feign as well as whether or not the participant had been coached.

Given the plethora of studies in this area, Ben-Porath (1994) focused on the ethical issues surrounding research in which investigators attempt to evaluate the effectiveness of various coping strategies to successfully elude the MMPI-2 Validity scales. Ben-Porath noted that the specific coping strategies detailed in these publications could be used in forensic settings to help individuals fake MMPI profiles in a manner that successfully avoids detection. Thus, this body of literature could be misused in a manner that compromises the integrity of the instrument. Underscoring this area of concern, Wetter and Corrigan (1995) conducted a survey of 70 attorneys and 150 law students that indicated that almost 50% of these attorneys and over 33% of the law students believed that their clients should typically or always be informed of validity scales on psychological tests.

Research by Archer et al. (1987) investigated the characteristics of fake-bad profiles among normal adolescents. The original form of the MMPI was administered to a group of 94 public high school students in four psychology classes, with the subjects ranging in age from 14 to 18 years and roughly equally divided in terms of gender and ethnic background (Black-White). Subjects were administered the MMPI with the following instructions:

We would like you to respond to the MMPI as you believe you would if you were experiencing serious emotional or psychological problems. By serious problems, we mean problems that were severe enough that hospitalization for treatment would be necessary. As you read the items in the MMPI, please respond to them as if you were seriously disturbed and in need of hospital treatment for psychiatric care.

(p. 508)

The mean profile produced by this group showed a grossly exaggerated picture of symptomatology that included a very elevated mean *F* scale value of T = 130, and clinical range elevations on all MMPI Clinical scales except *Mf* and *Si*. Data from the fake-bad administration was reprofiled, to derive MMPI-A norm-based T-score values. Figure 4.14, plotted on these MMPI-A norms, presents this fake-bad profile (the *TRIN* and *VRIN* scales cannot be derived from these data). Consistent with the findings by Archer et al. (1987) for the original MMPI, and the MMPI-2 results reported by Graham, Watts, et al. (1991) for college students, the fake-bad profile on the MMPI-A is characterized by extremely elevated *F* scale T-score values, and multiple clinical range elevations on the standard Clinical scales. These data indicate that adolescents will probably encounter

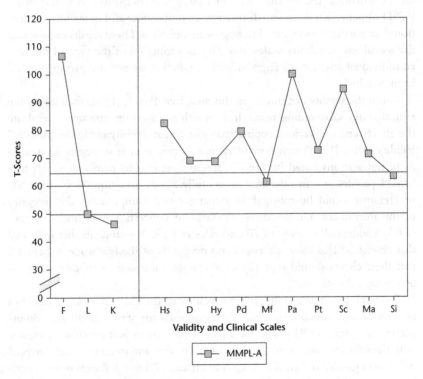

FIGURE 4.14 Fake-bad MMPI-A Validity scale profile.

substantial difficulty in successfully simulating psychiatric illness on the MMPI-A. The *TRIN* and *VRIN* raw score values for fake-bad and fake-good profiles, although not shown in Figures 4.13 and 4.14, would typically be within acceptable limits for response consistency, underscoring the difference between response inconsistency and response accuracy issues. Greene (2011) noted that individuals who attempt to underreport or overreport on the MMPI often produce highly consistent (although inaccurate and invalid) response patterns.

The *F* scale and Clinical scale criteria summarized here should serve to effectively screen for most adolescents who attempt to fake-bad on the MMPI-A.

1. *F* scale T-score value ≥ 90.
2. Presence of a floating profile characterized by clinical scale elevations within the clinical ranges (shaded zone or higher), with the exception of *Mf* and *Si* scale values.

The Validity scale and RC scale characteristics of MMPI-A-RF fake-bad profiles have been reported in the test manual (Archer et al., 2016a). Figures 4.15 and 4.16 present the MMPI-A-RF Validity scale and RC scale profiles for 127 adolescents instructed to overreport symptomatology in an MMPI-A research study by Stein, Graham, and Williams (1995). For these profiles, we computed the mean raw score for each scale and then presented the appropriate T-scores.

The guidance provided in the MMPI-A-RF manual (Archer et al. 2016a) on the identification of overreporting is as follows:

1. *F-r* T-scores in the range of 80–89 may reflect inconsistent responding or overreporting of psychiatric symptoms.
2. *F-r* scores ≥ 90 indicate invalid protocols.

A Conceptual Model for Validity Assessment

Greene (2000, 2011) presented a conceptual approach or model for understanding validity assessment issues, as well as a number of empirical criteria through which to assess the validity of MMPI profiles. Figure 4.17 provides an overview of Greene's model. This approach is applicable for evaluating protocol validity on the MMPI-A and the MMPI-A-RF.

Greene emphasized the use of sequential steps or stages in the validity assessment process.

Number of Omitted Iems

The first stage involves the determination of the number of omitted items (i.e., the *CNS* scale raw score value), with the omission of more than 29 items on the MMPI-A, or more than nine items on the MMPI-A-RF, related to invalid profiles potentially requiring test re-administration. Greene noted that excessive item omissions may reflect not only characteristics of the respondent, but can also serve as a signal of problems in the MMPI administration process.

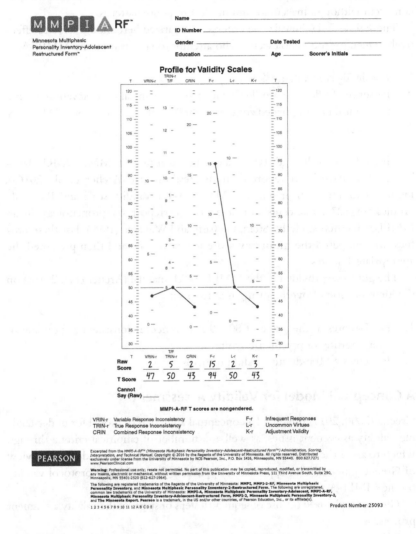

FIGURE 4.15 Fake-bad MMPI-A-RF Validity scale profile.

Source: MMPI-A-RF Administration, Scoring, Interpretation and Technical Manual by Archer, et al. Copyright © 2016 by the Regents of the University of Minnesota. Reproduced with the permission of the University of Minnesota Press. All rights reserved. "Minnesota Multiphasic Personality Inventory" and "MMPI" are trademarks owned by the Regents of the University of Minnesota.

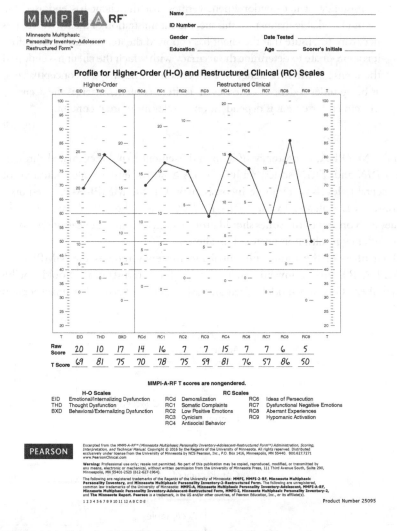

FIGURE 4.16 Fake-bad MMPI-A-RF *H-O* and *RC* scale pattern.

Source: MMPI-A-RF Administration, Scoring, Interpretation and Technical Manual by Archer, et al. Copyright © 2016 by the Regents of the University of Minnesota. Reproduced with the permission of the University of Minnesota Press. All rights reserved. "Minnesota Multiphasic Personality Inventory" and "MMPI" are trademarks owned by the Regents of the University of Minnesota.

Consistency of Item Endorsement

The next step in evaluating the validity of patients' responses involves an assessment of the consistency of item endorsement. As noted by Greene (2011):

Consistency of item endorsement verifies that the client has endorsed the items in a reliable manner for this specific administration of the MMPI-2. It is necessary to ensure that the client has endorsed the items consistently before it is appropriate to determine the accuracy with which the client has endorsed the items . . . the consistency of item endorsement (may be conceptualized) as being independent of or irrelevant to item content, whereas the accuracy of item endorsement is dependent on or relevant to item content.

(p. 48)

On the MMPI-A, consistency of item endorsement may be evaluated through the *VRIN* and *TRIN* scales, with T-scores ≥ 80 on either scale indicative of unacceptable levels of response inconsistency. On the MMPI-A-RF, response consistency is evaluated by the *VRIN-R*, *TRIN-r*, and the *CRIN* scales. T-score values ≥ 75 on any of the scales should prompt concerns about excessive response inconsistency resulting in protocol invalidity.

Regardless of the cause, substantial inconsistency renders the MMPI-A or MMPI-A-RF profile invalid and further profile interpretation should not be undertaken. Greene's model of validity assessment indicates that unacceptably

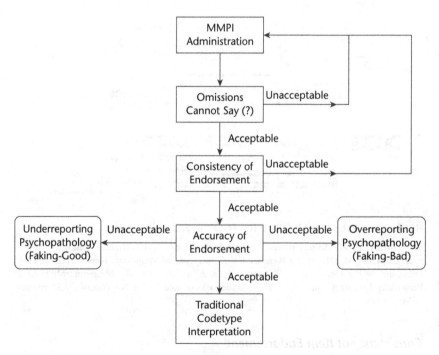

FIGURE 4.17 Greene's Stage Model of Validity Assessment.

Source: Roger L. Greene *MMPI-2: An Interpretive Manual (2nd Ed.)* © 2000. Printed and electronically reproduced with the permission of Pearson Education, Inc., New York, NY.

high levels of response inconsistency require re-administration of the MMPI in order to obtain interpretable clinical data.

Accuracy of Item Endorsement

The next step in the process of assessing MMPI-A or MMPI-A-RF validity is to derive an estimate of item endorsement accuracy. Greene (2011) noted several assumptions relevant to this stage of validity assessment. First, overreporting and underreporting represent a continuum, and any particular respondent may be placed at some point along this dimension. Second, attempts to overreport and underreport symptomatology tend to be generalized rather than specific. For example, adults who underreport tend to deny the presence of any type or dimension of psychopathology, and individuals engaging in overreporting tend to endorse psychopathology related to a wide variety of mental disorders. Third, Greene pointed out that the occurrence of overreporting or underreporting is relatively independent from the patient's actual psychopathology. It would be inappropriate to assume that evidence of underreporting or overreporting can be used to conclude that a patient does or does not have actual psychopathology. A patient may overreport *and* manifest actual and severe symptomatology, or substantially underreport and also be relatively free from actual symptomatology. Finally, Greene observes that the scales used to assess consistency of item endorsement (e.g., *VRIN* and *TRIN* on the MMPI-A; *VRIN-r*, *TRIN-r* and *CRIN* on the MMPI-A-RF) are not appropriate or useful in evaluating the accuracy of item endorsement.

Several indices have been used in determining response accuracy with the MMPI-2 that have also produced some research with the MMPI or MMPI-A with adolescents. These include the Wiener–Harmon Subtle-Obvious subscales (Wiener, 1948), and the Lachar–Wrobel (1979) Critical Item List. Because of the empirical method of scale construction used by Hathaway and McKinley in the development of the original form of the MMPI, the Clinical scales contain numerous *subtle* items that seem, or appear to be, unrelated to the construct that is the focus of measurement. Wiener and Harmon rationally developed Subtle and Obvious subscales for five of the MMPI clinical scales: *D, Hy, Pd, Pa,* and *Ma.* Greene (2000) noted that when individuals overreport symptomatology, scores on Obvious subscales would be expected to increase relative to Subtle scale values. Conversely, when individuals attempt to underreport symptomatology, Subtle scale values will become elevated in relation to Obvious subscale values.

Research on the Subtle-Obvious subscales in adult samples has been marked by controversial and mixed findings. Boone (1994, 1995) observed that the internal reliability estimates for the subtle scales are unacceptably low and that the inclusion of these items attenuates the reliability estimates for the Basic Clinical scales. Brems and Johnson (1991) explored the utility of the Subtle-Obvious scales as profile validity indicators in a sample of 291 psychiatric inpatients. These researchers found these scales useful in identifying individuals who tend to overreport symptomatology on the MMPI and other self-report measures. Dannenbaum and Lanyon (1993) requested groups of college undergraduates to take the MMPI under one of three instructional sets involving standard administration, faking-good, and faking-bad. As expected, faking-bad subjects scored significantly lower than subjects in the standard administration condition on the 100 most subtle items, a result interpreted as consistent with the presence of multiple items whose content relevance or face validity is opposite to the keyed direction of scoring on the subtle scales. These authors cautioned that although the subtle items have generally been shown to lack predictive ability, these items may prove useful in the detection of deception. Timbrook, Graham, Keiller, and Watts (1993) examined the MMPI-2 profiles of 49 psychiatric patients and 105 college students under various instructional sets to evaluate the degree to which the Subtle-Obvious subscales correctly classified faked versus accurate profiles. Although the authors found that the Subtle-Obvious subscales correctly classified a relatively high proportion of profiles, they also reported that information from the Subtle-Obvious subscales provided no incremental gain above that achieved through the use of scales *L* and *F* in accurately classifying profiles. Bagby, Buis, and Nicholson (1995) compared the MMPI-2 responses of participants asked to fake-bad with protocols from general psychiatric and forensic inpatient samples. In addition, these investigators examined the MMPI-2 responses of subjects asked to fake-good in comparison to the MMPI-2 protocols of college students responding accurately to the instrument. These investigators also found that scale *F* was superior to the Subtle-Obvious subscales in detecting fake-bad attempts, but reported that the Subtle-Obvious index and the *L* scale were equally effective in detecting efforts to fake-good. Finally, Hollrah, Schlottmann, Scott, and Brunetti (1995) reviewed the literature on the MMPI subtle items and concluded that the degree of support for the subtle items varies depending on the type of methodology employed by the investigators and the specific subtle subscale evaluated. These authors called for a clearer and more consistent research methodology to be employed across future studies in evaluating this important issue. They also concluded that the strongest current support for the Subtle-Obvious items lies in their apparent ability to detect fake-good profiles in psychiatric settings.

Graham (2012) has reached several conclusions critical of the use of the Subtle-Obvious subscales with the MMPI-2. First, he suggests that the subtle items were originally included in the MMPI Basic scales because item analyses and the selection process did not employ a cross-validation procedure. Second, he observed that Obvious, rather than Subtle items, are consistently related to extra-test behaviors. Third, he acknowledges that while individuals attempting to under or overreport on the MMPI and MMPI-2 may be evaluated through endorsement of subtle versus obvious items, the Subtle-Obvious subscales do not permit for accurate and consistent differentiation of valid from underreported or overreported profiles. Fourth, Graham notes that the standard Validity scales of the MMPI-2 appear to be as effective, or more effective, than the Subtle-Obvious subscales in detecting deviant response sets. Graham concludes that these and other problems with the Subtle-Obvious subscales led to the decision of the University of Minnesota Press to no longer include the Subtle-Obvious subscales in MMPI-2 test materials, interpretive reports, or scoring services.

Very little is known concerning the usefulness of the Wiener–Harmon Subtle-Obvious subscales in the assessment of adolescents. Herkov, Archer, and Gordon (1991) provided the only study of the Wiener–Harmon subscales in an adolescent sample. These investigators compared the use of the standard Validity scales in relation to the Wiener–Harmon subscales in terms of ability to accurately identify adolescents from four assessment groups. These groups included normal adolescents, psychiatric inpatients, normal adolescents instructed to fake-bad, and psychiatric inpatients instructed to fake-good. Table 4.19 presents the classification accuracy achieved by the use of the sum of the difference in T-score values between the Wiener–Harmon subscales (Obvious minus Subtle) in contrast to predictions based solely on the traditional Validity scales. Several points may be made in relation to these findings. First, the optimal Obvious minus Subtle subscale difference value used in identifying overreporting (≥ 140) and underreporting (≤ 0) differ substantially from

TABLE 4.19 Response Set Prediction Accuracy Based on the Wiener–Harmon Subtle-Obvious Subscales and Traditional Validity Indices of the Original *MMPI*

	Fake-Bad Versus Inpatient			Fake-Good Versus Normal	
	Predictors			Predictors	
Accuracy Measure	Obv.–Sub. $\geq +140$	F + K + Pa - Obv.	F $\geq$ T = 100	Obv.– Sub. ≤ 0	L $\geq T=55$
Hit Rate	84.7%	94.1%	93.5%	77.7%	89.3%
Sensitivity	71.9%	92.2%	92.2%	50.0%	71.4%
Specificity	92.5%	95.3%	94.3%	79.5%	90.4%
PPP	85.2%	92.2%	90.1%	13.5%	32.3%
NPP	84.5%	95.3%	95.2%	96.1%	98.0%

Source: Copyright © 1991 by the American Psychological Association. Reproduced with permission. Adapted from Herkov, Archer, and Gordon (1991). *MMPI response sets among adolescents: An evaluation of the limitations of the subtle-obvious susbscales*. Psychological Assessment: A Journal of Consulting and Clinical Psychology.

Notes
Obv.–Sub. = Obvious minus Subtle difference score
  Pa–Obv. = Obvious subscale for the Paranoia Basic scale
    PPP = Positive Predictive Power
    NPP = Negative Predictive Power

recommendations provided by Greene (1989a) and others for adult respondents. Additionally, it might be noted that the Subtle-Obvious subscales were of use in identifying various response sets, but were not as useful as simple prediction rules applied to the standard Validity scales to identify response sets. Specifically, predicting that adolescents who produced F scale T-score values ≥ 100 were overreporters, and that adolescents producing L scale T-score values ≥ 55 were underreporters, proved more accurate than predictions based on the Subtle-Obvious subscales. Based on these findings, combined with the observations offered by Graham (2012) concerning limitations of the Subtle-Obvious subscales, the use of these subscales is not recommended in clinical practice with the MMPI-A or MMPI-A-RF.

Critical Items

The Lachar and Wrobel (1979) critical items consist of 111 empirically selected MMPI items related to symptoms that may motivate individuals to seek psychological treatment, or symptomatology crucial in the clinician's diagnostic decision-making. Greene (2000) recommended that the total number of Lachar

TABLE 4.20 Distribution of the Total Number of Lachar and Wrobel (1979) Critical Items Endorsed on the Original MMPI in Psychiatric Samples Grouped by Age and Gender

Total Critical Item	Psychiatric Patients (Hedlund & Won Cho, 1979)			
	Adults		Adolescents	
	Male (N = 8,646)	Female (N = 3,743)	Male (N = 693)	Female (N = 290)
91+	0.3%	0.3%	0.7%	0.0%
81–90	1.8	1.4	2.6	1.7
71–80	3.9	3.2	4.8	4.2
61–70	6.9	7.3	6.6	11.7
51–60	10.7	12.7	13.0	13.8
41–50	14.3	18.0	16.2	19.3
31–40	18.6	18.7	16.7	15.2
21–30	20.3	19.3	21.7	14.4
11–20	17.3	14.1	13.9	16.9
0–10	5.9	5.0	3.8	2.8
Raw Score				
M	36.5	38.0	39.2	40.5
SD	19.3	18.3	19.5	19.3

Source: Greene, Roger L., *The MMPI-2/MMPI: An Interpretive Manual*, © 1991. Published by Allyn & Bacon, Boston, MA. Copyright © 1991 by Pearson Education. Adapted by permission of the publisher. Printed and electronically reproduced with the permission of Pearson Education, Inc., New York, NY.

and Wrobel critical items endorsed should be used as an index of accuracy of item endorsement. An individual who is attempting to overreport symptomatology, for example, might be expected to endorse a large number of these items, whereas a person underreporting psychopathology would be expected to endorse relatively few critical items.

Data on adolescent response patterns for the Lachar and Wrobel (1979) critical items on the original MMPI have been provided by Greene (1991), who reported the frequencies of the critical item endorsement produced by adolescents and by adults receiving services in the Missouri public mental health system. These data, shown in Table 4.20, indicate roughly comparable levels of critical item endorsement for these two groups.

Archer and Jacobson (1993) examined the item endorsement frequency of the Koss-Butcher (1973) and the Lachar–Wrobel (1979) critical items derived from normative and clinical samples for the MMPI-A and MMPI-2. Adolescents in both normal and clinical samples endorsed clinical items with a higher frequency than did normal adults. Further, whereas MMPI-2 clinical subjects consistently endorsed more critical items than adults in the MMPI-2 normative sample, similar comparisons between clinical and normative samples for the MMPI-A typically showed that adolescents in clinical settings did not endorse more critical items than did normal adolescents. Tables 4.21 and 4.22 provide the MMPI-2 and MMPI-A mean item endorsement percentages for male and female subjects for the Lachar–Wrobel critical categories as reported in Archer and Jacobson (1993). These findings underscore the difficulties inherent in creating a critical item list specifically for adolescents using the type of empirical methodology that has been employed with adults in which such items are selected based on item endorsement frequency differences found between comparison groups. Beyond the issue of technical difficulty in creating a critical item list for the MMPI-A, several conceptual issues were raised related to the application of critical items to the MMPI-A. Specifically, Archer and Jacobson noted that the concept of critical items has not been defined consistently throughout the history of the MMPI. Further, both the reliability and validity of critical items may be inherently limited in adolescent populations. The authors concluded that the commonly used MMPI/MMPI-2 critical item lists that have been developed based on adult samples may not be useful in the assessment of adolescents with the MMPI-A.

Forbey and Ben-Porath (1998) developed a set of critical items specifically for the MMPI-A and this list has now been formally incorporated into the MMPI-A as shown in the MMPI-A manual supplement (Ben-Porath, Graham, Archer, Tellegen, and Kaemmer, 2006). Their research attempted to address the inadequacies inherent in previous attempts to extend critical item lists generated for adults to use with adolescents. Item endorsement frequencies for boys and girls in the MMPI-A normative sample were examined, and any item that was endorsed in the scored direction by more than 30% of the

TABLE 4.21 MMPI-2 and MMPI-A Mean Item Endorsements for Males for the Lachar–Wrobel Critical Item Categories

Number of Items			MMPI-2			MMPI-A		
MMPI-2	MMPI-A	MMPI	Normal	Clinical	X^2	Normal	Clinical	X^2
Anxiety and Tension								
11	11	11	18.36	45.18	15.66***	35.25	34.01	0.00
Sleep Disturbance								
6	5	6	18.50	42.67	12.67***	29.26	29.26	0.02
Deviant Thinking and Experience								
10	10	10	17.50	35.20	6.78**	33.45	28.72	0.21
Antisocial Attitude								
9	9	9	28.11	49.67	9.27**	38.21	63.16	11.52**
Depression and Worry								
16	15	16	15.06	45.94	21.23***	27.92	30.42	0.02
Deviant Beliefs								
15	13	15	7.53	27.33	11.22***	19.67	19.25	0.00
Substance Abuse								
3	2	3	27.67	49.00	8.45**	26.00	43.85	6.35*
Family Conflict								
4	4	4	18.75	53.25	23.63***	42.85	60.45	5.12*
Problematic Anger								
4	4	4	23.25	37.75	4.62*	44.58	52.67	0.98
Somatic Symptoms								
23	22	23	12.74	32.91	10.19**	22.60	19.15	0.27
Sexual Concern and Deviation								
6	4	6	20.67	35.00	4.19*	23.80	14.90	2.04

* $p < .05$, ** $p < .01$, *** $p < .001$

Source: The item endorsement frequencies for the MMPI-2 normative and clinical samples are reported in Butcher et al. (1989), and are reported for the MMPI-A samples in Butcher et al. (1992). Adapted from Archer and Jacobson (1993). Copyright © 1993 by Lawrence Erlbaum Associates, Inc. Reprinted with permission.

normal sample was removed from the pool of potential critical items. Items that were endorsed 30% of the time or less in the keyed direction were then subjected to further analysis utilizing the response frequencies of adolescents in a clinical sample. Items differing in response frequency by more than 10 percentage points between the normative and clinical samples were then subjected to additional statistical and subjective item selection processes. Finally, all of the 81 items identified as having "critical" content in the previous steps were rationally examined by Forbey and Ben-Porath and placed into 15 item content groups. These groupings included Aggression, Anxiety, Cognitive Problems, Conduct Problems, Depression/Suicidal Ideation, Eating Problems, Family Problems, Hallucinatory Experiences, Paranoid Ideation, School Problems, Self-Denigration, Sexual Concerns, Somatic Complaints, Substance Use/Abuse,

TABLE 4.22 MMPI-2 and MMPI-A Mean Item Endorsements for Females for the Lachar–Wrobel Critical Item Categories

Number of Items			MMPI-2			MMPI-A		
MMPI-2	MMPI-A	MMPI	Normal	Clinical	X^2	Normal	Clinical	X^2
Anxiety and Tension								
11	11	11	20.00	39.22	16.24***	39.22	40.09	0.02
Sleep Disturbance								
6	5	6	24.83	38.52	11.35***	38.52	40.04	0.00
Deviant Thinking and Experience								
10	10	10	16.80	36.04	9.16**	36.04	27.53	1.13
Antisocial Attitude								
9	9	9	17.11	29.48	10.03**	29.48	48.37	6.84**
Depression and Worry								
16	15	16	16.94	33.09	20.51***	33.09	40.37	0.78
Deviant Beliefs								
15	13	15	6.53	17.05	16.05***	17.05	18.87	0.03
Substance Abuse								
3	2	3	18.67	38.33	7.95**	25.45	42.00	5.75*
Family Conflict								
4	4	4	22.50	53.75	19.43***	52.25	70.68	6.84**
Problematic Anger								
4	4	4	20.25	39.75	8.60**	45.88	48.30	0.04
Somatic Symptoms								
23	22	23	16.13	36.61	10.27**	27.30	25.31	0.03
Sexual Concern and Deviation								
6	4	6	20.17	41.83	10.31**	34.65	30.48	0.36

* p < .05, ** p < .01, *** p < .001.

Source: The item endorsement frequencies for the MMPI-2 normative and clinical samples are reported in Butcher et al. (1989), and are reported for the MMPI-A samples in Butcher et al. (1992). Adapted from Archer and Jacobson (1993). Copyright © 1993 by Lawrence Erlbaum Associates, Inc. Reprinted with permission.

and Unusual Thinking. The authors recommend a number of ways in which the MMPI-A critical item list may facilitate test interpretation and feedback, but also caution that adolescents' responses to individual test items should never be taken as psychometrically sound indicators of psychopathology or maladjustment. With this caution in mind, the authors note that the MMPI-A critical items may have been incorporated into the interpretive process to provide the clinician with a sense of the specific nature and severity of an adolescent's problems as revealed in self-report. For example, an inspection of the Depression/Suicidal Ideation content area may aid in the determination of whether a depressed adolescent has endorsed items suggestive of an increased risk for suicide. Further, the authors note that the MMPI-A critical items may be very usefully employed in feedback to the adolescent. For example, the test interpreter may identify critical items that have been endorsed in a manner that is seemingly inconsistent with the adolescents' history of current functioning, and invite the adolescent to provide further information and explanation of these responses.

A study of the use of the Forbey and Ben-Porath MMPI-A critical item set by Forbey, Ben-Porath, and Graham (2005) was generally supportive of the use of this list as a means of understanding the nature and severity of the adolescent's responses. Forbey and his colleagues examined the frequency of endorsement of MMPI-A critical items in large samples of adolescents in inpatient, outpatient, correctional, drug/alcohol treatment, general medical, and school settings. Results indicated that the pattern of endorsement of critical items was related to the setting of the adolescent. For example, adolescents receiving substance abuse treatment endorsed more items related to problems with drugs and alcohol, adolescents in forensic settings endorsed more behavioral and conduct disorder types of problems, while adolescents receiving inpatient treatment endorsed more problems related to affective and cognitive issues.

TABLE 4.23 Forbey and Ben-Porath Critical Item List for the MMPI-A and the MMPI-A-RF

MMPI-A		MMPI-A-RF	
Content Area	# of Items	Content Area	# of Items
Aggression	3	Aggression	2
Anxiety	6	Anxiety	4
Cognitive Problems	3	Cognitive Problems	2
Conduct Problems	7	Conduct Problems	7
Depression/Suicidal Ideation	7	Depression/Suicidal Ideation	7
Eating Problems	2	Eating Problems	2
Family Problems	3	Family Problems	2
Hallucinatory Experiences	5	Hallucinatory Experiences	3
Paranoid Ideation	9	Paranoid Ideation	6
School Problems	5	School Problems	4
Self-Denigration	5	Self-Denigration	2
Sexual Concerns	4		
Somatic Complaints	9	Somatic Complaints	6
Substance Use/Abuse	9	Substance Abuse/Use	5
Unusual Thinking	4	Unusual Thinking	1
	81		53

Based on the usefulness of the Forbey and Ben-Porath MMPI Critical Item List, this list has been adopted and incorporated into the development of the MMPI-A-RF (Archer et al. 2016a). Of the 81 items in the MMPI-A Forbey and Ben-Porath critical item list, 53 items were retained in the 241-item MMPI-A-RF, representing 14 content areas of the 15 MMPI-A critical content areas (sexual concerns did not retain enough items to be retained in the MMPI-A-RF). Table 4.23 shows the criteria categories, with the corresponding number of items in each category, for the Forbey and Ben-Porath MMPI-A and MMPI-A-RF Critical Item lists.

The MMPI-A and MMPI-A-RF critical item lists were not designed and are not recommended as a means to evaluate profile validity. These critical item sets, created for the MMPI-A and carried over into the MMPI-A-RF, certainly warrants substantially more research and empirical evaluation. The development of these critical item sets is well documented and the clinical uses recommended by Forbey and Ben-Porath appear both prudent and appropriate. As noted by Forbey and Ben-Porath, the alternative to using these critical item sets, from a practical standpoint, is that each clinician would select his or her own critical items and check the responses in the MMPI-A test booklet in order to allow these items to be useful for interpretive or feedback purposes. Forbey and Ben-Porath observe that searching through item responses to determine whether a client responded in the keyed direction to particular items is both inefficient and ineffective. Clearly, the use of a standard list of critical items identified through a series of empirical procedures such as those utilized by Forbey and Ben-Porath is preferable to individual clinician's reliance on nonstandard critical item selection.

Summary

This chapter has provided an overview of the MMPI-A and MMPI-A-RF Validity scales in the assessment of protocol validity, and reviewed a number of profile features produced by these instruments under various response sets. Further, emphasis was placed on the validity assessment model developed by Greene (1989a, 2000, 2011). In particular, a sequential approach to MMPI-A and MMPI-A-RF Validity assessment was presented, with particular attention to the distinction between the consistency of item endorsement and the accuracy of item endorsement. Within the Greene model, consistency of item endorsement may be viewed as a necessary, but not sufficient, component of valid response patterns.

Adolescents are most likely to overreport psychopathology as a conscious or unconscious plea for help in order to communicate their desire for attention and support. Conversely, adolescents are most likely to underreport symptomatology when they have been involuntarily placed in treatment by their parents or court officials, and wish to emphasize their assertion that they do not have any significant problems. Additionally, adolescents will often underreport or over-report on the MMPI-A as a result of inappropriate test instructions or testing procedures that influence the adolescent, either consciously or unconsciously, to distort the accuracy of their responses.

Overall, there are currently insufficient data to support the use of the Wiener–Harmon Subtle-Obvious subscales. The MMPI-A and MMPI-A-RF Advisory Committees did not recommend the creation of Subtle-Obvious subscale pro-file sheets because of the lack of empirical evidence supporting the use of these measures in adolescent populations. The use of the MMPI-A and MMPI-A-RF Validity scales, individually and configurally, is recommended for the evalua-tion of response accuracy on these instruments. As previously noted, elevations of original and revised versions of L and K, singly or in combination, in rela-tion to the F and F-r scales, have been related to conscious and unconscious efforts to underreport symptomatology. Further, elevations on F and F-r may be related to conscious or unconscious efforts to overreport symptomatology on the MMPI-A and MMPI-A-RF, respectively.

5

MMPI-A BASIC CLINICAL SCALE
AND CODETYPE CORRELATES
FOR ADOLESCENTS

Profile Elevation Issues and the MMPI-A
Profile "Shaded" Zone

As noted in previous chapters, adolescent MMPI-A responses should be interpreted exclusively through the use of age-appropriate adolescent norms. The conclusion that adolescent norm conversion is the most appropriate means of interpreting adolescent responses does not imply that such a procedure renders the evaluation of MMPI-A profiles to be either simple or straightforward. The most important difficulties that occur when interpreting adolescent responses scored on adolescent norms is that resulting profiles typically produce subclinical elevations, even for adolescents in inpatient psychiatric settings if a T-score value ≥ 65 is employed as the criterion for determining clinical range elevation. The inherent contradiction in interpreting a normal-range profile for an adolescent who exhibits evidence of serious psychopathology probably contributed to the inappropriate but widespread practice of using adult norms for adolescents on the original form of the MMPI. Thus, just as the application of adult norms to adolescent patterns tends to produce profiles that grossly overemphasize or exaggerate psychiatric symptomatology, so the application of adolescent norms, either on the original form of the MMPI or the MMPI-A, produces profiles that may often appear to underestimate an adolescent's psychopathology.

Normal-range mean profiles (e.g., mean T-score values < 70) for inpatient adolescent populations on the original form of the MMPI have been reported by Archer (1987b), Archer, Ball, and Hunter (1985), Archer, Stolberg, Gordon, and Goldman (1986), Ehrenworth and Archer (1985), and Klinge and Strauss (1976). The result of this phenomenon for adolescent MMPI profile interpretation on the original MMPI instrument was that the application of a T-score criterion of ≥ 70, traditionally found useful in defining clinical symptomatology for adult respondents, had substantially less utility with adolescents. Based on these observations, Ehrenworth and Archer (1985) recommended the use of a T-score value of 65 for defining clinical range elevations for adolescents on the original instrument. Employment of this criterion in inpatient and outpatient adolescent samples served to substantially reduce the frequency of normal-range profiles obtained for adolescents (Archer, 1987b). For example, Archer, Pancoast, and Klinefelter (1989) found that the use of clinical scale T-score values of 65 or greater (rather than ≥ 70) to detect the presence of psychopathology resulted in increased sensitivity in accurately identifying profiles produced by normal adolescents versus adolescents from outpatient and inpatient samples. Archer (1987b) speculated that the "within normal limits" T-score elevations typically found for adolescents on the original instrument were partially related to the absence of K-correction procedures as well as the high base rate of endorsement of clinical symptoms typically found in samples of normal adolescents. Alperin, Archer, and Coates (1996) showed, however, that the development of an MMPI-A K-correction procedure was not effective in significantly reducing the number of false negatives produced by this instrument.

Figure 5.1 presents the mean profile of normal adolescents, scored on the Marks and Briggs (1972) traditional adolescent norms, from eight studies conducted between 1947 and 1965, in contrast to the mean profile produced by normal adolescents in four studies conducted between 1975 and 1987 (Pancoast & Archer, 1988). These profiles (which present the validity scales

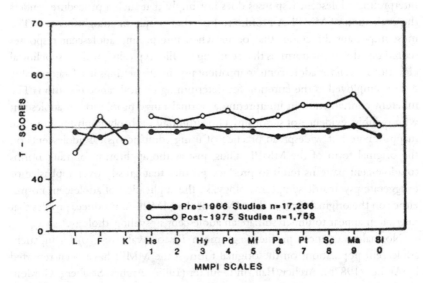

FIGURE 5.1 Mean values for normal adolescents from two time periods plotted on adolescent norms by Marks and Briggs (1972).

Source: Pancoast and Archer (1988). Copyright © by Lawrence Erlbaum Associates. Reprinted with permission.

in the traditional order) suggest that detectable changes have occurred in adolescent MMPI response patterns over the past 40 years, with these results lending support to the effort to create a contemporary adolescent MMPI norm set.

Figures 5.2 and 5.3 compare the post-1975 mean profile from the Pancoast and Archer (1988) review with the MMPI-A normative response patterns, separately by gender, as profiled on the Marks and Briggs (1972) adolescent norms. These data show that mean values from the MMPI-A normative sample are relatively consistent with other samples of normal adolescents that have been collected since 1975. Because the MMPI-A normative set is based on adolescent response patterns that have higher mean scale raw score values than do the original Marks and Briggs adolescent norms, a major effect of the MMPI-A norms is to reduce profile elevation for a given set of raw score values in comparison with the original Marks and Briggs norms. This is illustrated in Figures 5.4 and 5.5, which provide a comparison of the MMPI profile elevations produced for a group of female (N = 1,032) and male (N = 730) adolescent psychiatric patients as profiled on the traditional Marks and Briggs (1972) norms, and on the MMPI-A adolescent norms. A comparison of profile elevations in these figures

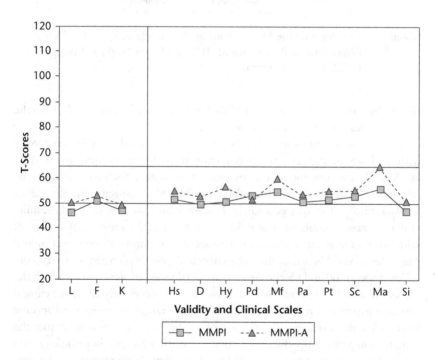

FIGURE 5.2   Males from the MMPI-A normative sample and post-1975 male
adolescents on the original MMPI: Profiles on Marks and Briggs
(1972) adolescent norms.

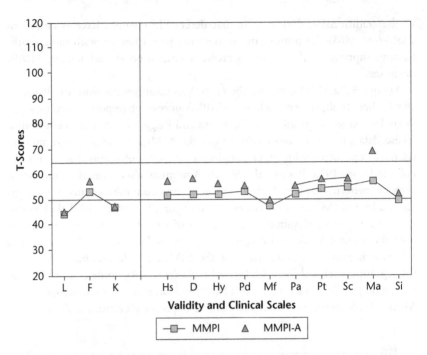

FIGURE 5.3 Females from the MMPI-A normative sample and post-1975 female adolescents on the original MMPI: Profiles on Marks and Briggs (1972) adolescent norms.

clearly demonstrates a reduction in MMPI scale T-score elevations related to the use of the more recent adolescent norm set.

In response to the profile elevation issues related to the use of the MMPI with adolescents, and the further reduction in profile elevations produced by the MMPI-A adolescent norms, an innovative strategy for determining clinical range elevations was developed for the MMPI-A. Specifically, the use of a "black line" value, that is, a single T-score value that denotes the beginning of clinical range elevations, was modified in favor of the creation of a range of values that serve as a transitional area or zone between normal-range and clinical range elevations. The use of this zone concept explicitly recognizes that T-score values between 60 and 65 constitute a marginal range of elevation in which the adolescent may be expected to show some, but not necessarily all, of the clinical correlate patterns or traits associated with higher range elevations for a specific MMPI-A scale. Conceptually, the use of a "shaded" zone recognizes that the demarcation point or dividing line between normalcy and psychopathology during adolescence may be less clear than during adult development. Adolescents who are not deviant in a statistical sense (i.e., who do not produce clinical range elevations in excess of a particular T-score value) may still display behaviors or

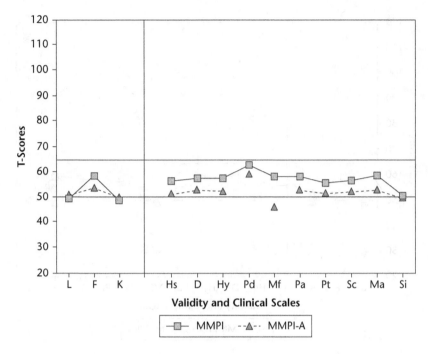

FIGURE 5.4   Male adolescent patients profiled on Marks and Briggs (1972) norms and MMPI-A adolescent norms.

report experiences disturbing enough to be labeled as clinically significant, and to require psychological intervention. As noted by Archer (1987b), the "typical" adolescent may experience sufficient psychological turbulence and distress during adolescent development such that relatively minor deviations in the course of normal development may warrant psychiatric intervention and response. Thus, in addition to the traditional categories of *within normal limits* and *clinical range* elevations that have been typically associated with MMPI responses, the MMPI-A included a new category of *marginally elevated* T-score values.

Studies on MMPI-A Profile Elevation Issues

Newsom, Archer, Trumbetta, and Gottesman (2003) sought to explore changes in adolescent self-presentation on the MMPI and MMPI-A over a 40 year period. The primary samples used for comparison in this study included 1,235 adolescents between the ages of 12 and 16, inclusive, derived from the MMPI-A normative sample collected in 1989 and 10,514 adolescents in the same age grouping collected between 1948 and 1954 as part of Hathaway and Monachesi's (1963) study of adolescent personality and behavior. Results showed a pattern of moderate to large changes in response frequencies between eras of data collection,

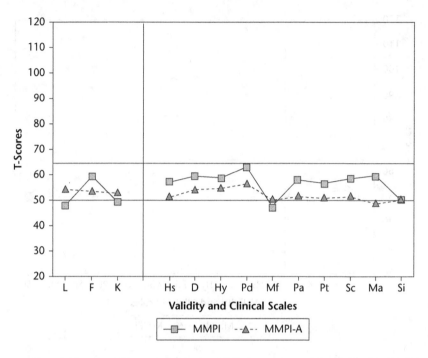

FIGURE 5.5 Female adolescent patients profiled on Marks and Briggs (1972) norms and MMPI-A adolescent norms.

with a substantially higher rate of endorsement of items in the pathological direction by adolescents in the contemporary MMPI-A normative sample. This study provided evidence of changes in mean raw score values for many of the MMPI Basic scales and Harris–Lingoes subscales, as well as reporting significantly higher rates of item endorsement for contemporary adolescents on the 393 items shared in common in the MMPI and MMPI-A. Overall, the results showed that contemporary normal adolescents not only endorse more psychopathological symptoms than do adults, but also endorse more pathology than did adolescents forty years ago.

Research by Archer, Handel, and Lynch (2001) compared the item endorsement frequencies for the MMPI-A normative sample with results from two adolescent clinical samples, and these results were also contrasted with the item endorsement frequencies reported for the MMPI-2 normative sample and a clinical sample of adult psychiatric inpatients. Figure 5.6 shows the mean MMPI-A Basic scale profile for 271 boys and 160 girls in inpatient settings reported in the MMPI-A manual. Results of this study showed that the MMPI-A contained a substantial number of items that do not show a significant difference in item endorsement frequency between normal and clinical samples. Furthermore, MMPI-A Basic and Content scales generally showed a much lower percentage

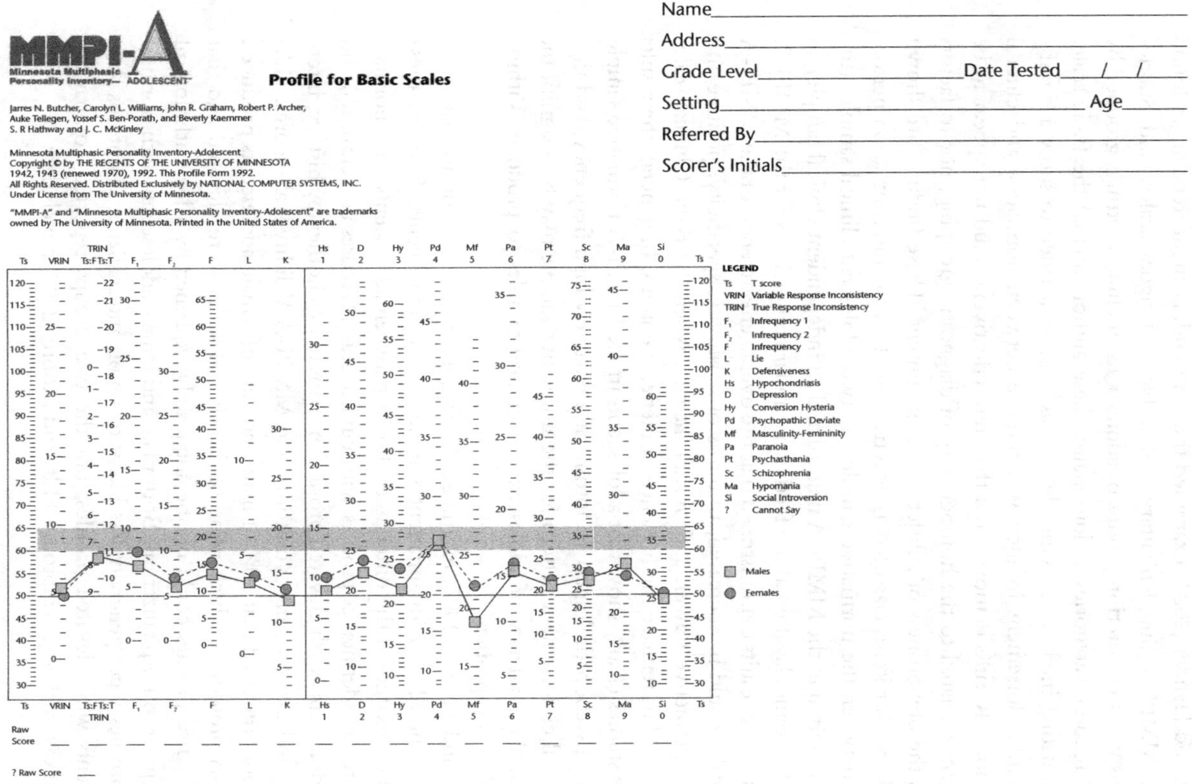

FIGURE 5.6 Mean MMPI-A Basic Scale Profile for 271 boys and 160 girls in inpatient settings.

Source: MMPI-A Profile for Basic Scales reproduced with permission. Minnesota Multiphasic Personality Inventory-Adolescent (MMPI®-A) Manual for Administration, Scoring, and Interpretation by Butcher, et al. Copyright © 1992 by the Regents of the University of Minnesota. Reproduced with the permission of the University of Minnesota Press. All rights reserved. "Minnesota Multiphasic Personality Inventory" and "MMPI" are trademarks owned by the Regents of the University of Minnesota.

of effective items than do corresponding scales of the MMPI-2. Archer et al. (2001) discussed these results as a possible factor in the relatively low-range MMPI-A profiles found for clinical samples.

Following up on the research by Archer and his colleagues (2001), Lynch, Archer, and Handel (2004) examined the item endorsement frequencies found for the MMPI-A Supplementary scales, Harris–Lingoes scales, and Subtle-Obvious items in criterion groups of adolescents in clinical settings grouped by gross diagnostic categories. Additionally, these authors revised the Basic scales by eliminating ineffective items, defined as items that failed to show a significant item endorsement frequency difference between normative and clinical populations. Results demonstrated that item effectiveness did not appear to be significantly related to the homogeneity of diagnostic grouping, nor to factors such as the obviousness or subtlety of item content. These findings are shown in Table 5.1 for items classified as effective based on the discrimination performance between the normative sample and two adolescent clinical samples (the sample reported in the MMPI-A manual and an independent clinical sample), as well as for items classified as ineffective in similar comparisons for the MMPI-2. Further, these results demonstrated that the overall effectiveness of the MMPI-A Basic scales could be increased, in terms of sensitivity, specificity, positive and negative predictive power, and overall hit rate, when the Basic Clinical scales were revised to remove the presence of ineffective items. In general, the results of these studies clearly show that adolescents in the MMPI-A normative sample endorsed psychopathological symptoms at a relatively high frequency, and that this overall endorsement pattern for the normative sample may be a significant factor in the tendency of adolescents in clinical samples to produce Within-Normal-Limits profiles.

Hilts and Moore (2003) examined the frequency base rates of normal-range MMPI-A profiles in an inpatient sample of 388 adolescents. Further, these researchers examined the differences shown between adolescents with normal-range profiles (defined as profiles with clinical scale T-scores all below 60) and those adolescents with elevated profiles in terms of psychotherapy history, internalizing and externalizing symptoms, and MMPI-A Validity scale scores. Hilts and Moore reported that 30% of male and 25% of female adolescents produced MMPI-A profiles in which none of the clinical scales were elevated and that normal-range profiles could not be adequately explained by a less pathological history prior to hospitalization. Both male and female adolescents with normal-range profiles were generally less likely to report internalizing symptoms than adolescents with elevated profiles, but the two groups reported comparable levels of externalizing symptoms. Hilts and Moore (2003) concluded:

> The present study has implications for both clinicians and researchers. Clinicians encountering MMPI-A profiles with no significant elevations should consider the hypotheses that the adolescents may not be experiencing

TABLE 5.1 MMPI-A Basic Scale Items Classified Based on Discrimination Performance Between the Normative Sample and Two Adolescent Clinical Samples, With Similar Item Comparisons for the MMPI-2 Normative Sample and an Adult Clinical Sample

	MMPI-A Percent Effective Items Normative/Clinical Samples		MMPI-A Percent Effective Items Normative/Independent Samples		MMPI-2 Percent Effective Items	
	Boys	Girls	Boys	Girls	Men	Women
Hs (1)	3% (1/32)	13% (4/32)	28% (9/32)	50% (16/32)	84% (27/32)	91% (29/32)
D (2)	28% (16/57)	40% (23/57)	40% (23/57)	54% (31/57)	70% (40/57)	66% (38/57)
Hy (3)	25% (15/60)	28% (17/60)	28% (17/60)	38% (23/60)	60% (36/60)	55% (33/60)
Pd (4)	63% (31/49)	71% (35/49)	69% (34/49)	67% (33/49)	72% (36/50)	72% (36/50)
Mf (5)	16% (7/44)	25% (11/44)	14% (6/44)	16% (7/44)	45% (25/56)	14% (8/56)
Pa (6)	30% (12/40)	33% (13/40)	48% (19/40)	23% (16/40)	73% (29/40)	70% (28/40)
Pt (7)	23% (11/48)	29% (14/48)	35% (17/48)	40% (19/48)	94% (45/48)	94% (45/48)
Sc (8)	18% (14/77)	30% (23/77)	45% (35/77)	44% (34/77)	92% (72/78)	97% (76/78)
Ma (9)	35% (16/46)	17% (8/46)	48% (22/46)	29% (14/46)	57% (26/46)	65% (30/46)
Si (0)	11% (7/62)	19% (12/62)	24% (15/62)	19% (12/62)	70% (48/69)	64% (44/69)

Source: Reprinted with the permission of the authors. Minnesota Multiphasic Personality Inventory-Adolescent (MMPI®-A) Manual for Administration, Scoring, and Interpretation by Butcher, et al. Copyright © 1992 by the Regents of the University of Minnesota. MMPI®-2 (Minnesota Multiphasic Personality Inventory®-2) Manual for Administration, Scoring, and Interpretation, Revised Edition. Copyright © 2001 by the Regents of the University of Minnesota. Reproduced with the permission of the University of Minnesota Press. All rights reserved. "Minnesota Multiphasic Personality Inventory" and "MMPI" are trademarks owned by the Regents of the University of Minnesota.

Note

Percentage figures reflect the total percentage of items within each scale that showed significant differences in item endorsement frequencies between the normative and clinical sample, that is, items classified as "effective" in terms of discrimination between samples. The first number within each parentheses indicates the number of "effective" items within the scale, and the second number reflects the total number of items in the scale.

feelings of distress or may not see themselves as having problems; a profile with no elevations may not mean that the adolescent is not having
problems in some area of his or her life. Future research should address
the issue of lack of apparent or acknowledged internal distress in some
adolescents who present with externalizing symptoms.

(p. 271)

Two studies have examined the usefulness of reducing the standard T-score
cutoff employed to define clinical range elevation on the MMPI-A from the
standard T ≥ 65 to the T ≥ 60 criterion used by Hilts and Moore. Janus, Toepfer,
Calestro, and Tolbert (1996) used a sample of 300 adolescents in a psychiatric
inpatient setting and reported no significant gender differences in frequency of
elevations on the MMPI-A when either the traditional or modified cutoff scores
were used. These authors did report, however, that defining Within-Normal-
Limits cases as adolescents producing T-scores < 60 on all Basic scales produced
a substantial reduction in the number of false-negative classifications for this
clinical population in comparison to the traditional T ≤ 64 criterion. In the
absence of a sample of normal adolescents, however, Janus, Toepfer et al. (1996)
were not able to evaluate the overall impact of reducing the T-score standard
used to define clinical range elevations on the occurrence of false positives, that
is, the misclassification produced by elevations on the MMPI-A Basic scales
for adolescents functioning normally. Fontaine, Archer, Elkins, and Johansen
(2001) were able to address this issue by examining MMPI-A profiles from a
sample of 203 adolescent inpatients in comparison with subsamples from the
MMPI-A normative group. Fontaine and her colleagues compared T-score
elevation criterion of T ≥ 60 and T ≥ 65 in defining clinical range elevations when the clinical base rate for actual psychopathology was 20% and under
conditions in which it was 50%. Classification accuracy analyses indicated that
T ≥ 65 resulted in higher levels of accurate identification, while minimizing misclassifications of both clinical and normal cases. Their results suggest that reducing
the T-score elevation for identifying clinical range elevations to a criterion of
T ≥ 60 to reduce the frequency of false-negative misclassifications of adolescents
in clinical samples may be problematic in reducing high false-negative rates at
the cost of increased false positive misclassification for normal adolescents.

In summary, the current literature indicates that the MMPI-A tends to produce
relatively low scores for adolescents in clinical settings. The evidence also suggests
that this issue is not effectively resolved by developing a K-correction procedure
for the MMPI-A. Findings indicate that the relatively high rate of endorsement
of items in the pathological direction by adolescents in the MMPI-A normative
sample may be one of the primary causes for the frequent Within-Normal-Limit
profiles found for adolescents in clinical settings. In this regard, Lynch, Archer,
and Handel (2004) noted that adolescents in the MMPI-A normative sample
were not excluded based on history of psychotherapy. Approximately 15% of

the adolescents in the normative sample responded yes to an item on a life events form asking if they had "been referred to a therapist or a counselor" within six months of the administration of the MMPI-A. This referral frequency is generally consistent with estimates of the national incidence of adolescent psychopathology reported in the first chapter of this text, and subsequent analyses by Lynch et al. found that Basic scale T-scores were significantly higher for this referral group in comparison with their counterparts in the MMPI-A normative sample who did not report being referred for therapy or counseling. Following up on this observation, Hand et al. (2007) removed the MMPI-A data for the 193 adolescents who reported referral for counseling from the normative sample and recalculated uniform T-score values for the remaining 1,427 adolescents. The frequency of Within-Normal-Limits profiles for adolescents in clinical settings were only marginally reduced by using these revised MMPI-A norms, with only minimal improvements obtained in classification accuracy analyses. Eliminating adolescents referred for counseling did not serve to reduce substantively the high frequency of Within-Normal-Range profiles for adolescents in clinical settings.

Uniform T-Score Transformation Procedures for the MMPI-A

As previously noted, the traditional adolescent norms developed by Marks and Briggs (1972), as well as the original MMPI norms for adults, utilized linear T-score transformations to convert raw score values to T-scores. As noted by Colligan, Osborne, and Offord (1980, 1984), and by Tellegen and Ben-Porath (1992) in their presentation of uniform T-scores, linear T-score values have presented problems in the interpretation of MMPI profiles because a given linear T-score value typically converts to differing percentile equivalents across the various MMPI scales. Thus, a given T-score value on the original Marks and Briggs (1972) norms may convert to a percentile equivalent value that ranges as much as 10 to 15 percentile points across the 10 MMPI Basic scales. This occurs because the raw score distribution for different MMPI scales varies in shape (e.g., in skewness), whereas a linear T-score transformation procedure will produce equivalent percentile values for a given T-score only if the raw score distributions for the Basic scales were each normally distributed. Because the Basic scales display varying degrees of skewness, the same linear T-score value will have a different percentile equivalency score across the different scales. Uniform T-scores represent composite or averaged linear T-scores, which serve to promote percentile equivalence across MMPI-A Clinical scales (excluding 5 and 0), and the Content scales. Uniform T-scores do not, however, have major effects on the underlying distribution of raw scores, and do not serve to "normalize" the underlying raw score distributions. This is important in that the "true" distribution of scores on the MMPI scales may in fact *not* be normal and, therefore, a normalizing procedure may actually serve to distort T-score values by artificially lowering those in the higher range (Tellegen & Ben-Porath, 1992). Table 5.2 shows the percentile values of uniform T-scores as derived for the Basic scales on the MMPI-A, and for the MMPI-2 as reported by Ben-Porath (1990). As shown in this table, uniform T-scores do not correct or normalize the underlying raw score distributions such that a T-score value of 50 equals a percentile value of 50. Rather, the uniform T-score procedure makes relatively small adjustments in individual scale raw score distributions, achieved by creating a composite or overall distribution across the affected scales. These adjustments permit comparable percentile equivalents to be assigned to T-score values such that a given T-score will yield equivalent percentile ranks across the eight Clinical scales and the Content scales. Edwards, Morrison, and Weissman (1993b) compared the effects of MMPI-2 linear versus uniform T-score transformations for a sample of 200 psychiatric outpatients. These authors reported that the differences created by the uniform technique were relatively slight and that observed differences between MMPI and MMPI-2 T-scores were mainly attributable to differences in response patterns in the normative sample rather than the use of uniform T-score transformation procedures.

TABLE 5.2 Percentile Values of Uniform T-scores for the MMPI-A and MMPI-2

T-score	MMPI-A	MMPI-2[a]
	Percentile	Percentile
30	0.6	0.2
35	4.2	3.7
40	15.1	15.1
45	36.5	34.2
50	59.1	54.9
55	76.0	72.3
60	85.7	84.7
65	92.2	92.1
70	95.8	96.0
75	98.3	98.1
80	99.4	99.3
85	99.9	99.8

Source: Minnesota Multiphasic Personality Inventory-Adolescent (MMPI®-A) Manual for Administration, Scoring, and Interpretation by Butcher, et al. Copyright © 1992 by the Regents of the University of Minnesota. MMPI®-2 (Minnesota Multiphasic Personality Inventory®-2) Manual for Administration, Scoring, and Interpretation, Revised Edition. Copyright © 2001 by the Regents of the University of Minnesota. Reproduced with the permission of the University of Minnesota Press. All rights reserved. "Minnesota Multiphasic Personality Inventory" and "MMPI" are trademarks owned by the Regents of the University of Minnesota.

Note
a MMPI-2 values reported by Ben-Porath (1990). Reprinted with permission.

Codetype Congruence Issues

A major area of controversy concerning the development of the MMPI-2 centered on the degree to which adult profiles produced by the revised instrument were comparable to, or congruent with, adult profiles derived from the original MMPI (Archer, 1992). For example, a series of articles by Dahlstrom (1992) and by Humphrey and Dahlstrom (1995) have suggested that the MMPI and MMPI-2 often produce substantially different profiles, whereas Tellegen and Ben-Porath (1993) and Ben-Porath and Tellegen (1995) responded with perspectives that stressed the comparability of profiles produced by these two instruments. This issue has received substantial focus because it relates to the degree to which the research literature available on the interpretation of the traditional MMPI may be generalized to the MMPI-2.

Empirical research has accumulated on the issue of congruence between the MMPI and MMPI-2. The MMPI-2 manual (Butcher et al., 1989) provides congruence data for two-point codes using MMPI-2 norms and the original test instrument norms in a sample of 232 male and 191 female psychiatric patients. These data indicate a congruence rate of approximately 70% for males and 65% for females when high points were defined as the most elevated clinical scale regardless of the magnitude of that elevation. Graham, Timbrook, Ben-Porath, and Butcher (1991) re-examined these data and reported that when two-point codetype elevations were "well defined," as reflected in at least a 5-point T-score difference between the second and third most elevated scales in the clinical scale codetype, the congruence rate increased to 81.6% for males and 94.3% for females. Edwards, Morrison, and Weissman (1993a), Husband and Iguchi (1995), and Morrison, Edwards, Weissman, Allen, and DeLaCruz (1995) reported congruence rates ranging from 60% to 94% for well-defined codetypes derived in clinical samples, with findings varying as a function of the definition of congruence employed in these studies. In general, it is possible to conclude that although the MMPI and MMPI-2 are not psychometrically equivalent forms, the two instruments are likely to produce similar profiles, particularly when a two-point codetype represents a well-defined configural pattern. For example, Clavelle (1992) asked experienced MMPI users to review pairs of MMPI and MMPI-2 profiles derived from the same test responses and to determine if these data yielded comparable clinical results. The 35 clinical psychologists in this study estimated that 92% to 96% of their diagnoses and 89% to 93% of their narrative interpretations would be essentially the same, or only slightly different, between the two instruments. Harrell, Honaker, and Parnell (1992) administered the MMPI, the MMPI-2, or both, in a counter-balanced repeated-measures design with adult psychiatric patients. Although MMPI-2 scores were generally lower than MMPI T-scores on several of the clinical scales, subjects were essentially equivalent in terms of rank ordering of T-scores and the dispersion of Basic scale scores. As the research literature on the MMPI-2 has grown over the past 25 years, the issue of codetype congruence has become less important since much of the interpretation of the MMPI-2 can now be based on research with that instrument.

Table 5.3 provides data from the MMPI-A manual (Butcher et al., 1992) on the congruence rate between profiles generated by normal adolescents, based on the Marks and Briggs (1972) original norms, and on the MMPI-A adolescent norm set. Table 5.3 also provides similar data, comparing MMPI and MMPI-A profile characteristics, for a group of adolescents in psychiatric treatment settings. Table 5.3 indicates that the overall congruence rate between profiles generated from the original test instrument and the MMPI-A is 67.8% for boys and 55.8% for girls, with the congruence rate increasing to 95.2% for boys and 81.8% for girls when the criterion for two-point codetype definition requires at least a 5-point T-score difference between the second and third most elevated scale. In the clinical sample of adolescents, the overall congruence rate is 69.5% for boys and 67.2% for girls, and reaches 95% for boys and 91% for girls employing well-defined codetype classification procedures. Table 5.3 also shows the very dramatic reductions that occur in the number of profiles classi-fied into two-point codetypes when the 5-point level of definition is required. These estimates for MMPI and MMPI-A congruence for adolescent samples are comparable to the congruence agreement rates reported for adults on the MMPI and MMPI-2 (Butcher et al., 1989; Graham, Timbrook et al., 1991). Thus, it seems reasonable to assume that much of the MMPI clinical research literature for adolescent samples is generalizable to the MMPI-A, but it is erroneous to assume that all adolescent patients will produce equivalent or congruent profiles across the two test instruments.

In the only study to explore the important issue of the relative accuracy of adolescents' MMPI versus MMPI-A profiles, Janus, Tolbert, Calestro, and Toepfer (1996) requested that clinicians blindly rate the accuracy of interpre-tive statements based on MMPI-A responses scored on (1) MMPI-A norms, (2) the Marks and Briggs adolescent norms for the original MMPI, and (3) adult K-corrected norms for the original MMPI. Both sets of adolescent norms (orig-inal and MMPI-A) produced higher accuracy ratings than did the use of adult norms, but the adolescent norms did not produce ratings that differed from each other. Janus, Tolbert et al. (1996) concluded that the MMPI-A profiles based on standard MMPI-A norms produced clinical utility (accuracy) that was equiv-alent to the Marks and Briggs adolescent norms for the original instrument. Table 5.4 provides data on the frequency of profile assignments to two-point codes as reported in the MMPI-A manual (Butcher et al., 1992) for samples of normal adolescents and psychiatric patients scored on the MMPI-A adolescent norms.

Table 5.5 provides data from Archer, Gordon, and Klinefelter (1991) on 1,762 adolescent inpatients and outpatients scored on the Marks and Briggs norms, and rescored on MMPI-A norms, presented separately by gender.

TABLE 5.3 Two-Point Codetype Congruence Rates as a Function of Codetype Definition for Profiles Scored on the MMPI-A Norms and the Marks, Seeman, and Haller (1974) Adolescent Norms

Definition[a]	Boys		Girls	
	N	%	N	%
Normal Sample				
0	805	67.8	815	55.8
1	692	71.7	703	57.8
2	518	81.1	521	64.1
3	384	87.8	379	70.4
4	288	92.4	277	76.9
5	208	95.2	203	81.8
6	152	94.7	125	88.0
7	116	95.7	89	88.8
8	81	97.5	63	90.5
9	63	96.8	41	90.2
10	43	100.0	23	95.7
Psychiatric Sample				
0	420	69.5	293	67.2
1	368	72.6	266	70.7
2	294	82.0	213	75.6
3	223	89.2	169	81.1
4	175	93.7	134	87.3
5	141	95.0	100	91.0
6	105	94.3	80	93.8
7	85	96.5	56	92.9
8	65	96.9	41	95.1
9	45	100.0	27	92.6
10	32	100.0	22	95.5

Source: Butcher et al. (1992). Reprinted with permission. Minnesota Multiphasic Personality Inventory-Adolescent (MMPI®-A) Manual for Administration, Scoring, and Interpretation by Butcher, et al. Copyright © 1992 by the Regents of the University of Minnesota. Reproduced with the permission of the University of Minnesota Press. All rights reserved. "Minnesota Multiphasic Personality Inventory" and "MMPI" are trademarks owned by the Regents of the University of Minnesota.

Note
a T-score difference between the second and third most elevated clinical scales in the MMPI codetype (using the Marks et al. norms).

The adolescents used in these analyses were 12 to 18 years old ($M = 16.19$ years; $SD = 1.51$) who completed the group booklet form of the MMPI, produced F scores of T < 100 on the Marks and Briggs norms, and omitted less than 30 responses. The data sources include psychiatric settings in Missouri, Minnesota, and Texas and they are described in Archer and Klinefelter (1991). Table 5.5 shows codetype frequency data for 45 codetype combinations and for *no-code profiles*. A no-code profile was defined as a profile containing no clinical scale

TABLE 5.4 Frequency Distribution of MMPI-A Codetypes With No Definition

Code type	Normative Boys	Normative Girls	Clinical Boys	Clinical Girls
	N = 805	N = 815	N = 420	N = 293
1-2/2-1	21	26	3	4
1-3/3-1	51	60	4	8
1-4/4-1	16	6	7	2
1-6/6-1	16	12	0	2
1-7/7-1	23	12	3	3
1-8/8-1	6	11	2	3
1-9/9-1	23	24	3	4
2-3/3-2	69	43	18	20
2-4/4-2	21	36	50	44
2-6/6-2	16	25	6	7
2-7/7-2	35	39	9	14
2-8/8-2	7	13	0	1
2-9/9-2	16	12	4	0
3-4/4-3	27	27	35	43
3-6/6-3	27	47	6	4
3-7/7-3	6	3	1	2
3-8/8-3	5	4	1	3
3-9/9-3	32	30	13	2
4-6/6-4	25	19	35	25
4-7/7-4	11	18	27	9
4-8/8-4	13	14	9	8
4-9/9-4	48	42	87	37
6-7/7-6	14	21	10	2
6-8/8-6	23	17	4	4
6-9/9-6	29	37	9	3
7-8/8-7	36	30	14	3
7-9/9-7	45	23	6	3
8-9/9-8	24	36	7	3

T-score value ≥ 65 for the Marks and Briggs norms, and no clinical scale T-score ≥ 60 for MMPI-A norms.

Basic Scale Reliability

The MMPI-A manual (Butcher et al., 1992) provides information concerning the internal consistency, test-retest reliability, and factor structure of the MMPI-A scales. The test-retest correlations for the MMPI-A Basic scales range from r = .49 for *F1* to r = .84 for *Si*, and in general these values are very similar to the test-retest correlations reported for the corresponding MMPI-2 Basic scales. Stein, McClinton, and Graham (1998) evaluated the long-term (one-year) test-retest reliability of MMPI-A scales and reported Basic Clinical scale values ranging from r = .51 for *Pa* to r = .75 for *Si*. Test-retest correlations for the Content scales, in contrast, ranged from r = .40 for *A-trt* to r = .73 for *A-sch*. The typical standard error of measurement for the MMPI-A Basic scales is estimated to be 2 to 3 raw score points (Butcher et al., 1992), which generally converts to 5 T-score points. Thus, it is possible to state, as noted by Archer and Krishnamurthy (2002), that if an adolescent is readministered the MMPI-A within a relatively short time interval, and without significant change in psychological functioning, his or her Basic scale T-scores would fall in a range of roughly ± 5 T-score points of their original score approximately 50% of the time. The standard error of measurement is very important when attempting to evaluate changes shown on the MMPI-A in terms of separating significant clinical changes from changes attributable to the standard error of measurement. In general, changes in T-score value ≤ 5 T-score points are more likely to reflect measurement error than reliable change.

The internal consistency of the MMPI-A Basic scales, as represented in coefficient alpha values, range from relatively low values on such scales as *Mf* and *Pa* (r = .60) to substantially higher values for other Basic scales such as *Hs* (r = .78) and *Sc* (r = .89). In contrast, internal consistency scores tend to be higher for other MMPI-A scales, such as content scales, because alpha coefficient estimates were utilized in the construction of these more recent MMPI-A scales. In addition to test-retest and internal consistency measures of reliability, the MMPI-A manual (Butcher et al., 1992) also provides information concerning the item endorsement frequencies and reading levels required by each of the MMPI-A items and the Principal Components Analysis (PCA) structure of the MMPI-A Basic scales using a varimax rotation procedure. Butcher et al. (1992) reported that a PCA of the MMPI-A Basic scales resulted in a four-factor solution, appropriate for both boys and girls, with a large first factor labeled General Maladjustment. The second factor was labeled Over Control and is marked by high loadings on *L* and *K*, and the third and fourth factors appear to be best described as non–clinical dimensions related to *Si* and *Mf*, respectively.

The Codetype Interpretation Approach

As noted by Graham (2012), configural approaches to the interpretation of the MMPI have been viewed as potentially the richest source of diagnostic and descriptive information that may be derived from this test instrument. The early writings on the MMPI (Meehl, 1951, 1956; Meehl & Dahlstrom, 1960) emphasized the interpretation of codetype information, and several of the early MMPI

TABLE 5.5 A Comparison of MMPI-A and MMPI Codetype Frequencies for 1,762 Adolescents Receiving Mental Health Services.

Codetype	MMPI-A				MMPI			
	Males		Females		Males		Females	
	N	%	N	%	N	%	N	%
1-2/2-1	9	0.9%	16	2.2%	14	1.4%	25	3.4%
1-3/3-1	23	2.2%	44	6.0%	33	3.2%	38	5.2%
1-4/4-1	16	1.5%	2	0.3%	21	2.0%	7	1.0%
1-5/5-1	4	0.4%	5	0.7%	12	1.2%	2	0.3%
1-6/6-1	12	1.2%	3	0.4%	14	1.4%	2	0.3%
1-7/7-1	7	0.7%	2	0.3%	13	1.3%	4	0.5%
1-8/8-1	9	0.9%	6	0.8%	19	1.8%	24	3.3%
1-9/9-1	6	0.6%	6	0.8%	13	1.3%	12	1.6%
1-0/0-1	7	0.7%	2	0.3%	4	0.4%	1	0.1%
2-3/3-2	25	2.4%	30	4.1%	25	2.4%	22	3.0%
2-4/4-2	52	5.0%	24	3.3%	38	3.7%	50	6.9%
2-5/5-2	12	1.2%	9	1.2%	25	2.4%	3	0.4%
2-6/6-2	8	0.8%	5	0.7%	4	0.4%	7	1.0%
2-7/7-2	11	1.1%	6	0.8%	9	0.9%	16	2.2%
2-8/8-2	1	0.1%	2	0.3%	5	0.5%	7	1.0%
2-9/9-2	0	0.0%	0	0.0%	2	0.2%	5	0.7%
2-0/0-2	19	1.8%	28	3.8%	9	0.9%	13	1.8%
3-4/4-3	51	4.9%	26	3.6%	41	4.0%	20	2.7%
3-5/5-3	10	1.0%	22	3.0%	34	3.3%	5	0.7%
3-6/6-3	6	0.6%	10	1.4%	4	0.4%	5	0.7%
3-7/7-3	0	0.0%	4	0.5%	2	0.2%	3	0.4%
3-8/8-3	1	0.1%	5	0.7%	0	0.0%	4	0.5%
3-9/9-3	7	0.7%	6	0.8%	6	0.6%	15	2.1%
3-0/0-3	1	0.1%	3	0.4%	0	0.0%	1	0.1%
4-5/5-4	17	1.6%	28	3.8%	37	3.6%	8	1.1%
4-6/6-4	64	6.2%	29	4.0%	58	5.6%	33	4.5%
4-7/7-4	25	2.4%	9	1.2%	18	1.7%	12	1.6%
4-8/8-4	29	2.8%	15	2.1%	21	2.0%	31	4.3%
4-9/9-4	104	10.1%	29	4.0%	82	7.9%	63	8.6%
4-0/0-4	24	2.3%	15	2.1%	7	0.7%	5	0.7%
5-6/6-5	5	0.5%	8	1.1%	20	1.9%	0	0.0%
5-7/7-5	1	0.1%	1	0.1%	5	0.5%	1	0.1%
5-8/8-5	1	0.1%	5	0.7%	7	0.7%	3	0.4%
5-9/9-5	3	0.3%	19	2.6%	29	2.8%	9	1.2%
5-0/0-5	3	0.3%	8	1.1%	4	0.4%	0	0.0%
6-7/7-6	14	1.4%	4	0.5%	16	1.5%	1	0.1%
6-8/8-6	33	3.2%	25	3.4%	25	2.4%	21	2.9%
6-9/9-6	22	2.1%	12	1.6%	22	2.1%	17	2.3%
6-0/0-6	3	0.3%	2	0.3%	1	0.1%	1	0.1%
7-8/8-7	19	1.8%	14	1.9%	21	2.0%	17	2.3%

7-9/9-7	18	1.7%	5	0.7%	16	1.5%	10	1.4%
7-0/0-7	13	1.3%	9	1.2%	4	0.4%	2	0.3%
8-9/9-8	16	1.5%	7	1.0%	12	1.2%	18	2.5%
8-0/0-8	2	0.2%	7	1.0%	1	0.1%	0	0.0%
9-0/0-9	6	0.6%	0	0.0%	4	0.4%	0	0.0%
No Code	314	30.4%	212	29.1%	276	26.7%	186	25.5%
Total	1,033		729		1,033		729	

Source: Adapted from Archer, R. P., Gordon, R. A., & Klinefelter, D. (1991). [Analyses of the frequency of MMPI and MMPI-A profile assignments for 1762 adolescent patients]. Unpublished raw data.

validity studies were focused on identifying reliable clinical correlates of MMPI two-point codetypes (e.g., Meehl, 1951).

A two-point codetype is usually referred to by the numerical designation of the two Basic Clinical scales that are most elevated in that profile, with convention dictating that the most elevated scale be designated first in the codetype sequence. Thus, if an adolescent produces his or her highest T-score elevations on scales *Pd* and *Ma* (in that order), the profile would result in classification as a *4-9* codetype. Throughout this text, individual MMPI-A scales have often been referred to by their names or alphabetic abbreviations rather than numerical designations. This procedure has been followed to minimize confusion in scale delineations for the novice MMPI-A user. In discussing codetype classifications, however, MMPI-A scales are referred to by their numerical designation in the manner consistent with the codetype literature. In addition to MMPI tradition, numerical designation of scales is the generally preferred practice among experienced MMPI-2 and MMPI-A users for a very important reason: The names that were originally given to clinical scales may be misleading and may serve as inadequate labels of what that scale is currently believed to measure. For example, the Psychasthenia scale was originally developed to measure symptomatology related to what was later referred to as obsessive-compulsive neurosis and now is termed obsessive-compulsive disorder. Psychasthenia is not a psychiatric label in common use today, and Graham (2012) noted that the *Pt* scale is currently thought of as a reliable index of psychological distress, turmoil, and discomfort, particularly related to symptoms of anxiety, tension, and apprehension.

Several codetype "cookbook" systems have been developed, such as those provided by Gilberstadt and Duker (1965) and Marks and Seeman (1963), which have employed very complex rules for classifying multiscale elevations. However, the more recent efforts regarding codetype descriptors have tended to employ much simpler two-point approaches to classify MMPI profiles. These systems, such as those exemplified in Friedman et al. (2015), Graham (2012), and Greene (2011), have typically interpreted codetypes based on the two scales with the highest clinical range elevation. Several investigations, such as research by Lewandowski and Graham (1972), demonstrated that reliable clinical correlates can be established for profiles that are classified based on the simpler two-point code systems. Data reported by Pancoast, Archer, and Gordon (1988) also indicate that assignments to simple codetype systems can be made with acceptable levels of reliability by independent raters. Additionally, diagnoses derived by the simpler MMPI classification systems provide comparable levels of agreement with clinicians' diagnoses as do those diagnoses derived from more complex methods of MMPI profile classification. The obvious advantage of using the two-point code system is that a much larger percentage of profiles can be classified in a typical clinical setting when numerous stringent criteria are not required for codetype assignments (Graham, 2012).

Of primary importance in employing codetype descriptors with any population is a clear understanding that the attribution of correlate descriptors to a particular client entails probability estimates. These estimates of accuracy may vary greatly based on the source of the descriptor statement (adequacy of research methodology, characteristics of the population sampled, statistical strength of findings) and the individual characteristics of the client being assessed (the base rate for similar symptoms/diagnoses in the general psychiatric population). Additionally, it is likely that the accuracy of descriptor statements will vary based on the degree of elevation and definition exhibited by a codetype (i.e., the degree to which the two-point code is clinically elevated, and elevated substantially above the remainder of the clinical scale profile). Even under optimal conditions in which cross-validated research has led to the derivation of clinical correlates from MMPI profiles highly similar to that of the individual being evaluated, a specific clinical correlate may be found not to apply to a specific individual. Thus, as Greene (2011) noted, MMPI cookbooks, even within adult populations,

> have not been the panacea that was originally thought. Increasing the specificity of a particular codetype helps by enhancing the homogeneity of the group and increasing the probability of finding reliable empirical correlates; however, it also substantially reduces the number of profiles that could be classified within a codetype.
>
> (p. 151)

Nevertheless, codetypes continue to serve as a valuable source of hypotheses concerning client characteristics when such cautions are borne in mind by the interpreter.

Deriving a Codetype Classification for Adolescents

In the adult codetype information provided by such sources as Graham (2012), Greene (2011), and Friedman et al. (2015), profiles are typically placed into two-point codetypes based on the two clinical scales that show the greatest degree of clinical range elevation. In these and most other systems, few high-point codes are provided that involve scales 5 and 0, because these scales have often been excluded from designation as clinical scales. These scales were also frequently excluded in codetype research in early MMPI investigations (Graham, 2012).

In general, two-point codes are used interchangeably; for example, 2-7 codetypes are seen as equivalent to 7-2 codetypes, unless differences are specifically noted. Furthermore, the absolute elevation of two high-point scales within the profile is typically not considered beyond the assumption that such elevations occur within clinical ranges. The relative elevation of the two highest scales in relation to the remaining profile is also not typically considered or discussed in codetype narratives. As previously noted, however, the degree to which the two-point code is well defined appears to be related to the short-term stability of the codetype (i.e., the degree to which profile characteristics are subject to change over relatively brief periods of time), and the degree to which clinical correlate patterns will be applicable for a codetype configuration. In standard codetype interpretation practice, if a profile does not fit any of the two-point codetypes presented, the clinician is generally advised to employ an interpretation strategy for elevated scores based on clinical correlates found for the individual MMPI scales.

Marks, Seeman, and Haller (1974) developed a classification system for adolescent MMPI profiles designed to increase the clinicians' flexibility in rendering codetype assignments. Once an adolescent's MMPI profile had been plotted, Marks et al. recommended that the resulting configuration should be compared to the codetype profiles provided in their 1974 text in terms of the two highest elevations occurring within that particular profile. If the codetype for the individual adolescent corresponded to one of the two-digit codetypes presented by Marks et al., the clinician was referred to the codetype descriptors appropriate for that configuration. If the respondent's codetype was not classifiable, however, the authors recommended dropping the second high-point scale and substituting the third-highest scale to produce a new two-point code. If this procedure then resulted in a classifiable codetype, the clinician was encouraged to interpret that profile based on the clinical correlate information provided for that code. If the profile remained unclassifiable following this "substitution and reclassification" procedure, Marks et al. suggested that their actuarial interpretation system should not be applied for that respondent. As commonly recommended in the interpretation of MMPI-2 profiles, these authors encouraged clinicians with unclassifiable profiles to employ a single-scale correlate interpretive strategy.

In terms of recommendations for the clinician deriving codetype assignments, it appears most appropriate to employ a simple codetype strategy that seeks to place an individual profile into a codetype classification based on the highest two-point characteristics occurring within clinical ranges for that profile.

The clinician should be mindful, however, that less elevated and less well-defined codetypes (the degree of elevation of the two-point code relative to the remainder of the profile) are likely to manifest fewer of the correlate features associated with that particular codetype. When classification does not result in an appropriate two-point codetype placement for which clinical correlate information is available from standard sources, it is suggested that the clinician interpret the profile based on single-scale correlates. The substitution and reclassification procedure suggested by Marks et al. (1974) is *not* recommended.

Single-Scale and Two-Point Codetypes

A substantial research literature has developed on the clinical correlate patterns exhibited by adolescents on the Basic MMPI scales. Hathaway and Monachesi (1963), for example, investigated high-point and low-point correlate patterns for approximately 15,000 ninth-graders who were administered the MMPI in the Minnesota public school system during 1948 and 1954. Lachar and Wrobel (1990) and Wrobel and Lachar (1992) later examined single-scale correlate patterns in a sample of adolescents from predominantly outpatient settings, with analyses conducted separately by gender. Information concerning the correlates of Basic MMPI scales for inpatient adolescents was examined in research studies by Archer et al. (1985), Archer and Gordon (1988), Archer, Gordon, Giannetti, and Singles (1988), Ball, Archer, Struve, Hunter, and Gordon (1987), and Williams and Butcher (1989a). Single-scale correlates for the MMPI-A Basic Clinical scales were reported in the manual for this instrument by Butcher et al. (1992) Handel, Archer, Elkins, Mason, and Simonds-Bisbee (2011), and in Veltri et al. (2009). Additionally, information concerning correlate patterns for various codetype configurations was presented by Archer (1987b), Archer and Klinefelter (1992), Archer and Krishnamurthy (2002), Marks et al. (1974), and Williams and Butcher (1989b). These research investigations and summaries serve as the primary sources of single-scale and codetype correlate data presented in this chapter.

In deriving the following codetype descriptors for adolescents, the 29 codetypes reported by Archer (1987b) were selected for presentation. In general, the core of this clinical correlate information is based on the Marks et al. (1974) data reported for high-point codetypes occurring within clinical ranges. This information was then supplemented with adult correlate information for these 29 high-point pairs from Friedman et al. (2015), Graham (2012), Greene (2011), and Lachar (1974). The typical narrative created by this method begins with statements found to be common across both the adolescent and adult descriptors for a particular MMPI configuration, based on the observations by Archer (1987b) and Archer et al. (1988) that MMPI scale descriptors found in studies of adolescents have typically been consistent with those found in adult studies. Further, when sources of adult correlate data were not available for a particular codetype, a relatively rare occurrence, this is noted in the first few sentences of the narrative. When marked or important differences occur between descriptors derived from adolescent and adult clinical populations, the interpretive implications of these discrepancies are presented. Finally, codetype frequency data for adolescents are based on our analyses of the codetype classification data for 1,762 adolescent patients shown in Table 5.5, as scored on MMPI-A norms.

In addition to the 29 codetype narratives, the following sections also contain information concerning characteristics of each of the 10 MMPI-A Basic Clinical scales. High and low single-scale correlates are suggested based on findings reported in studies of adolescent samples in normal and/or psychiatric settings. In the case of single-scale high-point correlates, this description is enriched by the MMPI-A correlate research reported in the test manual (Butcher et al., 1992). Much of the codetype correlate information provided in the following sections is based on research conducted with the original form of the MMPI utilizing the traditional adolescent norms as derived by Marks and Briggs (1972). This approach is similar to that taken by Graham (2012) and Greene (2011) in the generation of codetype findings for the MMPI-2. The generalization of MMPI findings to the MMPI-A appears to be supported in that the MMPI-A Clinical scales (except *Mf* and *Si*) have retained basically the same items as their counterparts in the original instrument. Further, as previously discussed in this chapter, the codetype congruence data for the MMPI and MMPI-A indicate that these instruments will produce similar or equivalent profiles in a majority of cases. Empirical research findings are still needed, however, concerning the degree to which codetype correlates found for adolescents on the original test instrument may be validly generalized to the MMPI-A. Examinations of MMPI-2 codetype correlates for adult psychiatric patients have found a striking degree of similarity in the descriptors identified for MMPI-2 based codetypes in inpatient (Archer, Griffin, & Aiduk, 1995) and outpatient settings (Graham, Ben-Porath, & McNulty, 1999) in relation to corresponding codes derived from the original MMPI. The issue of generalizability of findings from the original MMPI has become less important, however, as research projects have generated an additional correlate literature that is based directly on studies conducted with the MMPI-A.

Scale 1 (Hs: Hypochondriasis) Codetypes

Scale 1 originally consisted of 33 items developed to identify respondents who manifested a history of symptomatology associated with hypochondriasis. These symptoms include vague physical complaints and ailments and a preoccupation with bodily functioning, illness, and disease. One item was dropped from the original scale in the creation of the MMPI-A due to objectionable content, resulting in a revised scale length of 32 items. Graham (2012) reported that scale 1 appears to be the most unidimensional and homogeneous MMPI Basic Clinical scale in terms of item composition and content. All of the items on scale 1 relate to somatic concerns and complaints. Literature in adult samples has established that individuals who score high on scale *1* typically report many somatic symptoms and exaggerated complaints regarding physical functioning. Additionally, Graham (2012) noted that adults who produce elevated scale *1* MMPI profiles are not psychologically minded and often use physical complaints as a means of controlling or manipulating significant others in their environment.

Reports concerning physical functioning on scale *1* would also be expected to be influenced by the individual's actual physical condition - respondents with physical illness typically produce moderate subclinical elevations on this measure. For example, Ball et al. (1987) found subtle but detectable neurological differences between adolescent psychiatric inpatients with and without marked scale *1* elevations. MMPI profiles with scale *1* elevations have also been reported for adolescents with medical problems, including epilepsy (Dodrill & Clemmons, 1984), muscular dystrophy (Harper, 1983), nonprogressive physical impairments (Harper & Richman, 1978), Gilles de la Tourette Syndrome (Grossman, Mostofsky, & Harrison, 1986), sleep disorders (Monroe & Marks, 1977), surreptitious insulin administration among insulin-dependent diabetics (Orr, Eccles, Lawlor, & Golden, 1986), and rheumatic fever (Stehbens, Ehmke, & Wilson, 1982). Colligan and Osborne (1977) investigated the MMPI response features of 659 female and 534 male adolescents (ages 15 through 19) who presented at the Mayo Clinic for medical evaluation, and found these adolescents produced higher scores on the neurotic triad, which consists of scales *1*, *2*, and *3*. Profiles with elevations on scale *1* were unusual in the normal adolescent data collected by Hathaway and Monachesi (1963), although a larger number of these adolescents were classified as producing their lowest value on this scale.

High Scores on Scale 1

The following is a summary of descriptors for high scale *1* scores (T ≥ 60):

- Excessive somatic and bodily concerns that are likely to be vague in nature.
- Likely to display somatic responses to stress, which may include eating problems.
- Increased likelihood of problems related to neurotic diagnoses.
- Likely to be seen by others as self-centered, pessimistic, dissatisfied, and cynical.
- Demanding, critical, selfish, and whining in interpersonal relationships.
- Likely to display little insight in psychotherapy.
- Less likely to engage in delinquent behaviors.
- Likely to report school problems including academic and adjustment difficulties.

Low Scores on Scale 1

Low scale *1* scores have been associated with the following characteristics (T ≤ 40):

- Few physical symptoms and freedom from somatic preoccupation.
- Higher scores on tests of intelligence.
- More likely to come from urban than rural settings.
- Greater psychological sophistication and insight.

1-2/2-1 **Codetype.** Adolescent and adult clients with this codetype frequently complain of physical symptoms including weakness, fatigue, and tiredness. These individuals often show a consistent pattern of somatic preoccupation and overreactions to minor physical dysfunction. Marked affective distress appears to be associated with the *1-2/2-1* codetype and these individuals are often described as ruminative, tense, anxious, and insecure. There are also frequent reports of depression, social withdrawal, and isolation.

In both the adult and adolescent literatures, the *1-2/2-1* codetype has been associated with a very low probability of the use of acting out as a primary defense mechanism. There are often marked interpersonal concerns and unmet needs for attention and approval by others. Thus, individuals who produce this codetype have been described as fearful and hypersensitive in their interactions with others, and often as dependent and indecisive.

The *1-2/2-1* codetype occurred with a frequency of 0.9% for males and 2.2% for females in our sample of adolescent psychiatric patients scored on MMPI-A norms. Marks et al. (1974) reported that obsession and compulsion are the primary mechanisms of defense employed by adolescents with the *1-2/2-1* codetype. Adolescents with this codetype in the Marks et al. sample often complained of being teased by others during their childhood and indicated that they were afraid of making mistakes. They appeared to be quiet, depressed teenagers who established very few friendships and often manifested obsessional defenses. Although Graham (2012) reported that adults with the *1-2/2-1* profile often displayed excessive use of alcohol, the adolescents in the Marks et al. study with this codetype did not manifest significant drug or alcohol involvements. Finally, Marks and his colleagues noted that adolescents often had histories that included parental separation and divorce, academic problems including several cases of school phobias, and delayed academic progress.

1-3/3-1 **Codetype.** Both adult and adolescent sources of clinical correlate data indicate that individuals with the *1-3/3-1* codetype typically present themselves as physically or organically ill. Indeed, when scales *1* and *3* are greater than a T-score value of 65, and both of these scales exceed the T-score value for scale *2* by at least 10 points, this profile may be described as a classic *conversion V*. The types of physical complaints that have been noted in the general literature for the *1-3/3-1* codetype include headaches, dizziness, chest pain, abdominal pain, insomnia, blurred vision, nausea, and anorexia. It would be expected that these physical symptoms would increase in times of psychological stress, and the clinician might be advised to attempt to identify secondary gain characteristics associated with this symptomatology.

In the adult and adolescent literatures, the *1-3/3-1* codetype is associated more with neurotic and psychophysiological symptomatology rather than diagnoses related to psychoses. These respondents are frequently perceived as insecure and attention-seeking. Behaving in socially acceptable ways appears important to the *1-3/3-1* person. For the adult and adolescent *1-3/3-1*, there are problems in successfully establishing relationships with members of the opposite sex. Often, these problems are related to the lack of development of appropriate skills in these interpersonal areas. Primary defense mechanisms for this codetype consist of somatization, denial, and externalization.

As shown in Table 5.5, 2.2% of male and 6.0% of female adolescents in psychiatric settings produce the *1-3/3-1* codetype. Data unique to adolescent clinical sources for this profile indicate that the *1-3/3-1* teenagers are more frequently referred for treatment because of problems or concerns in their academic settings. The majority of adolescents in the Marks et al. (1974) sample indicated that they were afraid of receiving poor grades; a fear that appeared to be realistic in that 44% of this sample were a year behind their age-appropriate academic placement. In general, Marks et al. noted that adolescents with this codetype often displayed "diagnostic insight" into the descriptive features of their psychological problems. They were able to talk superficially about conflicts and were not evasive in psychotherapy. These features are in contrast to the descriptors in the adult literature indicating that *1-3/3-1* individuals typically display little willingness to acknowledge psychological factors in their life problems and little insight into their problems. Of the 20 patients in the Marks et al. (1974) 1970–1973 sample who produced a *1-3/3-1* codetype, over two-thirds had no history of drug abuse or drug involvement.

1-4/4-1 **Codetype.** The *1-4/4-1* codetype is relatively rare among adults, and it is found in approximately 1.5% of male and 0.3% of female adolescents in psychiatric settings. In both the adult and adolescent sources of clinical correlate information, the *1-4/4-1* individual appears to be defensive, negativistic, resentful, pessimistic, and cynical. Furthermore, research findings suggest these individuals may be described as self-centered and immature. The use of somatic complaints is a primary defense mechanism for both adolescents and adults, although this feature is more prevalent among adolescents producing a higher elevation on scale *1* in contrast to scale *4*.

In addition to these features, derived from the combined literature, a number of characteristics appear to be uniquely related to the adolescents' *1-4/4-1* codetypes. Specifically, more scale *4* features are reported as descriptive of adolescents with this codetype, including defiance, disobedience, and provocative behaviors. These problem areas are most likely to be manifested in the relationship between the adolescent and their parents. In the psychotherapy relationship, adolescents with this codetype have been described as superficial, cognitively disorganized, and moderately impaired in judgment. Therapists in the Marks et al. (1974) study rated adolescents with a *1-4/4-1* profile as manifesting an overall degree of psychiatric disturbance that was mild to moderate for most cases. In addition to the somatization, adolescents with this codetype often employ acting out as their primary defense mechanism. Therapists describe adolescent patients with this codetype as aggressive, outspoken, resentful, headstrong, and egocentric. Despite the use of acting out as a primary defense mechanism, adolescents with the *1-4/4-1* codetype in the Marks et al. sample were typically not found to be substance abusers.

1-5/5-1 Codetype. The *1-5/5-1* is a relatively infrequent codetype among adults, and is found for less than 1% of male and female adolescents in psychiatric treatment. In both the adult and adolescent literatures, the *1-5/5-1* is often accompanied by somatic complaints of a hypochondriacal nature and patients with this codetype often present as physically ill. Additionally, these individuals are often seen as passive, and the adolescent data indicate that boys with this codetype are unlikely to enter into open conflict or disagreement with their parents.

Teenagers with this codetype are often referred for treatment by parents and by school officials. Primary therapists view these adolescents as displaying mildly inappropriate affect, and compulsion appeared to be a primary defense mechanism distinctive to this codetype. Interestingly, many of these teenagers in the Marks et al. (1974) sample actually had experienced serious physical illnesses as children. Therapists described *1-5/5-1* adolescent patients as having difficulty in discussing their problems and conflict areas, and these teenagers were seen as unreliable in terms of the information they provided to their therapists. They were not generally liked by others and had difficulty in forming close relationships. Finally, teenage males with this profile type were described as effeminate.

1-6/6-1 Codetype. Of the adult sources reviewed, only Greene (2011) and Friedman et al. (2015) provide descriptive summaries for the *1-6/6-1* profile. Greene's brief description of this codetype emphasizes the occurrence of hypochondriacal symptomatology combined with hostile and suspicious traits related to elevations on scale *6*. Additionally, he noted that the personality structure of the adult *1-6/6-1* appeared resistant to change as a result of psychotherapy. In contrast, the results of investigation of adolescent *1-6/6-1* codetypes by Marks et al. (1974) produced a quite different descriptive picture. Confidence in any codetype descriptors for this configuration must be tempered, however, by awareness that little research has been done in adult settings and that the *1-6/6-1* codetype reported by Marks et al. was based on a very small sample size ($N = 11$). Among adolescent psychiatric patients, only 1.2% of males and 0.4% of females produced *1-6/6-1* codetypes (see Table 5.5).

Hypochondriacal tendencies and somatic complaints do not appear to be characteristics of adolescents with the *1-6/6-1* codetype. Rather, these adolescents were primarily referred for psychotherapy because of excessive emotional control. Therapists viewed these teenagers as evasive, defensive, and fearful of emotional involvement with others. More than half of these adolescents lived with their mothers in father-absent homes. When fathers were present in the family of these teenagers, their attitude toward the adolescent was reported to be rejecting. The *1-6/6-1* adolescent was viewed as egocentric and prone to rationalization as a defense mechanism. Data from the Marks et al. (1974) 1970-1973 sample indicated some drug abuse involvement for this codetype, but it was not widespread or characteristic of this code. Intense anger directed at parents was frequently displayed by this group, including occasional violent outbursts. Suicidal attempts, perhaps representing an internalization of rage and anger, were also characteristic of the *1-6/6-1* in the 1970–1973 adolescent sample.

1-8/8-1 Codetype.   Common features across the adolescent and adult literatures for the *1-8/8-1* codetype emphasize correlates commonly associated with both scales *1* and *8*. Patients with this profile type frequently present somatic concerns such as headaches and insomnia, and often perceive themselves as physically ill. There are additional data from adolescent sources to suggest that teenagers with this codetype were, in fact, often ill with serious health problems during their childhood. These adolescents also frequently reported histories of poor social adjustment and social inadequacy. Further, individuals with the *1-8/8-1* profile appear to have difficulty in forming and maintaining interpersonal relationships. There is evidence in both the adolescent and adult literatures that the *1-8/8-1* codetype is often associated with delusional or disordered thinking, including symptoms related to difficulty in concentration and thought processes. Adolescents with the *1-8/8-1* codetype often described themselves as distractible and forgetful.

Approximately 0.9% of male and 0.8% of female adolescents in psychiatric settings produce the *1-8/8-1* codetype. Several clinical descriptors are uniquely available for this codetype classification from the Marks et al. (1974) study. These adolescents frequently reported problems during childhood involving being teased and harassed by peers, and often had difficulty in academic performance, including reading. Overall, their adjustment appeared to be problematic both in and outside of school settings, and they experienced substantial difficulty in making friends. Nearly one-half of the *1-8/8-1* teenagers in the Marks et al. sample were a grade behind their expected academic placement.

Unique among the two-point codetypes involving scale *1*, the *1-8/8-1* adolescents in the Marks et al. data were likely to be involved in drug abuse, and over 50% of the sample reported a drug use history. Data from Archer and Klinefelter (1992) also indicate adolescents with this codetype frequently exhibit elevated values on the *MAC* scale. Additionally, attempted suicides frequently occurred among these adolescents, with 65% of adolescents with this codetype attempting to take their own lives. Finally, intense family conflict was present for a very high percentage of the *1-8/8-1* teenagers, which often involved fighting or overt conflict with their parents. Two-thirds of these adolescents were from families in which their parents were divorced.

Scale 2 (D: Depression) Codetypes

Scale *2* originally consisted of 60 items, of which 57 were retained in the MMPI-A scale *2*. The essential characteristics of this MMPI-A dimension include poor morale, lack of hope for the future, and general dissatisfaction with one's life status and situation (Hathaway & McKinley, 1942). The major content areas involved in this scale include lack of interest in activities or general apathy, physical symptoms such as sleep disturbances and gastrointestinal complaints, and excessive social sensitivity and social withdrawal. Graham (2012) described scale *2* as a sensitive measure of the respondent's life discomfort and dissatisfaction. He noted that although very elevated values on this scale are suggestive of clinical depression, more moderate scores have generally been seen as reflective of a life attitude or lifestyle characterized by apathy and poor morale. The content subscales derived by Harris and Lingoes (1955) for scale *2* include item groupings labeled *Subjective Depression (D_1), Psychomotor Retardation (D_2), Physical Malfunctioning (D_3), Mental Dullness (D_4), and Brooding (D_5).*

Scale *2* high points were very infrequent among adolescents in the Hathaway and Monachesi (1963) Minnesota sample. Profiles containing their lowest values on scale *2*, however, were relatively more common among these adolescents. Greene (2011) reported that adult psychiatric patients who produce elevations on scale *2* generally have characteristics of clinically depressed individuals including feelings of inadequacy, lack of self-confidence, guilt and pessimism, and self-depreciation. Greene also noted that individuals who produce spike *2* profiles tend to be good psychotherapy candidates, and often show significant improvement as a result of relatively brief psychiatric interventions. Consistent with this finding, Archer et al. (1988) found that high scale *2* inpatient adolescents were perceived by clinicians and psychiatric staff as more motivated to engage in psychotherapy and openly discuss their feelings and perceptions. They were also less likely than other adolescents to engage in rebellious, deceitful, manipulative, or hostile behaviors. In addition, Archer and his colleagues found that high scale *2* adolescents were described as more introspective, self-critical, guilty, ashamed, and more likely to have problems involving suicidal thoughts or ideations. Butcher et al. (1992), based on analyses of MMPI-A data, found that adolescent inpatients with scale *2* elevations were more likely to be characterized as depressed and more likely to have problems related to suicidal ideations and/or gestures. Archer and Gordon (1988), however, found no evidence of a significant relationship between scale *2* elevations among adolescent inpatients and clinicians' use of depression-related diagnoses, including dysthymia and major depression. Research by Nelson (1987) suggested that scale 2 may more accurately identify clinically depressed individuals when only face-valid or obvious Depression scale items are employed. Nelson and Cicchetti (1991) replicated and expanded these findings in an outpatient adult sample composed of individuals suffering from milder forms of maladjustment. Merydith and Phelps (2009) found that MMPI-A scale 2 scores were highly intercorrelated with MMPI-A Content scale Depression scores (r = .76) in a sample of 252 inpatient adolescents. Veltri et al. (2009) reported that scale 2 was correlated with higher ratings of anxiety, poor concentration, psychomotor retardation, and self-mutilation in a sample of 197 girls in a psychiatric inpatient sample. Handel et al. (2011) found MMPI-A scale 2 related to higher ratings of withdrawal and depression in a sample of 315 boys and 181 girls referred for court-ordered evaluations.

Although clinical lore holds that scale 2 results may be predictive of suicide attempts, the empirical literature does not appear to support this assumption. Marks and Haller (1977) examined groups of male and female adolescents who made suicide attempts in contrast with other emotionally disturbed adolescents without suicidal histories. The authors reported that MMPI scales 3 and 5 were significantly higher for male attempters, whereas scale 9 elevations were associated with suicide attempts among females. In contrast, Archer and Slesinger (1999) found single-scale elevations on scale 2 or 8, and co-elevations on the 4-8 and 4-9 codetypes, related to higher levels of suicidal ideation among adolescents. Spirito, Faust, Myers, and Bechtel (1988), however, found no significant differences in scale 2 mean elevations between female adolescent suicide attempters and a control group of female adolescents initially hospitalized for medical problems and referred for psychiatric consultation. Based on very similar profiles produced by these two groups, in conjunction with the largely negative findings in the adult literature, Spirito et al. (1988) concluded that, "primary reliance on the MMPI alone to determine suicidal risk seems non-judicious" (p. 210). Friedman, Archer, and Handel (2005) reviewed the literature on the MMPI-2 and MMPI-A and suicide. They noted that the primary problem inherent in attempting to predict suicide from any personality scale or measure is the limitations, discussed by Meehl and Rosen (1955), involved in the prediction to low base rate behaviors or events. This base rate issue makes the effective identification of suicidal ideation among adolescents a realistic objective (which occurs with a relatively high base rate among adolescents), but precludes the useful prediction of actual suicidal behaviors.

High Scores on Scale 2

The following is a summary of descriptors for high scale 2 scores (T ≥ 60):

- Feelings of dissatisfaction, hopelessness, and unhappiness.
- General apathy and lack of interest in activities.

- Presence of guilt feelings, shame, and self-criticism.
- Lack of self-confidence and a sense of inadequacy and pessimism.
- Social withdrawal and social isolation.
- A degree of emotional distress that may serve as a positive motivator for psychotherapy efforts.

Low Scores on Scale 2

The following are characteristics that have been associated with low scale 2 scores (T ≤ 40):

- Higher levels of intelligence and academic performance.
- Freedom from depression, anxiety, and guilt.
- Self-confidence and emotional stability.
- The ability to function effectively across a variety of situations.
- Alert, active, and competitive.
- Rebellious, argumentative, irresponsible, and manipulative when found for adolescent psychiatric patients.

2-3/3-2 Codetype. There is substantial overlap in the correlates of the 2-3/3-2 codetype for adolescent and adult psychiatric patients. They are characteristically described as emotionally overcontrolled, and unlikely to employ acting out as a primary defense mechanism. They typically have histories that reflect a lack of involvement or interest in relationships with others, and when relationships are established they tend to have dependent characteristics. Adjectives such as *passive*, *docile*, and *dependent* are frequently applied to individuals with the 2-3/3-2 profile, and they are often described as unassertive, inhibited, insecure, and self-doubting. Both adolescents and adults with the 2-3/3-2 code are very achievement oriented and set high goals for their own performance. These aspirations are often unrealistic and appear to be a contributor to their sense of inferiority and depression. Antisocial personality or psychopathic diagnoses are markedly rare for adolescents and adults who produce the 2-3/3-2 code. There is also little evidence of thought disorder or the presence of schizophrenic or psychotic diagnoses among these individuals. Defense mechanisms involving somatization and hypochondriasis appear to be central to the 2-3/3-2 code. In particular, weakness, fatigue, and dizziness appear to be common physical symptoms.

Among adolescent patients, the 2-3/3-2 codetype is relatively common and found in 2.4% of males and 4.1% of females (see Table 5.5). Data unique to the adolescent findings for the 2-3/3-2 code indicate that the majority of these adolescents were referred for treatment because of poor peer relationships. These adolescents were seen as socially isolated and lonely individuals. They have few friends inside the school environment and are loners outside of academic settings. The *2-3/3-2* adolescent reported a relatively passive, compliant, and obedient childhood that often involved an under-involved father in a professional occupation and a mother who may have been overinvolved with these children. Sexual acting out and drug abuse do not appear to be high-frequency problem areas for these adolescents, and 76% of the teenagers in the Marks et al. 1970–1973 sample reported no history of drug abuse. In research by Archer and Klinefelter (1992), the *MAC* scale raw scores for these adolescents were typically quite low. In the adult literature, the *2-3/3-2* codetype is more prevalent among female patients, and the majority of patients with this codetype are seen as psychoneurotic or reactive depressive. The *2-3* codetype was the modal pattern found for bulimia and anorexic adolescent patients in a study by Cumella, Wall, and Kerr-Almeida (1999).

2-4/4-2 Codetype.   Among teenagers and adults, high-point codes involving scales *2* and *4* are typically produced by individuals who have difficulty with impulsive control and often act without sufficient deliberation. They exhibit a marked disregard for accepted social standards, and problems with authority figures are manifested by inappropriate or antisocial behaviors and actions. Hypochondriacal and somatic defense mechanisms are not typically displayed by these individuals. Acting out, displacement, and externalization appear to be primary defense mechanisms. There is often a history of legal violations, including incidents of arrest, legal convictions, and court actions. Indeed, one-half of the adolescents in the Marks et al. (1974) sample had been placed on probation or held in detention.

In the adult and adolescent literatures, there are also frequent references to substance abuse and alcohol problems associated with this codetype. In the adult literature, the *2-4* profile is often the mean profile produced by samples of alcoholics (Greene & Garvin, 1988; Sutker & Archer, 1979). Marks et al. (1974) also noted that adolescents with the *2-4/4-2* codetype reported a wide variety of drug use, which included all pharmacological categories except narcotics. Indeed, Marks et al. found patterns indicating drug addiction, as well as drug abuse, among their *2-4/4-2* sample of adolescents. The *2-4/4-2* codetype was frequent in the findings shown in Table 5.5, reported for 5.0% of males and 3.3% of females in this sample. In hospital settings, adolescents with the *2-4/4-2* profile were often found to be elopement risks. They also had frequent histories of promiscuous sexual behavior, truancy, and running away from home. In general, the *2-4/4-2* adolescents indicated that much of their antisocial behaviors were attempts to escape or run away from what they perceived to be intolerable or highly conflicted home situations. In the adult literature, the *2-4/4-2* has been associated with a relatively poor prognosis for change. The major difficulty in treatment of adult psychiatric patients with this codetype is their tendency to terminate psychotherapy prematurely when situational stress has been reduced, but before actual attitudinal or behavioral change has occurred. Adolescents with this codetype are frequently referred for treatment because of difficulty with concentration. Further, these adolescents often perceive their parents as unaffectionate and inconsistent. The majority of adolescents in the Marks et al. (1974) sample stated that they had no one in their family with whom to discuss their personal concerns, feelings, and thoughts. Williams and Butcher (1989b) found that 2-4/4-2 adolescents were frequently described as depressed.

2-5/5-2 Codetype.   The 2-5/5-2 codetype is quite rare among adults, and is found for 1.2% of male and 1.2% of female adolescents in psychiatric settings. Among the commonly used MMPI-2 sources, Greene (2011) and Friedman et al. (2015) reported information concerning this codetype. Greene noted, based on findings from King and Kelley (1977) that male college students in outpatient psychotherapy who produced a 2-5/5-2 codetype were anxious, disoriented, and withdrawn and often had a history of somatic complaints. Further, the 2-5/5-2 college students displayed relatively poor heterosexual adjustment and dated infrequently.

Adolescents with this codetype were typically referred for treatment because of poor sibling relationships, indecisiveness, shyness, extreme negativism, hypersensitivity, and suspiciousness (Marks et al., 1974). As a group, these adolescents were seen to be quite vulnerable to stress, anxious, guilt-ridden, self-condemning, and self-accusatory. Similar to findings in the adult literature, these adolescents appeared to be quite anxious and indecisive and to have substantial difficulty in committing themselves to a definite course of action. The 2-5/5-2 adolescents typically displayed defense mechanisms involving obsession, manifested in perfectionistic and meticulous concerns, and intellectualization. They were described as depressed, socially awkward, and showed evidence of poor heterosexual adjustment. Individuals with the 2-5/5-2 profile were not described as athletic, and they performed poorly in sports. Males with this codetype were described as not masculine.

In general, teenagers with this codetype were interpersonally shy, passive, and unassertive. Unsurprisingly, drug use and abuse was not found to be associated with adolescents who produced this codetype. *MAC* raw scores for males with this codetype are typically below critical elevation levels (Archer & Klinefelter, 1992). Although many of these adolescents were seen to be intellectually and academically achieving at high levels, one-third of them were teased by their peers in school settings (Marks et al., 1974).

2-7/7-2 Codetype.   The 2-7/7-2 codetype occurs with a relatively high frequency in adult psychiatric patients, and appears to be less prevalent among adolescents in psychiatric settings, where it was found for only 1.1% of males and 0.8% of females. The adjectives and description for the 2-7/7-2 codetype, however, are quite consistent across both populations. Individuals with this profile type are anxious, tense, depressed, and highly intropunitive. They are often self-preoccupied and rigidly focused on their personal deficiencies and inadequacies. The adolescents in the Marks et al. (1974) *2-7/7-2* group consistently employed negative adjectives in their self-descriptions.

Individuals with the *2-7/7-2* codetype tend to employ obsessive-compulsive defenses. They typically do not come into conflict with others, and when interpersonal conflicts or difficulties do arise, they are handled by the *2-7/7-2* in a self-punitive and self-accusatory manner. These individuals are rigid in their thinking, and tend to be meticulous and perfectionistic in their everyday lives. They are seen by psychotherapists as self-defeating and behaviorally passive. Strong feelings of depression and anxiety frequently co-occur for these individuals, and there is often a history of overreaction or overresponse to minor life stress events. These individuals are frequently described as overcontrolled and unable to deal with or express their feelings in an open manner. In interpersonal relationships, there is often a pattern of dependency, passivity, and lack of assertiveness. Adolescents with a *2-7/7-2* codetype appear to have the capacity to form deep emotional ties with others, and typically report close relationships with family members. The primary reasons for referral among adolescents includes tearfulness, restlessness, anxiety, excessive worry, and nervousness. Acting-out behaviors such as drug use or school truancy were markedly low-frequency events for these teenagers. Roughly 40% of the adolescents in the Marks et al. (1974) sample with this codetype admitted or expressed suicidal thoughts. Roughly one out of four *2-7/7-2* teenagers were characterized as exhibiting severe depression.

2-8/8-2 **Codetype.** Both teenagers and adults with the *2-8/8-2* codetype are characterized by fearfulness, timidity, anxiety, and social awkwardness. This codetype appears with a frequency of less than 1% for both males and females in our clinical sample of adolescents. These teenagers appear to prefer a large degree of emotional distance from others, and are fearful and anxious concerning interpersonal relationships. Among adolescents, isolation and repression have been reported as primary defense mechanisms. Impaired self-concept and poor self-esteem are also associated with the *2-8/8-2* codetype. Kelley and King (1979) found that *2-8/8-2* female college outpatients were described with features related to affective distress and schizophrenic symptomatology, whereas *2-8/8-2* males were withdrawn and displayed flat or blunted affect. In the adult literature, individuals with a *2-8/8-2* codetype are often described as fearful of losing control, whereas the adolescent literature describes these individuals as highly emotional and characterized by deficits in the ability to moderate or modulate emotional expression. Further, adolescents with this codetype describe themselves as awkward and fearful of making mistakes. A high percentage of *2-8/8-2* adolescents in the Marks et al. (1974) study (44%) presented histories involving active suicide attempts. In the adult literature, the *2-8/8-2* codetype is associated with suicidal preoccupation, and Graham (2012) noted that adults with this codetype frequently have suicidal thoughts that are accompanied by specific plans for suicidal actions.

For adolescents and adults, the *2-8/8-2* codetype is also frequently associated with more profound psychiatric symptomatology, particularly when marked elevations occur on these two scales. Schizophrenic, schizoaffective, and manic depressive diagnoses are often attributed to adults with this codetype, and adolescents with these profile features have been found to display a higher-than-average frequency of such symptoms as hallucinations, preoccupation with bizarre or unusual concerns, and unusual sexual beliefs and practices. In the Marks et al. (1974) sample, over 25% of the *2-8/8-2* codetype adolescents were found to have vague and nonlocalized organic deficits such as minimal brain damage, or a history of seizure disorders, including epilepsy.

2-0/0-2 Codetype.   Among both teenagers and adults, the *2-0/0-2* high-point code has been associated with symptomatology including depression, feelings of inferiority, anxiety, social introversion, and withdrawal. These individuals are typically described as conforming, passive persons who are highly unlikely to engage in antisocial or delinquent behavior. Many *2-0/0-2* individuals show areas of social ineptitude and a general lack of social skills. Greene (2011) noted that social skills and assertiveness training may be beneficial in helping individuals with this codetype, as well as cognitive-behavioral approaches that focus on decreasing depressive cognitions.

The *2-0/0-2* codetype is found for 1.8% of male and 3.8% of female adolescents in psychiatric treatment settings (see Table 5.5), and occurs more frequently for adolescents on the MMPI-A, in contrast to the original test instrument. Adolescents with this codetype were typically referred for psychiatric treatment with presenting problems including tension and anxiety, apathy, shyness, lethargy, and excessive interpersonal sensitivity. As both children and adolescents, teenagers with the *2-0/0-2* codetype appear to be meek, socially isolated loners who conform to parental demands and who do not engage in alcohol or drug abuse. They typically expressed concerns to their therapists regarding feelings of inferiority, social rejection, and a self-perception of unattractiveness. They describe themselves as awkward, dull, gloomy, cowardly, shy, silent, and meek. Primary defense mechanisms include social withdrawal, denial, and obsessive-compulsive mechanisms. Psychotherapists in the Marks et al. (1974) study tended to view adolescents with a *2-0/0-2* codetype as schizoid, and individuals with this profile configuration produced a very low frequency of drug or alcohol abuse. Based on findings from the Marks et al. 1970–1973 sample, teenage girls with this profile reported that they wished to appear younger and less mature than their actual chronological age. Both boys and girls were seen as socially awkward, unpopular, and maintaining few significant friendships. Cumella et al. (1999) reported that the *2-0/0-2* codetype was associated with an increased frequency of eating disorders including bulimia and anorexia.

Scale 3 (Hy: Hysteria) Codetypes

The MMPI-A scale 3 consists of 60 items originally selected to identify individuals who utilize hysterical reactions to stressful situations. No items were deleted from this scale in the creation of the MMPI-A. The hysterical syndrome, as reflected in the item pool for scale 3, includes specific somatic concerns as well as items related to the presentation of self as well socialized and well-adjusted. Greene (2011) noted that although these two areas of item content are often unrelated or even negatively correlated in well-adjusted individuals, they tend to be positively correlated and closely associated for individuals with hysterical features. Graham (2012) noted that individuals who obtain a clinically elevated T-score value on scale 3 typically endorse a substantial number of items in both content areas.

The subscales derived by Harris and Lingoes (1955) for scale 3 include Denial of Social Anxiety (Hy1), Need for Affection (Hy2), Lassitude-Malaise (Hy3), Somatic Complaints (Hy4), and Inhibition of Aggression (Hy5). In the adult literature, marked elevations on scale 3 are typically associated with pathological conditions of hysteria. More moderate elevations have been found to be associated with a number of characteristics that include social extroversion, superficial relationships, exhibitionistic behaviors, and self-centeredness, but do not necessarily involve the classic hysterical syndrome.

Hathaway and Monachesi (1963) found that scale 3 profile high points (i.e., the highest elevation among the clinical scales) tended to occur with a greater frequency among Minnesota normal adolescents than scale 1 or scale 2 high points. They speculated that children who employ somatic complaints or "play sick" as a way of avoiding school and manipulating their parents would be expected to show elevations on scale 3. Further, these authors noted that moderate elevations on this scale might be expected among well-behaved and intelligent children who expressed what the authors referred to as "middle-class social conformity." In fact, Hathaway and Monachesi found that high scale 3 profiles were related to higher levels of intelligence and achievement and that these children often had parents in the professions. In contrast, scale 3 low-point profiles (i.e., the lowest clinical scale value) among normal adolescents were associated with lower academic achievement and lower socioeconomic background than high scale 3 adolescents.

Among adolescent psychiatric patients, Archer et al. (1988) found that high scale 3 adolescent inpatients were perceived by psychiatric staff as dependent, nonassertive, and prone to quickly modify their behaviors in order to meet social expectations and demands. Additionally, high scale 3 adolescents were described by treatment staff as more likely to express anxiety or stress through somatization and physical symptoms. Butcher et al. (1992) found that female adolescent patients with elevations on MMPI-A scale 3 manifested more somatic complaints and concerns than other adolescents, and Cumella et al.

(1999) found a relationship between Scale 3 elevations and various forms of eating disorders.

High Scores on Scale 3

The following is a summary of characteristics associated with high scale 3 profiles (T ≥ 60):

- Somatic concerns and preoccupations.
- Achievement oriented, socially involved, friendly.
- Patterns of overreaction to stress often involving development of physical symptoms.
- Self-centered, egocentric, and immature.
- Higher levels of educational achievement.
- Strong needs for affection, attention, and approval.
- Often from families of higher socioeconomic status.
- Psychologically naive with little insight into problem areas.

Low Scores on Scale 3

The following are characteristics of individuals who produce low scores on Scale 3 (T ≤ 40):

- Narrow range of interests.
- Limited social involvement and avoidance of leadership roles.
- Unfriendly, tough minded, realistic.
- School underachievement and lower socioeconomic status.
- Unadventurous and unindustrious.

3-4/4-3 Codetype. There appear to be at least three common features among adolescents and adults who exhibit the 3-4/4-3 codetype. First, these individuals often present hypochondriacal or somatic complaints, including symptoms of weakness, fatigue, loss of appetite, and headaches. Second, both teenagers and adults with 3-4/4-3 code tend not to perceive themselves as emotionally distressed, although they are often perceived as such by their therapists. Finally, individuals with this codetype in both age groups tend to manifest problems with impulse control and often report histories that include both antisocial behaviors and suicide attempts.

These problems in impulse control are often manifested in several ways. Sexual promiscuity appears to be relatively common among females with this codetype during adolescence and adulthood, and problems with substance abuse and dependence also appear prevalent. Adolescents with this codetype frequently have a history of theft, school truancy, and running away from home. As psychiatric inpatients, *3-4/4-3* adolescents often pose an elopement risk for the hospital unit. Drug use is also associated with this codetype, particularly among the adolescent sample. In the Marks et al. (1974) study, 63% of adolescents with this codetype reported a drug use history. Further, roughly one-third of these adolescents had made suicide attempts, a finding also characteristic of adults with *3-4/4-3* codes.

In the adult literature, the *3-4/4-3* individual is typically described as chronically angry, and harboring hostile and aggressive impulses. Particularly when scale *4* is higher than scale *3*, overcontrolled hostility may be manifested by episodic outbursts that could take the form of aggressive or violent behavior. Graham (2012) noted that prisoners with the *4-3* codetype frequently have histories of assaultive and violent crimes.

The *3-4/4-3* codetype is relatively common among adolescents, and was found for 4.9% of male and 3.6% of female adolescent patients (see Table 5.5). The *3-4/4-3* teenager is typically referred to treatment for sleep difficulties and for suicidal thoughts. They are often known as "roughnecks" in school, and their main problems and concerns relate to conflicts with their parents. Therapists of these teenagers frequently describe them as depressed, although also finding adequate ego strength among these teenagers. As Marks et al. (1974) noted, however, several of the descriptors associated with the *3-4/4-3* codetypes for adults may not apply to adolescents. The overcontrolled hostility syndrome that has been associated with the *3-4/4-3* codetype among adults, for example, does not appear to be applicable to teenagers with these MMPI features. In support of this observation, Truscott (1990) also reported that elevations on the Overcontrolled Hostility (*O-H*) MMPI special scale do not appear to be associated with the overcontrolled hostility syndrome for adolescents because adolescents do not typically employ repression or overcontrol as a defense mechanism.

3-5/5-3 Codetype.

This profile is extremely rare in the adult literature, and Greene (2011) reports that this pattern occurs with a frequency well below 1%. He notes that adults with this codetype are difficult to treat because they typically experience little emotional distress. No discussion of this codetype is available in either Graham (2012) or Lachar (1974), although Friedman et al. (2015) did briefly review it and reported that "There is limited empirical information on this codetype" (p. 313).

Among adolescents, this codetype was produced by 1.0% of males and 3.0% of females in psychiatric treatment (Archer, Gordon, & Klinefelter, 1991). Marks et al. (1974) were able to identify only 13 individuals who produced this codetype, all of whom were male. Among adolescents, the *3-5/5-3* codetype has many features that would be associated with individual scale high points for scales *3* and *5*. None of the adolescents in the Marks et al. *3-5/5-3* codetype were referred to treatment by court agencies or authorities, an unusual finding in adolescent psychiatric populations. Many of the teenagers with this codetype came from homes in which moral and religious values were firmly and often rigidly enforced, and the teenagers in this sample viewed the moral and ethical judgments of their parents as highly predictable. 3-5/5-3 adolescents were seen by their therapists as moderately depressed. Perhaps consistent with the scale 3 utilization of denial, however, several of these adolescents described themselves as "elated." A major symptom pattern connected with this codetype was one of withdrawal and inhibition. Although these adolescents were perceived as basically insecure and having strong needs for attention, they were also perceived as shy, anxious, inhibited, and socially uncomfortable. These teenagers were often found to be affectively shallow and their rate of speech was described as rapid. They did not employ acting out as a primary defense mechanism, and, in fact, tended to overcontrol their impulses. When adolescents with this codetype were involved with drug abuse, the substances employed were alcohol, marijuana, amphetamines, and sopors. Interestingly, 43% of the teenagers in the Marks et al. (1974) sample were found to have weight problems, including obesity and anorexia.

3-6/6-3 Codetype. There are a variety of characteristics commonly displayed by adolescents and adults who produce a 3-6/6-3 profile type. They tend to be generally suspicious and distrustful individuals who manifest poor interpersonal relationships and have substantial difficulty in acknowledging the presence of psychological problems and conflicts. In general, both teenagers and adults with this codetype utilize defenses of rationalization and projection, and often have difficulty in understanding why others are concerned about their behavior. Among adolescents, descriptors associated with suspicion and paranoia were often used to characterize these 3-6/6-3 teenagers. In general, individuals with this codetype appear difficult to get along with, self-centered, and distrustful and resentful of others. They maintain an egocentric and guarded stance concerning the world around them.

The 3-6/6-3 codetype was found among 0.6% of male and 1.4% of female adolescents receiving psychiatric services. Among adolescents, the most distinctive characteristic of this group was a relatively high incidence of suicide attempts, and one-third of adolescents in the Marks et al. (1974) study were seen for psychotherapy following such behaviors. In the Marks et al. 1970–1973 sample, this profile was associated with substance abuse, but not as extensively as other adolescent codetypes. In this sample, roughly 50% of these adolescents acknowledged drug involvement. Interestingly, 40% of this 3-6/6-3 codetype group were academically superior students.

Scale 4 (Pd: Psychopathic Deviate) Codetypes

This MMPI-A scale consists of 49 items, with one item deleted from the original Pd scale due to inappropriate content. Scale 4 was originally designed to identify or diagnose the psychopathic personality, referred to under the DSM-5 as *antisocial personality disorder*. As described by Dahlstrom, Welsh, and Dahlstrom (1972), the criterion group for scale 4 consisted largely of individuals who were court-referred for psychiatric evaluation because of delinquent actions including lying, stealing, truancy, sexual promiscuity, alcohol abuse, and forgery. The 49 items in the MMPI-A *Pd* scale cover a diverse array of content areas including family conflicts, problems with authority figures, social isolation, delinquency, and absence of satisfaction in everyday life. Scale 4 has a substantial degree of item overlap with many of the Validity and Clinical scales, and it contains an almost equal number of true and false responses that are keyed in the critical direction.

In the adult literature, individuals who score high on scale 4 are typically described in pejorative or unfavorable terms that include strong features of anger, impulsivity, interpersonal and emotional shallowness, interpersonal manipulativeness, and unpredictability. Thus, a marked elevation on scale 4 often indicates the presence of antisocial beliefs and attitudes, although Greene (2011) noted that such elevations do not necessarily imply that these traits will be expressed overtly. The degree to which antisocial behaviors are manifested is typically seen as related to the individual's standing on additional MMPI scales, including scales 9 and 0. Higher scale 9 and lower scale 0 values, in combination with an elevated scale 4, increase the likelihood for the overt behavioral expression of antisocial attitudes, beliefs, and cognitions. Harris and Lingoes (1955) identified five content subscales within scale 4, which are labeled *Familial Discord (Pd1)*, *Authority Problems (Pd2)*, *Social Imperturbability (Pd3)*, *Social Alienation (Pd4)*, *and Self-Alienation (Pd5)*.

Scores on scale 4 have been identified as varying in relationship to the respondent's age and race. Colligan et al. (1983) provided data from cross-sectional studies of 18- to 70-year-old adults that indicated that scale 4 values tend to decrease with age for both males and females. There is quite clear evidence that scale 4 values also differ as a function of adolescence versus adulthood in both normal and clinical populations (Archer, 1984). It has also been reported that African-American, Native American, and Hispanics subjects may score somewhat higher on scale 4 in contrast to Caucasians and Asian-Americans (Graham, 2012), based on findings from the MMPI-2 normative samples.

In normal samples, adolescents tend to endorse more scale 4 items in the critical direction than do adult respondents, and the mean scale 4 value for the MMPI-A sample would produce a T-score value of approximately 55 if scored using MMPI-2 norms. Research by Pancoast and Archer (1988) indicated that adolescents, in contrast to adults, are particularly likely to endorse items in the scale 4 content area labeled by Harris and Lingoes (1955) as Familial Discord (*Pd1*). Hathaway and Monachesi (1963) found that scale 4 was the most frequent high point for normal adolescents in the Minnesota statewide sample, with the highest frequency of scale 4 elevations found for girls and for adolescents from urban settings. The Minnesota data also indicated that scale 4 elevations increased as a function of severity of delinquent behavior. Further, high scale 4 profiles for both boys and girls were associated with higher rates of broken homes.

Within clinical samples, although codetypes involving scale 4 are relatively frequent in adult populations, they could be described as ubiquitous in adolescent settings. Nine of the 29 codetypes reported for adolescents by Marks et al. (1974) involved a scale 4 two-point code (i.e., scale 4 was one of the two scales most elevated in the profile), and nearly one-half of their clinical cases involved a high-point code that included scale 4. Similarly, in our analysis of MMPI profiles produced by adolescents in clinical settings, roughly 48% involved two-point codetypes that included scale 4 (Archer, Gordon, & Klinefelter, 1991).

Archer et al. (1988) found that adolescent inpatients who produced elevations on scale 4 were described by psychiatric staff members as evasive and unmotivated in psychotherapy. These adolescents were also found to be rebellious, hostile, and incapable of profiting from prior mistakes. Additionally, these adolescents had a high frequency of presenting problems involving drug and alcohol abuse, and nearly half received conduct disorder diagnoses. In the research by Archer and Klinefelter (1992), adolescent codetypes that involved scale 4 often produced substantially elevated mean raw score values on the *MAC* scale. Research by Gallucci (1997a; 1997b) also found the MMPI-A profiles of adolescent substance abusers often produced clinical range elevations on scales 4 and *MAC-R*. Butcher et al. (1992) found that adolescent boys and girls in their clinical sample with elevations on MMPI-A scale 4 were more likely to be described as delinquent and prone to exhibiting acting out or externalizing behaviors. In addition, girls who produced elevations on scale 4 were more likely to engage in sexual activity, and boys were more likely to exhibit incidents of running away. Veltri et al. (2009) reported that MMPI-A scale 4 elevations were related to higher levels of substance abuse and incidents of running away for adolescents in their acute care and forensic samples. Handel et al. (2011) found scale 4 associated with higher levels of rule-breaking, aggressive, oppositional-defiant, and conduct disorder behaviors for both boys and girls in a forensic sample.

High Scores on Scale 4

The following is a summary of characteristics for high scale 4 profiles (T ≥ 60):

- Poor school adjustment and problems in school conduct.
- Increased probability of delinquent, externalizing, and aggressive behaviors.
- Increased probability of a family history involving parental separation and divorce.
- Higher frequency of urban backgrounds.
- Difficulty incorporating or internalizing the values and standards of society.

- Rebelliousness and hostility toward authority figures.
- Increased likelihood of diagnoses involving conduct disorder and oppositional-defiant disorder.
- Inability to delay gratification.
- Poor planning ability and impulsivity.
- Low tolerance for frustration and boredom.
- Reliance on acting out as a primary defense mechanism.
- Increased probability of parent-adolescent conflicts and familial discord.
- Risk-taking and sensation-seeking behaviors, including use of drugs and alcohol.
- Selfishness, self-centeredness, and egocentricity.
- Ability to create a favorable first impression.
- Extroverted, outgoing interpersonal style.
- Relative freedom from guilt and remorse.
- Relatively little evidence of emotional/affective distress.

Low Scores on Scale 4

The following features have been associated with individuals who score low on scale 4 (T ≤ 40):

- Conventional, conforming, and compliant with authority.
- Lower probability of delinquency.
- Concerns involving status and security rather than competition and dominance.
- Accepting, passive, and trusting in interpersonal styles.
- Lower likelihood of delinquent behaviors.

4-5/5-4 Codetype.   The adult and adolescent literatures for the *4-5/5-4* profile codetype are substantially discrepant. Adults with these profile characteristics are typically discussed in terms of immaturity, emotional passivity, and conflicts centered on dependency. Friedman et al. (2015) noted that this codetype among adults is usually produced by male respondents as a result of the infrequency with which scale 5 is clinically elevated among females. Adults with this codetype are frequently rebellious in relation to social convention and norms, and this nonconformity is often passively expressed through selection of dress, speech, and social behavior. Because the scale selection serves to suppress aggressive acting out in men, the rebelliousness indicated with scale 4 more often takes the form of intellectual rebellion rather than aggressive delinquent acting out.

Although adults with these codetypes typically display adequate control, there are also indications that these individuals are subject to brief periods of aggressive or antisocial acting out. Sutker, Allain, and Geyer (1980) reported that the *4-5/5-4* codetype is found among 23% of women convicted of murder.

Among male college students, King and Kelley (1977) related this codetype to passivity, heterosexual adjustment problems, and both transient and chronic interpersonal difficulties. This sample did not display significant evidence of personality disorders, nor was homosexuality apparently characteristic of this group. Friedman et al. (2015) noted that detection of homosexual drive or behavior in adults with this codetype is difficult and "should the individuals want to conceal their homosexuality, they could do so readily without flagging any of the validity scales" (p. 299).

As shown in Table 5.5, the *4-5/5-4* codetype is found among 1.6% of male and 3.8% of female adolescents in psychiatric treatment settings. Marks et al. (1974) indicated that teenagers with this codetype appear to get along well with their peer group, and are gregarious and extroverted in their social interactions. In contrast to teenagers with other codetypes, the *4-5/5-4* adolescents were described by their therapists as better adjusted, easier to establish rapport with, and demonstrate greater ego strength. Further, therapists felt that teenagers with this codetype typically displayed relatively effective defenses in terms of protection of the adolescent from conscious awareness of depression or anxiety. The typical defense mechanisms utilized by these adolescents included acting out and rationalization. In contrast to *5-4s*, *4-5* adolescents appeared to have greater difficulty in controlling their tempers, and they described themselves as argumentative, opinionated, and defensive. Over half of the adolescents in the *4-5* codetype were rated by their therapists as having a good prognosis. In contrast to the adult literature, over 80% of the *4-5/5-4* adolescents in the Marks et al. study were engaged in heterosexual dating, a figure substantially higher than the base rate for other adolescent codetype groups.

Respondents with the *4-5/5-4* configuration in the Marks et al. 1970–1973 sample reported a relatively high frequency (72%) of drug abuse history. The drug use patterns found for these teenagers appeared to involve a broad variety of substances. In addition, adolescents in this sample had a high rate of antisocial behaviors, including shoplifting, auto theft, breaking and entering, and drug dealing. As a group, they were described as emotionally reactive and prone to temper tantrums and violent outbursts. Finally, teenagers in this sample also evidenced significant problems in school adjustment, including histories of truancy, school suspension, and failing academic grades.

4-6/6-4 Codetype. A relatively consistent picture emerges from the adolescent and adult literatures for individuals with the *4-6/6-4* codetype. They are uniformly described as angry, resentful, and argumentative. Adolescents with this codetype who are referred for treatment typically present symptomatology involving defiance, disobedience, and negativism. Treatment referrals for *4-6/6-4* adolescents are often made from court agencies, and Archer and Krishnamurthy (2002) have noted that several studies have associated elevations on these scales with delinquency.

4-6/6-4 individuals typically make excessive demands on others for attention and sympathy, but are resentful of even mild demands that may be placed on them in interpersonal relationships. They are generally suspicious of the motives of others, and characteristically avoid deep emotional attachments. Adolescents with this codetype appear to be aware of deficits in their interpersonal relationships and often reported that they were disliked by others. For both adults and teenagers, however, there is very little insight displayed into the origins or nature of their psychological problems. Individuals with this codetype tend to deny serious psychological problems, and they rationalize and transfer the blame for their life problems onto others. In short, they characteristically do not accept responsibility for their behavior and are not receptive to psychotherapy efforts. Although adolescents with this codetype are rated by others as aggressive, bitter, deceitful, hostile, and quarrelsome, they often appear to view themselves as attractive, confident, and jolly.

The *4-6/6-4* codetype is relatively common among adolescents and is found for 6.2% of male and 4.0% of female adolescents in psychiatric treatment settings (see Table 5.5). Among adolescents, the *4-6/6-4* codetype is almost inevitably associated with child-parent conflicts, which often take the form of chronic, intense struggles. These adolescents typically under-control their impulses and act without thought or deliberation. Williams and Butcher (1989b) found adolescents with this codetype were more likely to engage in acting-out behaviors, which included sexual acting out. Marks et al. (1974) reported that the *4-6/6-4* adolescent typically encountered problems with authority figures. Narcissistic and self-indulgent features appear prevalent in this codetype for both adolescents and adults. Therapists in the Marks et al. study described the *4-6/6-4* adolescent as provocative, and indicated that major defense mechanisms included acting out and projection. About half of the adolescents with this codetype in the Marks et al. sample reported a history of drug abuse, most frequently involving the use of alcohol.

4-7/7-4 Codetype.   The *4-7/7-4* codetype appears to be characteristic of adolescents and adults who employ acting out as their primary defense mechanism, but experience substantial feelings of guilt, shame, and remorse concerning the consequences of their behavior. Thus, they tend to alternate between behaviors that show a disregard for social norms and standards, and excessive and neurotic concerns regarding the effects of their actions. Underlying impulse control problems and tendencies to behave in a provocative and antisocial manner, these individuals appear to be insecure and dependent. They have strong needs for reassurance and attention.

The *4-7/7-4* codetype occurs in 2.4% of male and 1.2% of female adolescent psychiatric evaluations. In the Marks et al. (1974) research, the *4-7/7-4* teenager was described by therapists as impulsive, provocative, flippant, and resentful. At the same time, they demonstrated evidence of substantial conflicts concerning emotional dependency and sexuality. The majority of these adolescents exhibited substantial feelings of guilt and shame and were viewed by their therapists as guilt-ridden and self-condemning. Williams and Butcher (1989b) found that adolescents with the *4-7/7-4* codetype presented a mixed picture of internalizing and externalizing behaviors, and concluded that tension/nervousness, substance abuse, and acting-out behaviors were associated with this profile.

4-8/8-4 Codetype. The *4-8/8-4* codetype is associated with marginal social adjustments for both adolescents and adults. Marks et al. (1974) described the *4-8/8-4* adolescent as "one of the most miserable groups of adolescents we studied" (p. 218). They were frequently perceived as angry, odd, peculiar, and immature individuals who displayed impulse control problems and often exhibited chronic interpersonal conflicts. Only 16% of teenagers with this codetype were rated as showing a definite improvement as a result of psychotherapy, and only 9% were rated as showing a good prognosis for future adjustment. Adolescents with this codetype were often evasive in psychotherapy, and frequently attempted to handle their problems by denying the presence of any difficulties.

The *4-8/8-4* codetype is found with a frequency of 2.8% among male and 2.1% among female adolescent psychiatric patients. Teenagers with this profile typically display patterns of very poor academic achievement, and were often seen in psychotherapy as frequently as three times a week. Their family lives were described as chaotic, and unusual symptomatology such as anorexia, encopresis, enuresis, and hyperkinesia were often noted. Although excessive drinking and drug abuse are common among adults with this codetype, the *4-8/8-4* teenagers do not appear to be among the heavier drug abuser groups. Although the *8-4* adolescents were described as more regressed than the *4-8*s, the *4-8* adolescent was also noted to display thought patterns that were unusual and sometimes delusional. Thus, individuals with this codetype display antisocial features related to elevations on scale *4* in combination with schizoid or schizophrenic symptomatology characteristic of elevations on scale *8*. Williams and Butcher (1989b) reported that the *4-8/8-4* adolescents were more likely than other teenagers to have a history of sexual abuse, and Losada-Paisey (1998) reported that this codetype was associated with adolescent sex offenders. Archer and Slesinger (1999) found that adolescents with this codetype more frequently endorsed MMPI-A items related to suicidal ideation.

4-9/9-4 Codetype. A striking degree of similarity exists in the description of both teenagers and adults who produce a *4-9/9-4* codetype. These individuals almost always display a disregard for social standards and are likely to have difficulties in terms of acting out and impulsivity. They are characteristically described as egocentric, narcissistic, selfish, and self-indulgent and are often unwilling to accept responsibility for their own behavior. They are seen as high sensation-seekers who have a markedly low frustration tolerance and are easily bored. In social situations, the *4-9/9-4*s are often extroverted and make a positive first impression. They also, however, appear to manifest chronic difficulties in establishing close and enduring interpersonal relationships, and are highly manipulative and shallow in dealing with others. Classic features of the antisocial personality type are clearly relevant for adults with this codetype and adolescents with the *4-9/9-4* code often receive conduct disorder diagnoses.

The *4-9/9-4* is a frequently occurring codetype among adolescent psychiatric patients, but shows a substantial gender difference on the MMPI-A. Specifically, 10.1% of males and 4.0% of females produce this codetype, as shown in Table 5.5, when scored on MMPI-A norms. Huesmann, Lefkowitz, and Eron (1978) reported findings indicating that the summation of T-score values on scales *F*, *4*, and *9* serves as a viable predictor of aggression in older adolescents. In the Marks et al. (1974) research, the *4-9/9-4* adolescent was invariably referred for treatment because of defiance, disobedience, impulsivity, provocative behaviors, and truancy from school. In most cases, there were constant conflicts between the adolescents and their parents resulting from their history of misbehaviors. Intriguingly, fewer adolescents in the Marks et al. *4-9/9-4* codetype were raised in their natural homes than youngsters from any other codetype grouping. Specifically, 17% of adolescents with this codetype grew up in foster or adoptive homes, and 20% did not reside with their parents at the time of their evaluations in this study. As a group, these adolescents appeared to be socially extroverted and reported an earlier age of dating than other teenagers. Williams and Butcher (1989b) reported *4-9/9-4* teenagers were more sexually active than other adolescents. Nearly 50% of the subjects with this codetype in the Marks et al. study had a history of illegal behaviors that resulted in placements in detention or on probation. Ninety-three percent of these teenagers employed acting out as their primary defense mechanism, and problems with affective distress such as anxiety or feelings of inadequacy were not found for these teenagers. Archer and Krishnamurthy (2002) report that this codetype is frequent among adolescents with drug and alcohol abuse problems as well as male juvenile delinquents.

Therapists described adolescents with this codetype as resentful of authority figures, socially extroverted, narcissistic, egocentric, selfish, self-centered, and demanding. Further, this group was noted to be impatient, impulsive, pleasure-seeking, restless, and emotionally and behaviorally undercontrolled. Sixty-one percent of the adolescents with this codetype in the Marks et al. 1970–1973 sample reported a history of drug abuse. These teenagers, however, appeared to be selective in the substances they used and tended to avoid drugs such as hallucinogens or opiates. Archer and Klinefelter (1992) found that the *4-9/9-4* adolescents produced higher mean *MAC* scores than any other codetype group. This finding probably reflected the influence of a variety of factors, including the degree of item overlap between scales *4* and *9* and *MAC*, and the degree to which both the *4-9/9-4* codetype and the *MAC* scale commonly measure an extroverted, high sensation-seeking, risk-taking lifestyle. In the Marks et al. (1974) study, 83% of the *4-9/9-4*s were either chronically truant from school, had run away from home, or had run away from treatment settings. Many of these adolescents had engaged in all three of these activities. Marks et al. described these adolescents as provocative and seductive problem children with histories of lying, stealing, and other antisocial behaviors. These authors used the phrase "disobedient beauties" in reference to the *4-9/9-4* codetype. In the adult literature, these MMPI features have been repeatedly related to a poor prognosis for personality or behavioral change as a result of psychotherapy. It should be remembered, however, that adolescents who produce this codetype are likely to show substantially greater capacity for change and benefit from treatment than adults. In comparison to *4-9/9-4* features in adults, this personality structure is not as firmly entrenched and solidified during adolescence.

4-0/0-4 Codetype. As noted by Greene (2011), the *4-0/0-4* codetype is quite rare in adults (less than 1% frequency) and there is little empirical data on which to describe these individuals. Friedman et al. (2015) observed that individuals with this codetype rarely seek treatment. Conceptually, there is an inherent conflict presented by high-point elevations on both scales *4* and *0*. Whereas individuals who score high on scale *4* tend to be relatively comfortable around others, often show extroverted traits and are impulsive, high scale *0* respondents are often socially uncomfortable, introverted, and cautious. Thus, codetype elevations involving both scales would be an infrequent occurrence. Among adolescents in psychiatric settings, 2.3% of males and 2.1% of females produced the *4-0/0-4* codetype based on MMPI-A norms (Archer, Gordon, & Klinefelter, 1991). Marks et al. (1974) were able to identify 22 adolescents who produced the *4-0/0-4* codetype, evenly divided between high- and low-point codes.

Surprisingly, *4-0/0-4* adolescents appeared to display more features related to elevations on scale *6* than they did characteristics related to elevations on either scale *4* or scale *0*. They were described as suspicious and distrustful by their therapists. Additionally, they frequently expressed grandiose ideas and their main defense mechanism consisted of projection. These individuals were often resentful and argumentative adolescents who perceived themselves as shy and socially uncomfortable. Therapists described the *4-0/0-4* adolescent as quiet, passively resistant, and relatively under-involved in activities around them. They had few close friends, and establishing friendships tended to be one of their primary problem areas. Furthermore, they were judged to display moderate ego strength, and to demonstrate a pattern of overreaction to minor stressors.

Scale 5 (Mf: Masculinity-Femininity) Codetypes

Sixteen items were eliminated from the original MMPI *Mf* scale in the creation of the 44-item MMPI-A *Mf* scale. The content areas of scale *5* are heterogeneous, and include work and recreational interests, family relationships, and items related to fears and sensitivity. This scale was originally developed by Hathaway and McKinley to identify homosexual males, but the authors encountered difficulty in identifying or defining a clear diagnostic grouping to create a single criterion group. The primary criterion group eventually selected consisted of 13 homosexual males who were relatively free from neurotic, psychotic, or psychopathic tendencies. Items were assigned to the *Mf* scale, however, if they differentiated between high- and low-scoring men on an attitude interest test, or if the item showed a significant difference in endorsement between males and females. Dahlstrom et al. (1972) noted that an unsuccessful attempt was made by Hathaway and McKinley to develop a corresponding scale to identify female "sexual inversion," that is, an *Fm* scale. Martin and Finn (2010) have recently reviewed the development of the *Mf* scale on the MMPI-2 and MMPI-A, and discussed the underlying constructs and factor structure of the *Mf* scale.

Forty-one of the 44 items in the MMPI-A scale *5* are keyed in the same direction for both sexes. The three remaining items, which deal with overt sexual material, were keyed in opposite directions for males and females. T-score conversions are reversed for males and females so that a high raw score value for boys results in a high T-score placement, whereas a high raw score value for girls is converted to a low T-score value. Thus, the *Mf* scale represents a bipolar measure of gender role identification. The *Mf* scale and scale *0* constitute the two Basic scales for which linear T-score conversions were retained in the MMPI-A, rather than the uniform T-score procedures utilized for the remaining eight standard Clinical scales. Linear T-scores were employed for *Mf* and *Si* because the distributions for these scales were different than the remaining Basic scales, and more closely approximated a normal distribution.

Serkownek used item-factor loading patterns to construct six subscales for the *Mf* scale (Schuerger, Foerstner, Serkownek, & Ritz, 1987). The Serkownek subscales for *Mf* are *Mf1* (Narcissism-Hypersensitivity), *Mf2* (Stereotypic Feminine Interest), *Mf3* (Denial of Stereotypic Masculine Interests), *Mf4* (Heterosexual Discomfort-Passivity), *Mf5* (Introspective-Critical), and *Mf6* (Socially Retiring). Attempts to create a factor-analytically derived set of subscales for *Mf* were unsuccessful in the MMPI-2 Restandardization Project, and a similar attempt was not undertaken in the development of the MMPI-A.

Substantial controversy and debate has surrounded the meaning and interpretation of scale *5*, particularly in recent years. Graham (2012) noted that scores on scale *5* have been related to level of formal education, although this relationship appears more limited on the MMPI-2 than the original test instrument. As suggested by Greene (2011) and Friedman et al. (2015), elevations on the *Mf* scale may reflect the influence of a variety of factors in addition to sexual identification and orientation. Further, in the creation of both the MMPI-A and the MMPI-2, items directly related to sexual preferences were deleted, thereby essentially eliminating the usefulness of this scale as a measure of homosexuality. Finlay and Kapes (2000) compared scale *5* of the MMPI and the MMPI-A in a repeated-measures design with 60 emotionally disturbed adolescents. Test–retest results (with administration order balanced for the two test versions) showed generally higher scores for the original form of scale 5, and surprisingly low correlations between the two forms. The authors concluded that the deletion of 16 items and rewording of 6 additional in the creation of the MMPI-A scale 5 may have significantly altered measurement of the underlying construct. Greene (2011) noted that when scale 5 is the only clinical range elevation in an MMPI profile, those individuals are unlikely to be diagnosed as manifesting a psychiatric disorder. Mid-range elevations (T $\geq$ 40 and T $\leq$ 60) on the *Mf* scale have been difficult to interpret due to the variety of item endorsement patterns that may create this range of scores (e.g., a balance between masculine and feminine characteristics vs. low endorsement of both content areas may result in mid-range values).

Markedly low T-scores on the *Mf* scale for women appear to indicate a substantial identification with traditional feminine roles, which may include passivity, submissiveness, and the adaptation of many aspects of traditional femininity. Todd and Gynther (1988) found that low *Mf* females described themselves as tender and emotional. Low-scoring males have been described by Greene (2011) as displaying an "almost compulsive masculinity" in an inflexible and rigid manner (p. 128). Todd and Gynther found low *Mf* males described themselves as domineering and impersonal. T-scores of 60 or more on the *Mf* scale appear to be associated with women who are not interested in a traditional feminine role, and moderate elevations for men have been related to aesthetic interests. Todd and Gynther found that high-scoring *Mf* females describe themselves as self-confident and exploitive, and were rated by their peers as unsympathetic and bold. High *Mf* scores for males in this study were related to the perception of self as undemanding and shy, and clinical range elevations on scale 5 have also been related to passivity for males. Blais (1995) found elevated *Mf* scores among adult female psychiatric inpatients to be related to higher levels of anger, aggression, suspiciousness, and a tendency to be manipulative and egocentric in interpersonal relationships. Meunier and Bodkins (2005) reported that elevated *Mf* scores among girls in a residential treatment facility were associated with higher rates of failure to complete the treatment program, although this finding was criticized on methodological grounds by Brophy (2005). Long and Graham (1991) provided findings that do not support the usefulness of scale 5 in describing behaviors or personality characteristics for normal men, and the MMPI-A studies by Veltri et al. (2009) and Handel et al. (2011) did not yield meaningful correlates for *Mf* in their clinical and forensic adolescent samples, respectively.

On the original form of the MMPI, there was relatively little difference in the mean *Mf* raw score values found between normal male adolescents and adults, but there was a tendency for female adolescents to produce raw score values 2 to 3 points lower than adult females (Archer, 1987b). Data from Hathaway and

Monachesi (1963) indicated that the boys in their Minnesota normal sample who produced their highest values on scale 5 tended to be of higher socioeconomic status, with parents from professional and semi-professional occupations. These adolescents tended to have higher intelligence scores and academic grades. They also exhibited a lower frequency of delinquent and antisocial behaviors. In contrast, boys with low scale 5 scores tended to display patterns of school underachievement and delinquency, and produced lower intelligence test scores than high scale 5 boys. Similarly, female adolescents from the Minnesota normal sample who scored low on scale 5 were higher in terms of intelligence scores and displayed evidence of higher levels of academic achievement. Female adolescents scoring high on scale 5 were less clearly defined, but appeared to come from rural environments and did less well in school. Wrobel and Lachar (1992) found that male adolescents who scored high on scale 5 were more frequently described by their parents as fearful, and high scale 5 females were more frequently rated as aggressive. Williams and Butcher (1989a) reported that they were unable to find clinically relevant descriptors for scale 5 in their study of adolescent inpatients. In a reanalysis of these data for MMPI-A scales, however, Butcher et al. (1992) found high scores related to the occurrence of behavior problems for girls and fewer legal actions for boys.

High Scores on Scale 5

The following is a summary of descriptors for high scale 5 males (T ≥ 60):

- Intelligent, aesthetic interests, higher levels of academic achievement.
- Possible areas of insecurity or conflict regarding sexual identity.
- Emotional and comfortable in expressing feelings and emotions with others.
- Passive and submissive in interpersonal relationships.
- Lower likelihood of antisocial or delinquent behaviors.

The following is a summary of high scale 5 characteristics for females (T ≥ 60):

- Vigorous and assertive.
- Competitive, aggressive, tough minded.
- Greater problems in terms of school conduct.
- Increased frequency of behavioral problems.
- Interests in traditionally "masculine" academic areas and competitive sports.

Low Scores on Scale 5

The following is a summary of low scale 5 characteristics for males (T ≤ 40):

- Presentation of self with extremely masculine emphasis.
- Higher frequency of delinquency and school conduct problems.
- Overemphasis on strength, often accompanied by crude and coarse behaviors.

- Lower intellectual ability and academic achievement.
- Relatively narrow range of interests defined by traditional masculine role.

The following is a summary of low scale 5 characteristics for females (T ≤ 40):

- Presentation of self in stereotyped female role.
- Passive, yielding, and submissive in interpersonal relationships.
- Lower socioeconomic background.
- Higher levels of academic performance.
- Lower incidence of learning disabilities.

5-6/6-5 Codetype.

Friedman et al. (2015) and Greene (2011) provided the only available information concerning the 5-6/6-5 codetype among the commonly used guides to interpretation of adult profiles. Both sources indicate that little is known concerning this codetype among adults. The 5-6/6-5 codetype is found with a frequency of only 0.5% for males and 1.1% for females in treatment settings for adolescents (see Table 5.5). Marks et al. (1974) presented the 5-6/6-5 codetype based on findings from 11 adolescents. Thus, the 5-6/6-5 is a relatively rare codetype and very limited data are available concerning the characteristics of individuals who produce this MMPI configuration.

Most of the descriptors identified by Marks et al. (1974) for adolescents with the 5-6/6-5 profile appear to be related to the scale 6 elevation. Although teenagers with this codetype were able to acknowledge psychological problems with their therapists, they were often hesitant to establish deep or frequent contacts with them. In general, they were seen as fearful of emotional involvement with others. Of this group, 30.6% were given a good prognosis by their therapists, a percentage that is roughly three times higher than that found by Marks et al. for therapists' ratings for other codetypes. The 5-6/6-5 adolescents were described as resentful and insecure, and acting out was their primary defense mechanism.

The majority of teenagers in this small codetype grouping had a history of drug abuse, which entailed a variety of psychoactive drug classes. Additionally, a history of violent actions appeared to be associated with the 5-6/6-5 adolescent. Legal actions and arrests were reported for such offenses as assault and battery and assault with a deadly weapon. Marks et al. (1974) described this group as preoccupied with themes of death, murder, and brutality.

5-9/9-5 Codetype.

Like the previous codetype, the 5-9/9-5 profile has received little research attention in the adult literature. A summary of the literature on this configuration may be found in Friedman et al. (2015) and in Greene (2011). This codetype is found with a frequency of only 0.3% for male and 2.6% for female adolescent psychiatric patients (Archer, Gordon, &

Klinefelter, 1991). Marks et al. (1974) identified 10 teenagers with the 5-9 code and 10 teenagers with the 9-5 code in their clinical samples used to develop codetype descriptors.

In general, teenagers who produced the 5-9/9-5 code appeared to display substantially less psychopathology than adolescents from other codetype groups. Their overall degree of disturbance was typically judged to be mild to moderate. Primary defense mechanisms for this code appear to be rationalizations for the 5-9 group, and denial for the 9-5 codetype. Psychotherapists found that conflicts regarding emotional dependency and assertiveness were primary problems among these adolescents. One-third of the adolescents in the Marks et al. (1974) sample reported that they were raised by their mothers in a single-parent household.

A slight majority of 5-9/9-5 adolescents (56%) were found to have a history of drug abuse in the 1970–1973 Marks et al. sample. In contrast to adolescents from other codetype groups, members of the 5-9/9-5 group typically did well in school. None of these teenagers had been suspended or expelled from school, and in general they appeared to value academic achievement and emphasize aesthetic interests. Nevertheless, the parents of the teenagers with this codetype reported that they were unmanageable and rebellious. Family conflicts, rather than peer conflicts, appear to be most characteristic of this group.

5-0/0-5 **Codetype.** Consistent with the other high-point codes involving scale 5, little information is available on adults with the 5-0/0-5 codetype and what data are available are summarized in Friedman et al. (2015) and in Greene (2011). This configuration is found in 0.3% of male and 1.1% of female adolescents evaluated in clinical settings. The Marks et al. (1974) 5-0/0-5 codetype was created based on a sample of only 11 adolescents.

Consistent with the elevations on scales 5 and 0, adolescents with the 5-0/0-5 codetype in the Marks et al. (1974) study were seen as cautious, anxious, and inhibited teenagers who were fearful of emotional involvement with others. They did not employ acting out as a defense mechanism, generally exhibited few problems in impulse control, and did not report histories of antisocial behaviors. In fact, teenagers with this codetype typically exhibit overcontrol and are ruminative and overideational. Slightly more than one-third of the teenagers in the 5-0/0-5 codetype were involved in special education classroom settings, including classes for emotionally disturbed children.

The majority of adolescents with the 5-0/0-5 codetype perceive their major problems as social awkwardness and difficulty in forming friendships. In general, they describe themselves as awkward, shy, timid, inhibited, cautious, and submissive. Therapists tended to view these adolescents as manifesting severe anxiety. Major conflicts for these adolescents typically involve sexuality and difficulties in assertive behavior. The general picture that emerges for this codetype group is that of adolescents who retreat into personal isolation rather than reaching out to others in interpersonal relationships.

Scale 6 (Pa: Paranoia) Codetypes

Scale 6, in both the MMPI and the MMPI-A, consists of 40 items that were created to assess an individual's standing in relation to symptomatology involving ideas of reference, suspiciousness, feelings of persecution, moral self-righteousness, and rigidity. Although many of the items in scale 6 deal with overt psychotic symptoms such as ideas of reference and delusions of persecution, there are also large groups of items dealing with interpersonal sensitivity, cynicism, and rigidity that are not necessarily psychotic markers or symptoms. Further, Graham (2012) noted that it is possible to achieve an elevated T-score value on scale 6 without endorsing overtly or blatantly psychotic symptomatology. Harris and Lingoes (1955) identified three subscale areas for scale 6 that include *Persecutory Ideas (Pa$_1$), Poignancy (Pa$_2$),* and *Naivete (Pa$_3$).*

Although individuals who produce marked clinical elevations on scale 6 usually present paranoid symptomatology, some paranoid patients are able to achieve within-normal-limits values on this scale. Greene (2011), for example, noted that normal-range T-score values on scale 6 are typically produced by individuals in two categories: First, respondents without paranoid symptomatology, and, second, individuals who have well-established paranoid symptomatology but maintain sufficient reality contact to avoid critically endorsing obvious items on this dimension. Unfortunately, little research has been focused on this latter group, and most of the information concerning these individuals is based on MMPI clinical lore.

Adolescents have traditionally scored somewhat higher on scale 6 than adults on the original form of the MMPI (Archer, 1987b). Pancoast and Archer (1988) found that normal adolescents (in contrast to adults) endorsed more scale 6 items related to the Harris–Lingoes *Pa1* (Persecutory Ideas) content area, reflecting the belief that one is misunderstood and unjustly punished or blamed by others. Data from Hathaway and Monachesi (1963), based on Minnesota normal adolescents, indicated that boys who scored high on scale 6 are more likely to drop out of school, perhaps as a function of their interpersonal sensitivity in the school environment. In contrast, girls who scored high on scale 6 in this sample tended to have higher IQ scores and better academic grade averages, and were considered well-adjusted by others. Hathaway and Monachesi observed that moderate elevations on scale 6 appear to be an academic and social asset for girls, whereas boys with elevations on scale 6 tended to get into greater academic and social difficulties, perhaps reflecting increased aggressiveness for the males. Hathaway, Monachesi, and Salasin (1970) reported, in a follow-up study of the Hathaway and

Monachesi (1963) sample, that elevations on scales 6 and 8 were associated with poor academic and social outcomes primarily among adolescents with average or lower levels of intelligence. Lachar and Wrobel (1990) found that outpatient adolescent males who produced high scale 6 scores were more likely to be described as distrustful and suspicious, and more likely to manifest delusions of persecution or paranoia. Butcher et al. (1992) found scale 6 elevations related to neurotic/dependent and hostile/withdrawn behaviors for male adolescent inpatients. Overall, it appears that clinically relevant scale 6 descriptor patterns for female adolescents have been difficult to identify in these research investigations, and that more is known concerning the correlate patterns for teenage boys.

High Scores on Scale 6

The following is a summary of characteristics for individuals who produced marked elevations on scale 6 (T ≥ 70):

- Anger, resentment, hostility.
- Use of projection as primary defense mechanism.
- Disturbances in reality testing.
- Delusions of persecution or grandeur.
- Ideas of reference.
- Diagnoses often associated with the manifestation of thought disorder as exhibited in psychosis or schizophrenia.
- Social withdrawal.

The following are features usually associated with moderate elevations on scale 6 (T = 60 to 69):

- Marked interpersonal sensitivity.
- Suspicion and distrust in interpersonal relationships.
- Tendencies toward hostility, suspiciousness, resentfulness, and argumentativeness.
- Problems in school adjustment.
- Increased disagreements with parents.
- Difficulty in establishing therapeutic relationships due to interpersonal guardedness.

Low Scores on Scale 6

The following are associated with low scale 6 features (T ≤ 40):

- Lower levels of intelligence and academic achievement.
- Presentation of self as cheerful and balanced.

- Cautious and conventional.
- Interpersonally insensitive, unaware of the feelings and motives of others.
- If psychiatric patient, possibility of overcompensation for paranoid symptoms.

6-8/8-6 Codetype. The *6-8/8-6* codetype is indicative of serious psychopathology for both teenagers and adults. This codetype has clearly been associated with paranoid symptomatology, including delusions of grandeur, feelings of persecution, hallucinations, and outbursts of hostility. Individuals with this codetype appear to be socially isolated and withdrawn, and their behavior is frequently unpredictable and inappropriate. Difficulties in thought processes are often apparent, ranging from deficits in concentration to bizarre and schizophrenic ideation. It would appear that the *6-8/8-6* individual frequently has difficulty in differentiating between fantasy and reality, and will often withdraw into autistic fantasy in response to stressful events.

The *6-8/8-6* codetype occurs with a frequency of 3.2% for male and 3.4% for female adolescents in psychiatric settings (see Table 5.5). Adolescents with this codetype are typically referred for treatment in response to the occurrence of bizarre behaviors or excessive fantasy. As children, this group appear to have been subjected to physical punishment as a primary form of discipline. Nearly half of the adolescents with this codetype in the Marks et al. (1974) sample had received beatings as punishment for misbehaviors. Additionally, the majority of these adolescents had fathers who had committed either minor or major legal offenses, and 30% of these teenagers had attended five or more school settings within their elementary education years.

The *6-8/8-6* adolescents often have a violent temper and, when angry, these teenagers may express their feelings directly (e.g., by hitting others or throwing objects). They are not liked by their peers and they often perceive their peer group as "picking on" them or teasing them. In general, these adolescents were preoccupied with their physical appearance, and ratings by their psychotherapists indicated that they were, indeed, below average in appearance. The predominant affective distress for these teenagers included moderate depression and feelings of guilt and shame. Adolescents with this codetype were frequently delusional and displayed grandiose ideas. In the Marks et al. 1970–1973 sample, slightly over half of these teenagers had used drugs, although some of their drug use was connected with suicide attempts. As might be expected for a group of adolescents who produced this codetype, these teenagers typically displayed little or no insight into their psychological problems.

Scale 7 (Pt: Psychasthenia) Codetypes

Scale 7 in both the MMPI and MMPI-A consists of 48 items designed to measure psychasthenia, a neurotic syndrome that was later conceptualized as obsessive-compulsive neurosis and most recently labeled obsessive-compulsive disorder. Such individuals are characterized by excessive doubts, compulsions, obsessions, and high levels of tension and anxiety. Because this symptom pattern is more typically found among outpatients, the original criterion group employed by McKinley and Hathaway in the development of this scale was restricted to a relatively small group of 20 inpatients with this condition. McKinley and Hathaway were reluctant to use outpatients in their criterion groups because of their inability to confirm diagnoses for patients in this setting (Greene, 2000). The content areas of scale 7 cover a wide array of symptomatology including unhappiness, physical complaints, deficits in concentration, obsessive thoughts, anxiety, and feelings of inferiority and inadequacy. Harris and Lingoes (1955) did not identify subscales for scale 7, perhaps reflective of the relatively high degree of internal consistency (as reflected in Cronbach coefficient alpha) typically found for this MMPI Basic scale.

In general, those who score high on scale 7 have been described as anxious, tense, and indecisive individuals who are very self-critical and perfectionistic. At extreme elevations, there are often patterns of intense ruminations and obsessions constituting disabling symptomatology. Low scores on this scale are frequently indicative of self-confident, secure, and emotionally stable individuals who are achievement and success oriented. Greene (2011) noted that females typically endorse two to three more scale 7 items than men. Data from normal adolescents as reported by Hathaway and Monachesi (1963) showed that scale 7 high-point elevations were more common in adult than adolescent profiles, although scale 7 was the most frequently elevated neurotic scale in adolescent MMPI profiles. Scale 7 has also been reported to be a relatively rare high point among adolescent profiles in clinical settings (Archer, 1989). Data for adolescent outpatients, reported by Lachar and Wrobel (1990), indicated that high scale 7 males and females were described as overly self-critical, anxious, tense, nervous, and restless. Wrobel and Lachar (1992) reported that high scale 7 scores for male and female adolescents were related to an increased frequency of nightmares. Butcher et al. (1992) found that a clinical sample of girls who produced elevations on MMPI-A scale 7 were more likely to be described as depressed and to report an increase in disagreements with their parents. Veltri et al. (2009) reported that both boys and girls who produced higher scale 7 scores were more likely to report suicidal ideation, and Handel et al. (2011) reported increased anxiety and depression for both boys and girls with scale 7 elevations in forensic settings.

High Scores on Scale 7

The following is a summary of characteristics associated with high scale 7 scores (T ≥ 60):

- Anxious, tense, and apprehensive.
- Self-critical, perfectionistic approach to life.

- Feelings of insecurity, inadequacy, and inferiority.
- Emotionally overcontrolled and uncomfortable with feelings.
- Introspective and ruminative.
- Lacking in self-confidence and ambivalent in decision-making situations.
- Rigid, moralistic, conscientious.
- At marked elevations, obsessive thought patterns and compulsive behaviors.

Low Scores on Scale 7

The following are features associated with low scale 7 scores (T ≤ 40):

- Lack of emotional distress and freedom from anxiety and tension.
- Capable and self-confident in approach to problems.
- Perceived as warm, cheerful, and relaxed.
- Flexible, efficient, and adaptable.

7-8/8-7 Codetype. The 7-8/8-7 profile appears to be related to the occurrence of inadequate defenses and poor stress tolerance for both adults and adolescents. These individuals are frequently described as socially isolated, withdrawn, anxious, and depressed. There is also evidence that individuals with the 7-8/8-7 codetype feel insecure and inadequate. They have substantial difficulty in modulating their feelings and expressing their emotions in appropriate ways.

The 7-8/8-7 codetype is found among 1.8% of male and 1.9% of female adolescents in psychiatric settings (Archer, Gordon, & Klinefelter, 1991). Among adolescents, this profile configuration appears to be related to the presence of substantial tension resulting from failing defenses. These adolescents were typically described as anxious and depressed. They were also inhibited and conflicted in terms of their interpersonal relationships, particularly those involving aspects of emotional dependency. Many of these teenagers expressed fears of failure in school, and Marks et al. (1974) reported that roughly one-half of this sample had failed at least one academic grade.

In the adult literature, the relationship in elevation between scales 7 and 8 is frequently cited as a highly significant factor in interpretation of this profile. Scale 7 is seen as a suppressor of scale 8 symptomatology such that profiles displaying higher elevations on scale 7 (relative to scale 8) are seen as more neurotic, whereas profiles containing higher elevations on scale 8 (relative to scale 7) are frequently seen as indicative of more schizophrenic symptomatology. Marks et al. (1974) noted that there is no evidence of this phenomenon among the adolescents in their 7-8/8-7 codetype. Specifically, based on their data from the 1970–1973 sample, they observed that 7-8s and 8-7s were both quite deviant in thought and behavior, and nearly one-half of these adolescents had experienced either auditory or visual hallucinations.

7-9/9-7 **Codetype.**   Across both adult and adolescent respondents, the *7-9/9-7* codetype appears to be associated with tension, anxiety, and rumination. Over three-fourths of the adolescents with this codetype were characterized by their therapists as worriers who were vulnerable to both real and unrealistic threats and fears. For adults with this codetype, Greene (2011) recommended that the possibility of manic features be investigated and that psychopharmaco-logical medications be considered for the reduction of high levels of anxiety, agitation, and excitement.

Among adolescents in clinical settings, the *7-9/9-7* codetype occurs with a frequency of 1.7% for males and 0.7% for females (Archer, Gordon, & Klinefelter, 1991). Adolescents with this codetype were described by Marks et al. as insecure. These adolescents also tended to have strong needs for atten-tion, conflicts involving emotional dependency issues, and fears of losing control. They were tense and had difficulty "letting go," but did not show evidence of scale *9* manic characteristics such as elation. In general, these teen-agers appeared to be defensive when discussing their psychological problems, and very sensitive to demands placed on them by others. Within the adoles-cent sample, scale *7* correlates were more predominant for this codetype than scale *9* characteristics.

7-0/0-7 **Codetype.**   The *7-0/0-7* codetype appears to be rare among adults, and is found with a frequency of 1.3% for male and 1.2% for female adolescents in clinical settings (Archer, Gordon, & Klinefelter, 1991). Marks et al. (1974) were able to identify only 11 adolescents with this codetype in their research sample. For both adolescents and adults, this codetype appears related to the presence of neurotic symptomatology, including excessive anxiety, tension, social introversion, and shyness.

The predominant presenting problems for the *7-0/0-7* adolescents consisted of shyness and extreme sensitivity. Although defiant and disobedient behaviors were relatively common for this group, these characteristics tended to occur with a base rate frequency that was lower than that of many other adolescent codetype groups. Interestingly, almost one-half of these adolescents had family members with a his-tory of psychiatric disorder. Psychotherapists responded positively to adolescents with the *7-0/0-7* codetype and indicated that they displayed moderate motiva-tion for treatment, good treatment prognosis, and good cognitive-verbal insight. These teenagers performed well in academic settings and maintained high needs for achievement. Reaction formation and isolation appear to be the predomi-nant defense mechanisms for the *7-0/0-7* adolescent. These individuals become intropunitive in response to stress or frustration, and have a decided tendency toward emotional overcontrol. Marks et al. (1974) noted that these adolescents are basically insecure and tend to have conflicts regarding emotional dependency and assertion.

Scale 8 (Sc: Schizophrenia) Codetypes

Scale 8 consists of 77 items and constitutes the largest MMPI-A scale. One item, related to sexuality, was deleted from the original scale 8 in the modification of this measure for the MMPI-A. Scale 8 was developed to identify patients with schizophrenia, and deals with content areas involving bizarre thought processes, peculiar thoughts, social isolation, difficulties in concentration and impulse control, and disturbances in mood and behavior. Harris and Lingoes (1955) identified six subscales within the schizophrenia scale: *Social Alienation (Sc1); Emotional Alienation (Sc2); Lack of Ego Mastery, Cognitive (Sc3); Lack of Ego Mastery, Conative (Sc4); Lack of Ego Mastery, Defective Inhibition (Sc5); and Bizarre Sensory Experiences (Sc6).*

Individuals who score high on scale 8 are typically described as alienated, confused, and delusional. They often display psychotic features, and are socially isolated, withdrawn, shy, and apathetic. Extreme elevations on scale 8, particularly T-score values in excess of 100 for adults and 90 for adolescents, are typically produced by clients who are not schizophrenic but are experiencing intense, acute situational distress. Greene (2011) noted that an adolescent undergoing a severe identity crisis may frequently score in this extreme range. Individuals who score markedly low in scale 8 have typically been described as conventional, cautious, compliant persons who may be overly accepting of authority and who place a premium on practical and concrete thinking. Comprehensive reviews of the MMPI literature on schizophrenia in adult populations were provided by Walters (1983, 1988).

Research on scale 8 has shown a large degree of difference in the mean raw score endorsement patterns between adolescent and adult normals, with adolescents typically endorsing substantially more scale 8 items than their adult counterparts (Archer, 1984, 1987b; Pancoast & Archer, 1988). Hathaway and Monachesi (1963) found that boys were more likely than girls to have profiles that exhibited scale 8 as the highest point. Further, both male and female adolescents who produced high scale 8 scores were likely to be lower in intelligence and in academic achievement than other adolescents. High scale 8 girls were also more likely to drop out of school. Archer et al. (1988) found that high scale 8 adolescent inpatients were described as mistrustful, vulnerable to stress, interpersonally isolated, and socially withdrawn. Often, these adolescents had presenting problems that included impaired reality testing. Archer and Gordon (1988) found that scale 8 scores were significantly associated with schizophrenic diagnoses in an adolescent inpatient sample. Employing a criterion of a T-score value of ≥ 75 to identify schizophrenia, an overall hit rate of 76% was obtained. This result is comparable to Hathaway's (1956) original finding for this scale in adult samples. Butcher et al. (1992) found MMPI-A scale 8 elevations to be associated with higher levels of acting out, schizoid, and psychotic behaviors among adolescent male inpatients. They also reported an association between scale 8 elevations and histories of sexual abuse for both male and female inpatients. In addition to schizophrenia, adolescent scale 8 elevations may reflect a teenager's drug use history, particularly previous experiences with hallucinatory drugs (Archer, 1989). Interpretation of elevated scale 8 values, therefore, require the clinician's awareness of the adolescent's drug-taking history and behaviors (Archer & Krishnamurthy, 2002). Review of critical item endorsements and Harris–Lingoes subscales may often be used as a vehicle through which to determine whether an adolescent's scale 8 elevation represents a result of drug-taking experiences or actual schizophrenic symptomatology. Lachar and Wrobel (1990) found high scale 8 scores among adolescent inpatients to be related to frequent experiences of frustration, and Wrobel and Lachar (1992) found high scale 8 adolescents were often rejected and teased by other children. Handel et al. (2011) reported scale 8 scores related to total number of problems and social problems for boys and girls in the forensic sample, and Veltri et al. (2009) found high scale 8 scores related to a history of physical abuse for boys.

High Scores on Scale 8

The following are characteristics associated with high scale 8 scores (T ≥ 60):

- Withdrawn, seclusive, and socially isolated.
- Confused and disorganized.
- Presence of schizoid features.
- Feelings of inferiority, incompetence, low self-esteem, and dissatisfaction.
- Feelings of frustration and unhappiness.
- Rejection and teasing by peers.
- Poor school adjustment and performance.
- Vulnerable and easily upset.
- Reluctance to engage in interpersonal relationships, including psychotherapy relationships.
- Nonconforming, unconventional, and socially deviant.
- Poor reality testing.
- At marked elevations (T ≥ 70), associated with delusions, hallucinations, and other schizophrenic symptoms.

Low Scores on Scale 8

The following are characteristics of low scale 8 scores (T ≤ 40):

- Conforming, conventional, and conservative.
- Logical, practical, and achievement oriented.
- Unimaginative and cautious in approaches to problem solving.
- Responsible, cooperative, and dependable.

8-9/9-8 **Codetype.** The occurrence of an *8-9/9-8* codetype in either adolescence or adulthood appears to be related to the presence of serious psychopathology. Individuals who produce this MMPI configuration have been referred to as immature, self-centered, argumentative, and demanding. Although these individuals seek a great deal of attention, they are resentful and hostile in interpersonal relationships and display little capacity to form close relationships with others. Acting out, often of an unpredictable nature, is a salient defense mechanism for this codetype.

As shown in Table 5.5, the *8-9/9-8* codetype is found for 1.5% of male and 1.0% of female adolescents in psychiatric settings. Many of the respondents with this codetype display evidence of thought disorder, including grandiose ideas, as well as evidence of hyperactivity and a very rapid personal tempo. Marks et al. (1974) noted that adolescents with a *9-8* codetype appear to "think, talk, and move, at an unusually fast pace" (p. 239). For both adolescents and adults, this codetype has been associated with the presence of both schizophrenic and paranoid symptomatology. Within the Marks et al. 1970–1973 sample, this codetype was not particularly associated with substance abuse or addiction. In the Archer and Klinefelter (1992) study, however, the *8-9/9-8* code was related to significantly higher MAC scale elevations for female adolescent psychiatric patients. In a study by Archer and Slesinger (1999), this codetype was associated with a higher frequency of report of suicidal ideation on the suicide-related MMPI-A items (items 177, 283, and 399).

Scale 9 (Ma: Hypomania) Codetypes

Scale *9*, in both the original MMPI and the MMPI-A, consists of 46 items developed to identify patients manifesting hypomanic symptomatology. The content areas covered in this scale are relatively broad and include grandiosity, egocentricity, irritability, elevated mood, and cognitive and behavioral overactivity. Harris and Lingoes (1955) identified four content subscales contained within the hypomania scale: *Amorality (Ma1), Psychomotor Acceleration (Ma2), Imperturbability (Ma3), and Ego Inflation (Ma4)*.

Greene (2011) noted that scale *9* elevations are often difficult to interpret in isolation. In this sense, elevations on scale *9* are often seen as facilitating or moderating the expression of qualities or characteristics identified by elevations on other clinical scales, particularly scales *D* and *Pd*. High scores on scale *9* have been related to impulsivity, excessive activity, narcissism, social extroversion, and a preference for action in contrast to thought and reflection. In addition, individuals who score high on this scale may display manic features such as flight of ideas, delusions of grandeur, and hyperactivity. Lumry, Gottesman, and Tuason (1982), however, demonstrated that individuals with bipolar disorder provide very different MMPI profiles depending on the phase of the disorder during which the patient is assessed. For example, patients in the depressed phase produced a profile characterized by elevations on scales 2 and 7, whereas patients assessed during the manic phase produced spike 9 profiles. These findings indicate that the accurate diagnosis of bipolar disorder may require a longitudinal series of MMPI administrations because of the state dependency nature of MMPI assessment. Markedly low scores on scale 9 (T-score values below 44) have been related to lethargy, apathy, listlessness, and decreased motivational states (Greene, 2011).

Normal adolescents typically endorse substantially more scale 9 items than do adults (Archer, 1984, 1987b). Pancoast and Archer (1988) showed that adolescents are particularly likely to endorse scale 9 items related to the Harris–Lingoes content area of Psychomotor Acceleration, which measures feelings of restlessness and the need to engage in activity. Hathaway and Monachesi (1963) found low scores on scale 9 in their sample of normal adolescents to be associated with lower rates of delinquency. In general, the teenagers who scored low on this scale in the Minnesota sample were well-behaved and conforming, and demonstrated high levels of achievement in the academic setting.

In adolescent psychiatric outpatient samples, Lachar and Wrobel (1990) reported that elevations on scale 9 are related to the occurrence of temper tantrums. Boys who score high on scale 9 were described as hostile or argumentative, and girls were found to display rapid mood shifts and a tendency not to complete tasks that they undertake. Archer et al. (1988) reported that high scale 9 adolescent inpatients were described as impulsive, insensitive to criticism, and unrealistically optimistic in terms of their goal setting and aspirations. Archer and Klinefelter (1992) found that elevations on scale 9 were associated with higher scores on the MAC scale. Butcher et al. (1992) found high MMPI-A scale 9 scores among adolescents in inpatient settings to be associated with amphetamine abuse for boys and more frequent school suspensions for girls. Veltri et al. (2009) found that girls in an inpatient sample who produced higher scale 9 scores were rated as more oppositional, and Handel et al. (2011) found that both boys and girls in their court-referred sample who produced higher scale 9 scores were rated as more rule-breaking and externalizing, and reported more conduct problems.

High Scores on Scale 9

The following features are associated with high-point elevations on scale 9 (T ≥ 60):

- Accelerated personal tempo and excessive activity.
- Preference for action rather than thought and reflection.
- Impulsivity, restlessness, and distractibility.
- Lack of realism, and grandiosity in goal setting and aspirations.
- Outgoing, socially extroverted, and gregarious.
- Talkative and energetic.
- Egocentric, self-centered, insensitive, self-indulgent.

- Greater likelihood of school conduct problems and delinquent behaviors.
- Emotionally labile.
- Flight of ideas, euphoric mood, grandiose self-perceptions.

Low Scores on Scale 9

The following are characteristics or features associated with low scale 9 scores (T ≤ 40):

- Low energy level.
- Quiet, seclusive, withdrawn, depressed.
- Overcontrolled, inhibited, overly responsible.
- Decreased probability of acting out or delinquent behaviors.
- Depressed, lethargic, and apathetic.

Scale 0 (Si: Social Introversion) Codetypes

The MMPI-A Si scale consists of 62 items, reflecting the deletion of eight items from the original Si scale. Additionally, two items retained on the MMPI-A Si scale are keyed in the opposite direction from traditional scoring for this scale. These abbreviated items are:

No. 308 Bothered by trivial thoughts. (Scored in *true* direction on MMPI-A, *false* direction on original MMPI.)

No. 334 People often jealous of my ideas. (Scored in *true* direction on MMPI-A, *false* direction on original MMPI.)

The scoring direction of these items was modified for the MMPI-A because of the belief that the original scoring was both counterintuitive and incorrect. The Si scale was originally developed by Drake (1946) based on the responses of college students who produced extreme scores on a social introversion/extroversion measure. Elevated T-scores on the Si scale reflect greater degrees of social introversion. Although Harris and Lingoes did not attempt to create specific subscales for the social introversion scale, three Si subscales were created for the MMPI-2 and the MMPI-A based on a factor analytic approach. The MMPI-A Si subscales are discussed in the next chapter of this text. Graham (2012) indicated that the Si scale contains two broad clusters of items. These groups consist of items related to social participation and items related to neurotic maladjustment and self-depreciation. Graham noted that high scores on scale 0 can occur by the endorsement of either, or both, of these content areas.

Individuals who produce elevated scores on scale 0 are likely to be socially introverted, insecure, and markedly uncomfortable in social situations. They tend to be shy, timid, submissive, and lacking in self-confidence. When high scores occur for scale *0*, the potential for impulsive behaviors and acting out is decreased, and the likelihood of neurotic rumination and introspection is increased. Individuals who produce low scores on the *Si* scale are described as socially extroverted, gregarious, friendly, and outgoing. These individuals appear to have strong affiliation needs and are interested in social status, acceptance, and recognition. Low scorers may be subject to impulse control problems, and their relations with others may be more superficial than sincere and long enduring.

Greene (2011) noted that adolescents and college students typically scored toward the extroverted pole of the *Si* scale, and that *Si* scores tend to decrease somewhat with increasing years of education. Hathaway and Monachesi (1963) found an interesting pattern of correlates for scale *0* scores in their sample of Minnesota normal adolescents. Social introversion was a relatively frequent finding among boys and girls from rural farm settings, whereas social extroversion was characteristic of adolescents from families with parents in professional occupations. Intriguingly, low scale *0* profiles were found for children with higher intelligence levels but with spotty records of academic achievement. Hathaway and Monachesi interpreted these findings as indicating that there was a potential conflict between an adolescent's social interest and success, and his or her academic achievement.

Among psychiatrically disturbed adolescents, Lachar and Wrobel (1990) found that outpatients who produce high values on scale *0* are described as having few or no friends, and as being very shy. These teenagers often avoided calling attention to themselves and they did not initiate relationships with other adolescents. Butcher et al. (1992) found adolescent inpatients with elevations on scale *0* were described as socially withdrawn and manifesting low self-esteem. In addition, female adolescents with elevated scale *0* scores had lower levels of delinquency, acting out, and drug or alcohol use. Handel et al. (2011) found scale *0* related to higher levels of anxiety and depression in their forensic sample, and Veltri et al. (2009) reported similar results in their recent MMPI-A study.

High Scores on Scale 0

The following are features that have been associated with adolescents who score high on scale *0* (T $\geq$ 60):

- Social introversion and social discomfort.
- Low self-esteem.
- Reserved, timid, socially retiring.
- Decreased probability of delinquent or acting out behaviors.
- Submissive, compliant, accepting of authority.
- Insecure and lacking in self-confidence.
- Overcontrolled, difficult to get to know, interpersonally hypersensitive.

- Reliable, dependable, cautious.
- Lacking in social skills.

Low Scores on Scale 0

The following are features associated with adolescents who score low on scale *0* (T ≤ 40):

- Sociable, extroverted, gregarious.
- Intelligent, with a possible history of academic underachievement.
- Active, energetic, talkative.
- Interested in social influence, power, recognition.
- Socially confident and competent.

Factors Potentially Affecting Codetype Interpretation

A substantial amount of research literature has established that demographic variables such as race, gender, and age *may* significantly influence the MMPI profiles of adult respondents (Dahlstrom et al. 1975). In this regard, Schinka, Elkins, and Archer (1998) used multiple regression analyses to examine the effects of age, gender, and ethnic background on variance in MMPI-A raw scores for adolescents in normal and clinical settings. The analyses were designed to measure the incremental contribution of demographic variables to scale variance beyond that explained by the presence of psychopathology. All of the MMPI-A Validity and Clinical scales were characterized by small (< 10%) amounts of incremental variances in MMPI-A scores accounted for by demographic variables. Similarly, the MMPI-A Content and Supplementary scales did not appear to be meaningfully influenced by an adolescent's age, gender, or ethnic background. Before leaving this topic, however, each of these areas is examined in more detail in terms of the probable effects of these variables on codetype interpretation practices for the MMPI-A.

Race/Ethnic Factors

Gynther (1972) reviewed the literature on the influence of race on adults' MMPI scores and concluded that distinctive racial differences reliably occur that reflect variations in respective cultural and environmental backgrounds of Black and White respondents. In particular, Gynther interpreted findings from the analyses of item differences as indicating that the high scores for Blacks on scales *F*, *Sc*, and *Ma* reflected differences in perceptions, expectations, and values rather than differential levels of psychological adjustment. He called for the development of MMPI norms for Black respondents in order to allow for more accurate assessment of psychopathology in Black populations. Later, Gynther (1989) reevaluated the literature on comparisons of MMPI profiles from Blacks and Whites and concluded that, in the absence of studies employing unbiased criterion measures to evaluate potential racial differences, "definite conclusions to the racial bias question may be exceptionally difficult to reach" (p. 878).

The early studies that investigated the variable of subject race within adolescent populations appeared to support Gynther's 1972 position regarding the presence of racial differences in MMPI scale values. Ball (1960) examined MMPI scale elevations for a group of 31 Black and 161 White ninth-graders and found that Black males tended to score higher on scale *Hs* than White male students, and that Black female students produced significantly higher elevations on scales *F*, *Sc*, and *Si* than did White females. Similarly, McDonald and Gynther (1962) examined the MMPI response patterns of Black and White students within segregated high school settings. These findings indicated that Black students produced higher scores than their White counterparts on scales *L*, *F*, *K*, *Hs*, *D*, and *Ma*. Further, Black female students had significantly higher scores on all MMPI scales, with the exception of *K* and *Sc*, than did White female students.

Research results have suggested that when Blacks and Whites have experienced common cultural influences and socioeconomic backgrounds, racial differences are less likely to be found in MMPI profile elevations. Klinge and Strauss (1976) and Lachar, Klinge, and Grissell (1976) reported no significant MMPI differences between samples of Black and White adolescents. These results were attributable to the observation that the Black and White respondents in these investigations had been raised and educated in similar or equivalent environments. Bertelson, Marks, and May (1982) matched 462 psychiatric inpatients (of whom 144 were adolescents) on variables such as gender, age, residence, education, employment, and socioeconomic status. No significant MMPI differences were found for the matched racial samples in this study. Archer (1987b) reported evidence of minimal racial differences between groups of Black and White male and female adolescents from a predominantly middle-class public high school setting.

Marks et al. (1974) included 61 Black subjects in the clinical population they used to derive correlate descriptors of adolescent codetype profiles. These subjects were part of their Ohio State University Health Center sample. The authors found few Black–White differences among the descriptors generated for their adolescent codetypes, and statements regarding race of subject are seldom made in the Marks et al. (1974) text. Green and Kelley (1988) investigated the relationship between MMPI scores and external behavioral and interview criteria in 333 White and 107 Black male juvenile delinquents. They reported that as the apparent objectivity of the criterion increased, evidence of racial bias decreased (i.e., the predictability of the criteria did not differ as a function of race).

Figures 5.7 and 5.8 show the MMPI-A profile findings for Black, White, and other male respondents in the normative sample for this instrument, and

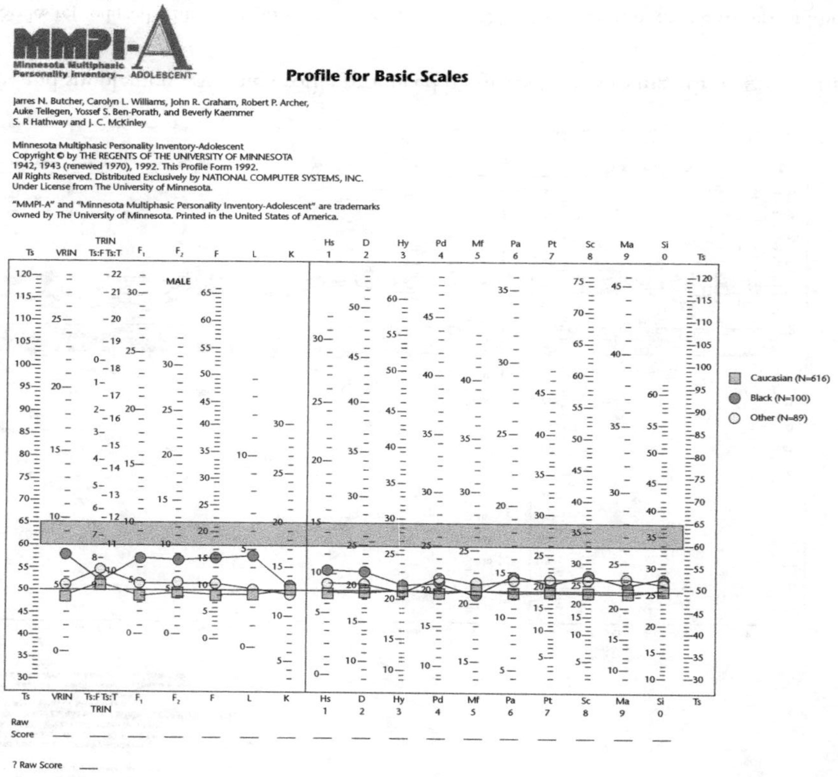

FIGURE 5.7 MMPI-A basic scale profiles produced by males from varying ethnic groups in the MMPI-A normative sample.

Source: MMPI-A profile for Basic Scales reproduced with the permission. Copyright © 1992 by the Regents of the University of Minnesota.

Note: TRIN T-score values were calculated for this profile based on conversions from the mean raw score value for each sample.

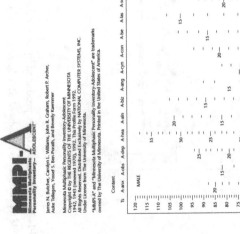

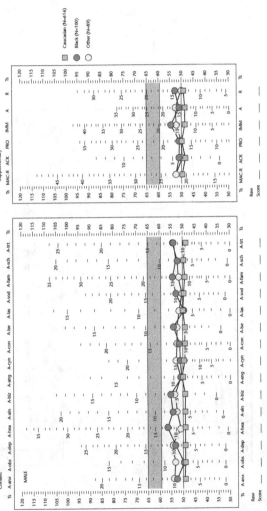

FIGURE 5.8 MMPI-A content and supplementary scale profile produced by males from varying ethnic groups in the MMPI-A normative sample.

Source: MMPI-A profile for Basic Scales reproduced with the permission. Copyright © 1992 by the Regents of the University of Minnesota.

Figures 5.9 and 5.10 show comparable data for females. These profiles show racial or ethnic differences of about 3 to 5 T-score points across MMPI Clinical scales L, F, 4, 6, 7, 8, and 9. Demographic data for this sample, however, indicate a significant socioeconomic difference between these three ethnic groupings as reflected in adolescents' reports of parental occupation and socioeconomic status. Thus, the relatively limited profile differences found between these groups reflect both ethnic and socioeconomic effects.

Greene (1980, 1987) surveyed the literature on the issue of racial differences in MMPI response patterns. His review of studies examining Black–White differences within normal samples failed to reveal any MMPI scale that consistently demonstrated racial differences across 10 independent investigations. A similar conclusion has also been reached in a review by Pritchard and Rosenblatt (1980). Greene noted that scales F and Ma were most frequently affected by race, but that significant differences were not found for scale Sc, which had been reported by Gynther (1972) as one of the scales typically elevated among Black populations. Further, Greene noted that the actual mean differences in studies reporting significant differences between Black and White respondents typically were ≤ 5 T-score points, a range comparable to the largest racial differences found for the MMPI-A normative sample. Greene (2011) recently updated his review in this area and observed that the potential role of moderator variables, including socioeconomic status (SES), education, and intelligence, are critical in evaluating any research on MMPI-2 or MMPI-A ethnic group differences. He concluded that based on the existing literature on Black-White, Hispanic-White, Black-Hispanic, Native-American-White, and Asian-American-White, no reliable or consistent pattern of ethnic differences has been established for any group, either in mean T-score values or empirical correlates. Dahlstrom, Lachar, and Dahlstrom (1986) provided a comprehensive review of the relationship between ethnic status and MMPI response patterns that included data from both adolescent and adult samples. These authors concluded that this literature supports the use of the MMPI in the assessment of psychological functioning for Black clients, "since the relative accuracy of these scores were as good or better for this ethnic minority as it was for White clients" (p. 205). Goldman, Cooke, and Dahlstrom (1995) reported on the MMPI and MMPI-2 profiles of undergraduate college students who varied in terms of ethnic background, gender, and socioeconomic status. The findings from this investigation indicated that the MMPI-2 showed patterns of fewer racial or ethnic differences than the original MMPI, a result attributable to the inclusion of a significant number of Black subjects in the MMPI-2 normative sample. Timbrook and Graham (1994) examined racial or ethnic differences by analyzing the responses of 75 Black and 725 White men and 65 Black and 742 White women who were part of the MMPI-2 normative sample. The authors reported that mean differences on MMPI-2 Basic scales between

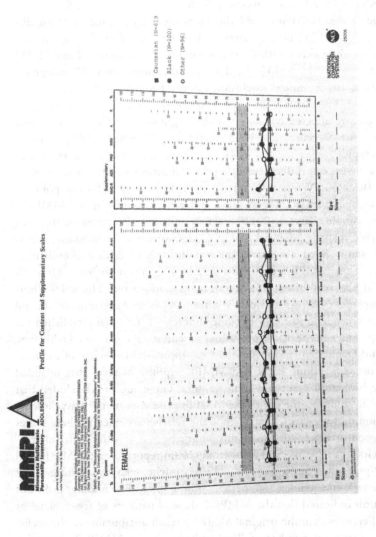

FIGURE 5.9 MMPI-A basic scale profiles produced by females from varying ethnic groups in the MMPI-A normative sample.

Source: MMPI-A profile for Basic Scales reproduced with the permission. Copyright © 1992 by the Regents of the University of Minnesota.

Note: TRIN T-score values were calculated for this profile based on conversions from the mean raw score value for each sample.

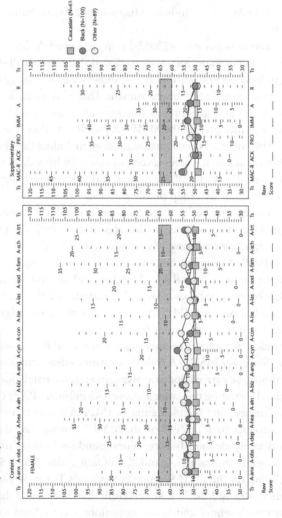

FIGURE 5.10 MMPI-A content and supplementary scale profile produced by females from varying ethnic groups in the MMPI-A normative sample.

Source: MMPI-A profile for Basic Scales reproduced with permission. Copyright © 1992 by the Regents of the University of Minnesota.

ethnic groups were small for both genders and when subjects were matched for age, education, and income, fewer MMPI-2 mean scale differences were observed. In a crucial component of this study, MMPI-2 Basic scale T-score values were correlated with personality ratings derived for these subjects. Findings did not indicate a systematic difference in the accuracy of these correlates for Black versus White subjects. The authors cautioned that the degree to which these findings may be generalized to other ethnic minorities, including American Indians, Hispanics, or Asian–Americans, is currently unknown.

Archer and Krishnamurthy (2002) briefly reviewed the literature on MMPI-A responses of ethnic minorities and concluded that the MMPI-A may be used in assessing individuals from various ethnic minority groups using the standard adolescent norms available for this instrument. They also noted, however, that given the relatively limited literature in this area, clinicians should be "appropriately conservative in interpreting the MMPI-A profiles of ethnic minority adolescents (p. 148)." They offered several further cautions including the observation that the bulk of MMPI research studies involving ethnicity have dealt with comparisons of profiles from Black and White groups, and that relatively little is known concerning other minority group profile patterns.

A number of studies, however, have been conducted examining MMPI-A profiles of Hispanic adolescents. Corrales et al. (1998), for example, has provided a comprehensive listing of research studies conducted with the MMPI-2 and the MMPI-A using U.S. Latino samples, including Puerto Ricans. This bibliography includes a total of 52 studies, and six additional resources, since 1989. Gumbiner (2000) has provided a critique of the limitations in ethnic research studies on the MMPI-A, noting that most investigators have simply compared the mean scale scores from two or more ethnic groups. Gumbiner recommended that greater research attention should be focused on the external correlates found for MMPI-A scales for various ethnic minorities, and that data analyses should be carried out to analyze findings separately for male and female adolescents. Illustrating this latter approach, Gumbiner (1998) compared Validity, Clinical, Content, and Supplementary MMPI-A scores from male and female Hispanic adolescents as profiled on the MMPI-A normative data. Analyses indicated moderately elevated T-score values found for boys on the L, F, F_1, and F_2 Validity scales, Basic scales *1*, *2* and *8*, Content scales *A-hea*, *A-biz*, *A-lse*, *A-las*, and *A-sch*, and on the *IMM* Supplementary scale. For girls, T-score values were not elevated on any MMPI-A scales. Gumbiner speculated that Hispanic boys' discomfort with school and lower aspirations were related to the lower educational and employment levels of their fathers, and that their scores from the *IMM* scale may prove useful in identifying adolescent boys "at risk" of dropping out of school.

Negy, Leal-Puente, Trainor, and Carlson (1997) investigated the MMPI-A responses of 120 Mexican-American adolescents based on the observation that

Hispanic adolescents were proportionally under-represented in the MMPI-A normative sample. Adolescents in this study completed the MMPI-A, a short demographic questionnaire, and a measure of acculturation designed for Mexican-Americans. Results indicated that the MMPI-A responses of these adolescents differed minimally from the MMPI-A normative group, and their performance varied as a function of socioeconomic status and level of acculturation.

Butcher et al. (2007) have provided a guide to assessing Hispanic clients with the MMPI-2 and MMPI-A. They noted that the MMPI instruments are the most extensively used research personality assessment tests with Spanish-speaking clients, and provided a comprehensive review of this research including the development of the Spanish language version of the MMPI-A used within the United States. Several studies have examined the performance of Hispanic adolescents in cross-national research studies. Scott, Butcher, Young, and Gomez (2002) administered the MMPI-A translation developed for use with Spanish-speaking adolescents in the United States to 385 Spanish-speaking adolescents in Columbia, Mexico, Peru, Spain, and the United States. The results of this study showed a high degree of similarity across the five countries on the MMPI-A Basic, Content, and Supplementary scales. Most scales were within 5 T-score points of the US Hispanic mean scores, and no group produced scale elevations greater than T = 65. Scott et al. concluded that their study indicated that the Hispanic MMPI-A, with its established norms, is appropriate for adaptation in Spanish-speaking countries other than the United States. Scott, Knoth, Beltran-Quiones, and Gomez (2003) reported on their use of the Hispanic MMPI-A to assess potential psychopathology in a group of 59 adolescent earthquake victims in Columbia in comparison to a control group of 62 Columbian adolescents with similar socioeconomic, educational, and ethnic backgrounds. The results of this study demonstrate the utility of the Hispanic MMPI-A in evaluating psychopathology, including evidence of post-traumatic stress disorder, in an Hispanic adolescent sample outside of the United States. Scott and his colleagues noted:

> The strength of this study is the use of the MMPI-A as the measure of psychological damage. Internationally, the MMPI-2 and the MMPI-A are the most widely recognized and most valid and clinically useful instruments to assess psychopathology. The Spanish versions of these tests are now being adapted for use throughout Latin America, including Columbia. This is the first study to use the recently released Hispanic MMPI-A to investigate the psychological effects of a natural disaster. Additional research is needed to further refine the instrument's appropriateness with disaster victims as well as other cross-national populations.
>
> (p. 55)

Scott et al. (2003) assessed the psychological functioning of 59 adolescent earthquake victims in Columbia, in contrast to a control group of 62 Columbian adolescents, using a Hispanic form of the MMPI-A. Zubeidat, Sierra, Salinas, and Rojas-Garcia (2011) evaluated the Spanish version of the MMPI-A in two samples of 939 and 109 Spanish adolescents and provided extensive reliability and validity data. Scott and Mamani-Pampa (2008) compared a Peruvian normative group of 348 adolescents to the standard MMPI-A Hispanic U.S. normative sample and found few clinically significant differences. The authors concluded that the Spanish adaptation of the MMPI-A based on U.S. norms appeared appropriate for use in Peru.

In summary, the literature on ethnic or racial effects on the MMPI-A has provided mixed findings, and does not permit for firm conclusions. If ethnic differences, independent of socioeconomic factors, do occur on MMPI-A profiles, however, it appears likely that the interpretive significance of such differences is relatively limited in terms of the standard or basic clinical profile. As is discussed in the following chapter covering supplementary scales, however, there is evidence that the *MAC* (MacAndrew, 1965) and *MAC-R* scales may be less useful with Black populations (i.e., produces more false positive errors) than with White respondents.

Gender

Hathaway and Monachesi (1963), in their Minnesota statewide sample, identified gender differences in item endorsement patterns, and in the frequency of occurrence of high-point codetypes. The authors identified the presence of 63 items in which the difference in percentage of *true* endorsement by boys and girls was 25 points or more. Regarding this pattern of item endorsement differences, Hathaway and Monachesi (1963) stated that:

> It is informative to imply generalized adjectives like "sensitive" or "fearful" or "candid." Such adjectives organize the pattern of correlated items expressing the feminine role, while "inquisitive" or "desirous of active outdoor activities" or "aggressive" may better characterize the male role.
>
> (p. 41)

Table 5.6 provides the MMPI-A abbreviated items that show the largest degree of difference in percentage of *true* responses by boys and girls in the normative sample. In general, this pattern of gender-related item differences is consistent with those found by Hathaway and Monachesi for the original form of the MMPI. In total, roughly 100 items showed an endorsement rate difference of at least 10% in the MMPI-A normative sample when data were analyzed separately by gender. The issue of gender differences in item endorsement frequency on the item level, and the interpretation of such differences, has been the subject of considerable controversy. Lindsay and Widiger (1995), for example, noted the presence of several MMPI items that appear to be systematically related to

TABLE 5.6 Fifteen MMPI-A Items Showing the Greatest Gender Differences in Percentage of Endorsement as True

MMPI-A Item		% True	% True
No.	Content	Male	Female
61	Like romances.	19.0	77.8
131	Keep a diary.	19.3	73.5
59	Wish was a girl or happy that am.	9.3	60.5
139	Cry readily.	16.9	55.5
254	Never liked to play with dolls.	53.5	16.0
21	Uncontrolled laughing and crying.	30.2	63.8
64	Like poetry.	37.6	70.1
1	Like mechanics magazines.	34.5	4.0
114	Like collecting plants.	15.2	43.2
121	Very sensitive to criticism.	34.5	61.3
60	Feelings not hurt easily.	49.6	23.4
190	Like hunting.	32.0	7.1
241	Would like to be a sports reporter.	55.2	31.4
319	Love going to dances.	47.5	69.9
19	Wanted to leave home.	47.3	69.6

Source: MMPI-A abbreviated items reproduced with permission. MMPI®-A Booklet of Abbreviated Items. Copyright © 2005 by the Regents of the University of Minnesota. Reproduced with permission of the University of Minnesota Press. All rights reserved. "Minnesota Multiphasic Personality Inventory" and "MMPI" are trademarks owned by the University of Minnesota.

the gender of the respondent but not to personality dysfunction or psychopathology. The authors concluded that items producing such correlate patterns displayed evidence of gender bias. Additionally, significant gender differences have traditionally been found in the number of items omitted on the original form of the MMPI by adolescent respondents. Although religion and sex were the content areas of items most frequently omitted by both boys and girls, items related to sex were more often left unanswered by female than male respondents (Archer, 1987b).

In terms of codetype profiles on the original form of the MMPI, girls more frequently displayed peak elevations on scale Si whereas boys were more likely to have high scale Sc. Hathaway and Monachesi (1963) noted that these gender differences were likely to be more marked when adolescents were viewed against the backdrop of adolescent norms in contrast to adult norms. Interactional effects between gender of respondent and type of norms utilized to score the profile (adolescent vs. adult) on the original form of the MMPI were also reported by Ehrenworth (1984), Klinge and Strauss (1976), and by Lachar et al. (1976). The direction and meaning of these interactional findings, however, have been complex and inconsistent. In the study by Ehrenworth, for example, T-score values for male adolescent inpatients on scales F, Pt, and Sc were significantly higher than female values when adult norms were employed, but nonsignificant when adolescent norms were used. In contrast, females produced higher *Si* T-scores than males using adolescent norms, with a less marked scale difference using adult norms.

Moore and Handal (1980) examined the MMPI profile elevations of 16- and 17-year-old male and female volunteers from school settings in the St. Louis area. These data were analyzed by gender of respondent for adult *K*-corrected T-scores. They reported substantial evidence that males tended to score significantly higher than females on scales *F, Pd, Mf, Pt, Sc,* and *Ma.* MMPI gender differences were more prevalent in this sample than racial differences, with males producing MMPI profiles suggestive of greater impulsivity, problems with authority, identity confusion, and rebelliousness than their female counterparts. Similarly, Ehrenworth and Archer (1985) examined the MMPI profiles of adolescents in psychiatric treatment and found that males produced higher T-score elevations than females on several scales when adult norms were employed. Differences in profile elevations by gender were minimal, however, when adolescent norms were used in this sample. Equivalent profiles for males and females were also reported by Archer (1984) for inpatient samples employing adolescent norms. When the data presented in Table 5.5 for MMPI-A codetype frequencies were analyzed separately by gender, the *4-9/9-4* and the *4-6/6-4* codetypes were the most frequent for males, whereas the *1-3/3-1* and *2-3/3-2* codetypes were most frequent for females.

On the two-point codetype level, Marks et al. (1974) stated they found no significant differences between males and females relative to clinical correlates of codetype descriptors. The Marks et al. text, therefore, provided codetype narratives that were not differentiated by gender. Williams and Butcher (1989a) analyzed correlate data for individual scales separately by gender and concluded that:

> Our results, in most respects, show a rather limited impact of gender on MMPI descriptors for adolescents from clinical settings when using established procedures for determining MMPI behavioral correlates. Further research, especially studies using T-scores, could combine male and female subjects when sample size is a critical issue and when studying adolescents in treatment settings.
>
> (p. 259)

In contrast, Wrobel and Lachar (1992) and Lachar and Wrobel (1990), in their studies of adolescent outpatients, found substantial evidence of gender-related differences in single-scale correlates. Their findings indicated that the majority of significant correlates were gender-specific, and indicated that gender may play an important role as a moderator variable in the interpretation of MMPI findings from adolescents. As previously noted in the discussion of ethnicity, Gumbiner (2000) has recently called for analyzing data from boys and girls separately in investigations of ethnic influences on the MMPI-A.

In summary, it is clear that significant gender differences occur in item endorsement patterns for adolescent respondents, and that these differences were reflected in the perceived need for the development of separate T-score conversions for male and female respondents in the MMPI-A norms. Significant gender differences in mean raw score values can also be shown for MMPI-A special scales. For example, boys produce higher mean values than girls on the *MAC-R* and *IMM* scales. The degree to which gender differences occur following T-score conversions, however, is currently unclear. Most importantly, the research by Lachar and Wrobel (1990) and Wrobel and Lachar (1992) suggest that significant gender-related differences in correlate patterns for MMPI scales may exist, and certainly underscore this area as one in crucial need of future, systematic research. As discussed in more detail in Chapter 7, however, it can be argued that the non-gendered norms developed for the MMPI-A-RF are more appropriate if important gender differences do occur in the measurement of constructs of clinical interest. Until more research is completed, however, firm conclusions cannot be drawn concerning the degree to which reliable gender differences occur in the correlate patterns of adolescents and the most appropriate course for researchers would be to conduct analyses capable of detecting gender effects whenever possible (i.e., analyses based on obtained raw score values).

Age

Differences between adult and adolescent MMPI response patterns were briefly discussed in the first chapter of this book. It was evident that numerous items show dramatic differences in endorsement frequency as a function of whether the respondent is an adolescent versus an adult. Further, on the item level, Hathaway and Monachesi (1963) identified 24 items that showed more than 39% instability in the direction of item endorsement from the time of assessment in the ninth grade to reevaluation during the senior year of high school. Additionally, 29 items for boys and 30 items for girls were identified as showing more than 17% change in endorsement direction between the 9th and 12th-grade assessments. The authors noted that these item endorsement shifts may be the result of item instability as well as true changes in personality that occurred across this three-year period of adolescent development. Finally, these changes in item endorsement were found to be specifically related to the gender of the respondent; that is, no common items appeared on the lists for both males and females. In general, those items that were most likely to shift in endorsement direction tended to involve personal attitudes or perceptions rather than biographical information.

Herkov, Gordon, Gynther, and Greer (1994) examined the influence of age and ethnicity on perceived item subtlety in the MMPI. Sixty-seven White and 54 Black subjects were asked to rank items from scales *F* and *9* to indicate how strongly that item indicated the presence of a psychological problem. Results indicated that adolescents often perceived MMPI item subtlety in a manner that differed significantly from that of adults and reflected discernable developmental influences. Although differences in subtlety ratings were also found between Black and White adolescents on scale *F*, these differences were relatively small and substantially less than those accounted for by age. Based on these findings, the authors recommended that the Wiener–Harmon Subtle-Obvious subscales should not be used with adolescents, and should be used cautiously with minorities.

A central question concerns the degree to which MMPI scale values are related to the age of the adolescent respondent. McFarland and Sparks (1985), for example, showed that the internal consistency of a variety of personality measures is related to age and educational level in a sample of adolescents and young adults ranging in age from 13 to 25. The traditional adolescent norms created by Marks et al. (1974) provided separate adolescent T-score conversions for age groupings of 17, 16, 15, and 14 and below, suggesting that age-related raw score differences might affect adolescents' response patterns. In contrast, Colligan and Offord (1989) found little evidence of age-related effects on MMPI raw score values in their sample of 1,315 adolescents between the ages of 13 and 17, inclusive. Based on this observation, these authors produced a contemporary set of adolescent norms for the original form of the MMPI that collapsed across age groupings. In the development of the MMPI-A, there was evidence that adolescents under the age of 14 produced response patterns that differed significantly from adolescents within the age grouping of 14 through 18. Based on this observed pattern of differences, the MMPI-A norms were collapsed across ages 14 through 18, and excluded 12- and 13-year-old adolescents from the normative sample. Thus, the age differences that occurred in MMPI-A Basic scale raw score values were primarily manifested in the comparison of younger adolescents (ages 12 and 13) versus adolescents 14 years of age and older. Janus, de Grott, and Toepfer (1998), however, examined the profiles of 56 13-year-old and 85 14-year-old psychiatric inpatients. They reported no significant differences by age in mean T-scores, nor did they find evidence of age effects in frequency of occurrence of elevated profiles.

A final question concerns the degree to which MMPI profiles of adolescents at different age groups yield differences in interpretive accuracy and validity. Three studies have produced findings relevant to this issue. Findings by Lachar et al. (1976), Ehrenworth and Archer (1985), and Wimbish (1984) indicated no evidence of significant age effects for clinical accuracy ratings of narrative MMPI reports for adolescents. Lachar et al. (1976) did find, however, significant age differences when comparing accuracy ratings produced from MMPI profiles using adolescent norms versus adult *K*-corrected norms. Specifically, the authors found that interpretations of profiles from adolescent norms produced more accurate ratings than statements for adult norms for adolescents in the 12- to 13-year-old age group. These norm-related differences were not significant for accuracy ratings for adolescents in the mid-adolescent and later adolescent groupings. Examination of mean values show that although accuracy ratings remain relatively constant for adolescent norms across the three age groups (12 to 13, 14 to 15, and 16 to 17), ratings for profiles based on adult norms were substantially more inaccurate for the 12- to 13-year-old period than for the other two age groupings.

In summary, there are known and substantial differences in item endorsement patterns as a function of age when the responses of adults are contrasted with those of adolescents on the MMPI. Within adolescent age groups, however, the developers of adolescent norms have dealt with possible age-related differences in a variety of ways. In terms of the MMPI-A, and more recently the MMPI-A-RF, a major factor in excluding normative data from 12- and 13-year-old adolescents involved the degree to which the responses from this age group appeared to be substantially different than those produced by adolescents in the 14- to 18-year-old age group. Thus far, findings suggest that the accuracy of MMPI correlate statements based on profiles using adolescent norms tend to be relatively unaffected by the age of the adolescent.

6

BEYOND THE BASIC SCALES: INTERPRETING ADDITIONAL MMPI-A SCALES AND SUBSCALES

In addition to the standard or Basic Validity and Clinical scales, many supplementary or special scales were created for the MMPI. Dahlstrom, Welsh, and Dahlstrom (1972, 1975), for example, noted that more than 450 special scales have been developed for the test instrument. Butcher and Tellegen (1978) observed that there may be more MMPI special scales than there are statements in the MMPI item pool! Clopton (1978, 1979, 1982), Butcher and Tellegen (1978), and Butcher, Graham, and Ben-Porath (1995) provided critical reviews of the methodological problems encountered in the construction of MMPI special scales. Several texts have been published specifically in the area of MMPI special scale use with the original instrument. Caldwell (1988) provided interpretive information on 104 supplementary scales based on his extensive clinical experience with these measures. Levitt (1989) and Levitt and Gotts (1995) provided an overview of special scale interpretation that includes discussions of the Wiggins (1966) Content scales and the Harris–Lingoes (1955) subscales. Ben-Porath et al. (2006) have provided a guide to the Content Component subscales, the Personality Psychopathology Five (PSY-5) scales, and critical items in a supplement to the MMPI-A manual.

The MMPI-A special scales appear on several separate profile sheets. Fifteen Content scales are placed on the Profile for Content Scales, as shown for females in Figure 6.1. In addition, 28 Harris–Lingoes subscales and three *Si* subscales appear on the Profile for Harris–Lingoes and *Si* subscales, shown for males in Figure 6.2. Six Supplementary scales and the Personality Psychopathology Five (PSY-5) scales appear on a separate profile sheet shown in Figure 6.3. The Harris–Lingoes and Social Introversion subscales, and Content Component scales, are presented in the MMPI-A Score Report by Pearson. The purpose of this chapter is to review these MMPI-A special scales, beginning with the Content scales.

Content and Content Component Scales

As noted by Butcher, Graham, et al. (1990), several approaches have been taken to the analysis of the content of MMPI responses. On the individual item level, a variety of "critical item" lists have been constructed that are composed of items believed to have a special significance in the task of clinical assessment. Grayson (1951), for example, employed a rational construction strategy to identify 38 items believed to serve as markers of significant symptomatology. Other critical item lists have also been constructed to analyze individual item responses, including those by Caldwell (1969), Koss and Butcher (1973), and Lachar and Wrobel (1979). Forbey and Ben-Porath (1998) also developed a set of 82 critical items for the MMPI-A organized into a series of 15 content areas.

A second approach to content analysis is exemplified by the work of Harris and Lingoes (1955). Because most of the MMPI Basic scales contain a variety of content areas (i.e., the scales are heterogeneous), it is often difficult to infer what area of scale content was actually endorsed by a respondent in the production of a particular T-score elevation. This issue is particularly pronounced for T-scores representing marginal clinical range elevations. To deal with this problem, Harris and Lingoes developed subscales for Basic scales 2, 3, 4, 6, 8, and 9 by rationally grouping similar items into homogeneous content areas for each of these scales. The resulting 28 subscales have been carried over into the MMPI-2 and the MMPI-A. In addition, three subscales for the *Si* scale are available for the MMPI-A, based on the work of Ben-Porath, Hostetler, Butcher, and Graham (1989).

On a separate and third level of content analysis, the MMPI may be discussed and interpreted in relation to a number of content dimensions represented by the total item pool. Because Hathaway and McKinley utilized external criterion groups to create the original MMPI Basic scales, these clinical groups served to define the measurement focus of the inventory. Such a development method, however, made no effort to use the full item pool in deriving the maximum number of meaningful dimensions of psychopathology in construction of clinical scales. Indeed, the Basic MMPI scales utilized only about half of the total item pool (Nichols, 1987). Wiggins (1966) offered an approach to MMPI scale construction and measurement that was based on a more complete utilization of this item pool. Beginning with the 26 content categories described by Hathaway and McKinley (see Chapter 1 for a description) to classify the total content array of all MMPI items, Wiggins derived 13 homogeneous content scales using a combination of rational and statistical scale construction methods. Nichols provided a 1987 monograph concerning the use of the Wiggins content scales in clinical interpretation of the original MMPI, and Kohutek (1992a, 1992b) and Levitt, Browning, and Freeland (1992) identified the Wiggins content scale items that were retained in the MMPI-2. Correlate patterns for the Wiggins content scales in adolescent samples were reported by Archer and Gordon (1991b), Wrobel

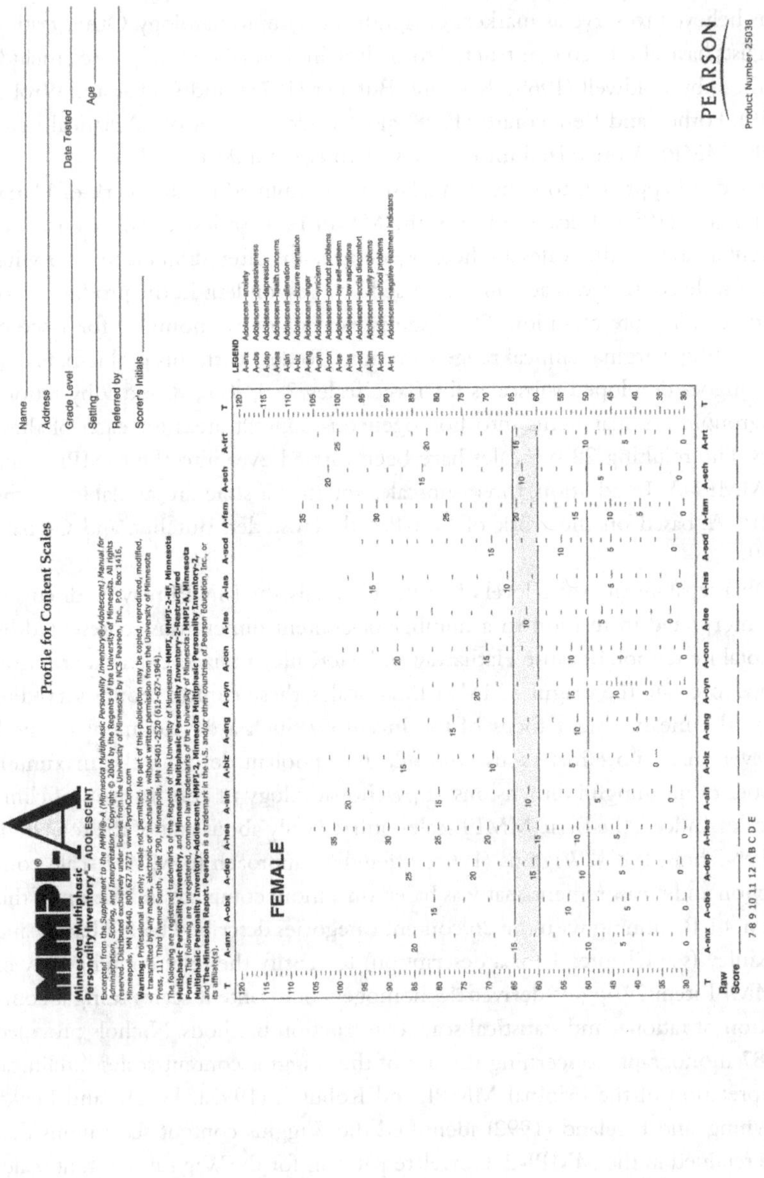

FIGURE 6.1 Profile for Content scales (female).

Source: Reproduced with permission of the University of Minnesota Press. All rights reserved. "Minnesota Multiphasic Personality Inventory®-Adolescent" and

(1991), Wrobel and Gdowski (1989), and Wrobel and Lachar (1995). Based on a recognition of the usefulness of the Wiggins scales, content scales were developed for the MMPI-2 by Butcher et al. (1990) and for the MMPI-A by Williams, Butcher, Ben-Porath, and Graham (1992). The MMPI-A Content scale profile for girls is shown in Figure 6.1.

Sherwood, et al. (1997) noted that although the content scales were developed to measure homogeneous constructs, it was useful to identify different dimensions or salient components for most of these scales. Using a series of PCAs, these authors produced a total of 31 subscales for 13 of the 15 MMPI-A Content scales as shown in Table 6.1. Sherwood et al. (1997) were not able to identify meaningful item clusters for the Anxiety and the Obsessiveness Content scales. The following section examines the analysis of content in the MMPI-A, as represented by the MMPI-A Content and Content Component scales, and by the Harris–Lingoes and *Si* subscales.

Several investigations have focused on the degree to which the MMPI-2 Content scales provide incremental gains in information beyond that provided by the Basic Clinical scales. Ben-Porath, McCully, and Almagor (1993), for example, evaluated the incremental contributions of MMPI-2 Content scales to the prediction of scores on self-report measures of personality and psychopathology in a sample of 596 college undergraduates. Results indicated that the inclusion of Content scales did add incrementally to the prediction of SCL-90-R score variance beyond prediction levels achieved solely by the Basic Clinical scales. Ben-Porath, Butcher, and Graham (1991) examined the contribution of MMPI-2 Content scales to differential diagnosis of schizophrenia and major depression in an inpatient psychiatric sample. Results from this study indicated that both Content scales and Clinical scales provided information that was useful in the differential diagnosis of these psychiatric categories. Specifically, findings from a stepwise hierarchical regression analysis indicated that the *DEP* and *BIZ* content scales contributed significantly to the differential diagnosis for males and the *BIZ* content scale added to diagnostic discrimination for female patients. Archer, Aiduk, Griffin, and Elkins (1996) examined the MMPI-2 Basic and Content scales in relation to the ability of these measures to predict to SCL-90-R scores and clinician ratings of psychopathology in a sample of 597 adult psychiatric patients. The findings from this study also demonstrated that the MMPI-2 Content scales added incrementally, although modestly, to the prediction of variance in outcome measures of psychopathology.

Several studies have specifically focused on the potential incremental utility of the MMPI-A Content scales. Forbey and Ben-Porath (2003) examined the MMPI-A Content scales in an evaluation of 335 adolescents receiving mental health services at a residential treatment facility. Regression analyses were utilized to identify the additional or incremental amount of variance accounted for by the Content scales (in contrast with the Clinical scales) in predicting

TABLE 6.1 MMPI-A Content Component Scales

Depression
A-dep$_1$: Dysphoria (5 items)
A-dep$_2$: Self-Depreciation (5 items)
A-dep$_3$: Lack of Drive (7 items)
A-dep$_4$: Suicidal Ideation (4 items)

Health Concerns
A-hea$_1$: Gastrointestinal Complaints
  (4 items)
A-hea$_2$: Neurological Symptoms (18 items)
A-hea$_3$: General health Concerns (8 items)

Alienation
A-aln$_1$: Misunderstood (5 items)
A-aln$_2$: Social Isolation (5 items)
A-aln$_3$: Interpersonal Skepticism (5 items)

Bizarre Mentation
A-biz1: Psychotic Symptomatology
  (11 items)
A-biz2: Paranoid Ideation (5 items)

Anger
A-ang$_1$: Explosive Behavior (8 items)
A-ang$_2$: Irritability (8 items)

School Problems
A-sch$_1$: School Conduct Problems
  (4 items)
A-sch$_2$: Negative Attitudes (8 items)

Cynicism
A-cyn$_1$: Misanthropic Beliefs (13 items)
A-cyn$_2$: Interpersonal Suspiciousness
  (9 items)

Conduct Problems
A-con$_1$: Acting-Out Behaviors
  (10 items)
A-con$_2$: Antisocial Attitudes (8 items)
A-con$_3$: Negative Peer Group
  Influences (3 items)

Low Self-Esteem
A-lse$_1$: Self-Doubt (13 items)
A-lse$_2$: Interpersonal Submissiveness
  (5 items)

Low Aspirations
A-las1: Low Achievement Orientation
  (8 items)
A-las2: Lack of Initiative (7 items)

Social Discomfort
A-sod$_1$: Introversion (14 items)
A-sod$_2$: Shyness (10 items)

Family Problems
A-fam$_1$: Familial Discord (21 items)
A-fam$_2$: Familial Alienation (11 items)

Negative Treatment Indicators
A-trt$_1$: Low Motivation (11 items)
A-trt$_2$: Inability to Disclose (8 items)

Source: Sherwood et al. (1997). Reproduced with permission. The MMPI-A Content Component Scales: Development, Psychometric Characteristics and Clinical Application by Sherwood, et al. Copyright 1997 by the Regents of the University of Minnesota. Reproduced with the permission of the University of Minnesota Press. All rights reserved. "Minnesota Multiphasic Personality Inventory" and "MMPI" are trademarks owned by the Regents of the University of Minnesota.

clinician's ratings of psychological symptomatology. Several of the MMPI-A Content scales demonstrated significant, although relatively limited, incremental validity beyond the Clinical scales in predicting clinician's ratings of adolescent behavior and personality characteristics. The Clinical scales also demonstrated incremental validity in reference to the Content scales, indicating that both Content and basic scales provide useful and complementary information in assessing adolescent personality and psychopathology. McGrath, Pogge, and Stokes (2002) evaluated the incremental validity of the MMPI-A Content scales in a sample of 629 adolescent psychiatric inpatients using criteria based on clinician's ratings, admission and discharge diagnosis, and chart-review data.

Results from hierarchical multiple and logistic regression analyses indicated that Content scales provided incremental information beyond that obtained through the Clinical scales. McGrath and his colleagues concluded that the use of the Content scales as an adjunct to the traditional Basic scales appeared to be supported by their findings. Finally, Rinaldo and Baer (2003) also evaluated the incremental contributions of the MMPI-A Content scales to the prediction of scores on other self-report measures of psychopathology in a sample of 62 adolescents receiving inpatient treatment and a non-clinical sample of 59 community adolescents. A series of hierarchical regression analyses indicated that the Content scales held incremental validity beyond the clinical scales in predicting variance in the criterion measures used in this study. Similar to the results by Forbey and Ben-Porath, Rinaldo and Baer also found that the Clinical scales demonstrated incremental validity in relationship to the Content scales when the order of entry of variables was reversed in the hierarchical design. Rinaldo and Baer concluded that their findings suggested that both Clinical and Content scales from the MMPI-A provide significant contributions to the assessment of adolescent psychological functioning. In summary, the results from these three MMPI-A studies are strikingly consistent in suggesting that both Basic and Content scales provide important information, and that the content scales are capable of providing a modest incremental gain when contrasted with data restricted solely to the basic Clinical scales.

MMPI-A Content Scales

The 15 MMPI-A Content scales exhibit a substantial degree of overlap with many of the MMPI-2 Content scales, as well as several of the Wiggins content scales. As described in the MMPI-A manual (Butcher et al., 1992), the MMPI-A Content scales were created in a series of five stages. The first stage involved an initial identification of those MMPI-2 Content scales (and items within MMPI-2 Content scales) that were appropriate for adaptation to the MMPI-A. Stage two of the development process involved the refinement of MMPI-A Content scales by the addition or deletion of specific items designed to improve the psychometric properties, including reliability and validity coefficients, of these scales. The third stage included a rational review and examination of scale content in order to evaluate item relevance in terms of the target construct. Stage four involved further statistical refinement of the scales, including the elimination of items that showed higher correlations with Content scales other than the Content scale on which the item was scored. The final stage involved the selection of narrative descriptors for each content scale utilizing a combination of empirical findings and logical inferences based on the item content of the scale. In addition to the MMPI-A normative sample, Williams et al. (1992) utilized a clinical sample of 420 boys and 293 girls from Minneapolis treatment facilities to refine the MMPI-A Content scales and to identify correlate patterns for these measures.

Several general statements may be made concerning the MMPI-A Content scales. These points may be listed as follows:

1. The interpretation of MMPI-A Content scales requires the administration of all 478 items in the MMPI-A booklet. The administration of the first stage of the MMPI-A booklet (i.e., the first 350 items) will not be sufficient to score the Content scales.

2. Most of the MMPI-A Content scales are predominantly composed of items from the original MMPI instrument. The School Problems (*A-sch*) scale and the Negative Treatment Indicators (*A-trt*) scale, however, consist primarily of items that do not appear on the original test instrument. In contrast, the Cynicism (*A-cyn*) scale consists entirely of items derived from the original form of the MMPI.

3. Eleven of the 15 MMPI-A Content scales heavily overlap with MMPI-2 content scales in terms of item membership and the constructs that are the focus of measurement. The Content scales unique to the MMPI-A form are Alienation (*A-aln*), Low Aspiration (*A-las*), School Problems (*A-sch*), and Conduct Problems (*A-con*).

4. Uniform T-score transformation procedures are consistently used in converting MMPI-A Content scale raw score totals to T-score values. Thus, the Content scales and eight Basic Clinical scales (*1*, *2*, *3*, *4*, *6*, *7*, *8*, and *9*) were the only MMPI-A scales to receive uniform T-scores.

5. The *true* response is typically the deviant endorsement direction for MMPI-A Content scales, with the exception of Health Concerns (*A-hea*) and Low Aspirations (*A-las*). The MMPI-A Obsessiveness (*A-obs*) and Cynicism (*A-cyn*) Content scales, for example, consist entirely of items scored in the *true* direction, and the Bizarre Mentation (*A-biz*) and Anger (*A-ang*) scales each contain only one item scored in the *false* direction. Most MMPI-A Content scales, therefore, involve the affirmation of the occurrence or presence of various psychiatric symptoms.

6. MMPI-A Content scales, similar to the MMPI-2 and the Wiggins content scales, are composed of items that are face-valid and obvious in terms of their relevancy to psychopathology. The MMPI-A Content scales, therefore, are easily influenced by an adolescent's tendency to underreport or overreport symptomatology. The MMPI-A interpreter should carefully evaluate the validity of the adolescent's responses, particularly the accuracy component of technical validity, prior to interpreting MMPI-A Content scales.

7. The MMPI-A Content scales, like their counterparts on the MMPI-2, exhibit relatively high internal reliability as reflected in alpha coefficient values (range .55 to .83). This characteristic might be expected given the scale construction method employed to develop these measures. Nevertheless, most of the MMPI-A Content scales contain two or more content subcomponents. Sherwood et al. (1997) have provided content component

subscales for 13 of the MMPI-A Content scales in a manner similar to that used by Ben-Porath and Sherwood (1993) in developing component sub-scales for the content scales of the MMPI-2.

8. MMPI-A Content scale results may be used by interpreters to supplement, augment, and refine the interpretation of the MMPI-A Basic Clinical scales. The Content scales are most useful when interpreted within the context of full array of data provided by the test instrument rather than interpreted independently.

Empirical information is available concerning the interpretation of the MMPI-A Content scales. Research-derived content scale descriptors are reported by Williams et al. (1992) for a clinical sample of 420 male and 293 female adolescents and by Archer and Gordon (1991b) in an independent sample of 64 male and 58 female adolescent psychiatric inpatients. Veltri et al. (2009) provided empirical correlates for the Content and Supplementary scales based on samples of 157 boys from a forensic setting and 197 girls from an acute psychiatric inpatient setting. Most recently, Handel, Archer, Elkins, Mason, and Simonds-Bisbee (2011) reported external correlates for the Content and Supplementary scales in a forensic sample of 315 boys and 181 girls, with findings presented separately by gender. In addition, the examination of content component scores within the MMPI-A Content scales can offer some inferences concerning the characteristics of individuals who produce elevated scores on these measures. Interpretive statements for the MMPI-A Content Component scales are provided in the MMPI-A Manual Supplement by Ben-Porath et al. (2006).

As with most other MMPI-A scales, T-scores $\geq$ 65 on MMPI-A Content scales may be regarded as clinical range scores, and T-score values between 60 and 64, inclusive, may be described as marginally elevated. As additional research has been conducted with the content scales, it has become possible to provide fuller descriptions of the clinical correlate patterns for these measures. Principal factor analyses by McCarthy and Archer (1998) shows that the 15 MMPI-A Content scales are generally accounted for by two broad factors labeled General Maladjustment and Externalizing Tendencies. The former factor was quite robust and identified by strong relationships to *A-trt*, *A-dep*, *A-aln*, *A-anx*, *A-lse*, and *A-hea*. The second factor accounted for much less total variance and was marked by loadings on *A-cyn*, *A-con*, and *A-ang*. Table 6. 2 provides the intercorrelations for MMPI-A Content scales in the normative sample.

Tables 6.3, 6.4, 6.5, and 6.6 provide the correlational values of these measures with the MMPI-A basic scales and the Wiggins content scales by gender, respectively. As shown in Tables 6.5 and 6.6, there is a very high degree of interrelationship between eight of the Wiggins content scales and seven counterparts on the MMPI-A. Specifically, the following Wiggins scale–MMPI-A Content scale pairs produced correlations of $r = .79$ or greater for both genders: Depression and *A-dep*; Poor Health and *A-hea*; Organic Symptoms and *A-hea*; Family Problems

TABLE 6.2 Raw Score Intercorrelations of MMPI-A Content Scales for 815 Females and 805 Males in the MMPI-A Normative Sample

Females

Scale	A-anx	A-obs	A-dep	A-hea	A-aln	A-biz	A-ang	A-cyn	A-con	A-lse	A-las	A-sod	A-fam	A-sch	A-trt
A-anx		.69	.74	.56	.61	.56	.51	.54	.41	.62	.32	.31	.53	.41	.62
A-obs	.66		.61	.42	.48	.51	.54	.60	.44	.57	.31	.24	.44	.39	.64
A-dep	.73	.55		.53	.70	.56	.43	.50	.47	.74	.42	.42	.57	.50	.71
A-hea	.50	.27	.48		.50	.56	.33	.34	.37	.46	.26	.29	.41	.45	.48
A-aln	.62	.46	.69	.47		.55	.38	.42	.50	.63	.37	.54	.61	.52	.74
A-biz	.54	.45	.56	.53	.53		.44	.49	.52	.48	.24	.26	.45	.44	.53
A-ang	.50	.52	.41	.23	.40	.36		.52	.54	.38	.27	.15	.47	.43	.49
A-cyn	.43	.57	.37	.07	.54	.37	.51		.52	.45	.22	.23	.46	.40	.61
A-con	.36	.44	.40	.22	.38	.41	.50	.47		.45	.37	.17	.53	.58	.56
A-lse	.60	.55	.68	.47	.62	.53	.36	.35	.37		.49	.48	.48	.51	.69
A-las	.36	.22	.39	.39	.39	.32	.16	.10	.30	.45		.31	.35	.53	.48
A-sod	.43	.26	.47	.35	.55	.33	.14	.14	.03	.49	.33		.28	.30	.47
A-fam	.53	.43	.59	.48	.61	.51	.44	.35	.50	.51	.41	.28		.52	.58
A-sch	.46	.40	.53	.48	.53	.50	.40	.31	.56	.52	.48	.29	.60		.57
A-trt	.60	.58	.64	.42	.67	.56	.43	.49	.48	.67	.48	.45	.56	.58	

and *A-fam*; Authority Conflict and *A-cyn*; Hostility and *A-ang*; Psychoticism and *A-biz*; and Social Maladjustment and *A-sod*. Two of the Wiggins content scales, however, including Feminine Interests and Religious Fundamentalism, produced consistently low correlations with MMPI-A Content scales, and three other Wiggins scales (Poor Morale, Phobias, and Hypomania) produced moderate to high correlations involving several MMPI-A scales. With the exception of the Religious Fundamentalism scale, the Wiggins content scales have retained a majority of scale items in the MMPI-A, with seven scales maintaining over 80% of their item pools. Table 6.7 provides an overview of the status of the Wiggins content scale within the structure of the MMPI-A.

Adolescent-Anxiety (A-anx) Scale

The MMPI-A Anxiety Content scale consists of 21 items, 20 of which also appear on the MMPI-2 Anxiety scale. Adolescents who score high on this measure report symptoms of anxiety, including tension, apprehension, and rumination, and the self-perception of being overwhelmed by stress. Most *A-anx* scale items involve cognitions and attitudes related to the experience of anxiety, with relatively few items related to physiological expression of anxiety symptoms. As shown in Tables 6.3 through 6.6, the *A-anx* scale is highly correlated with scale 7 of the basic profile, and also correlates highly with the Wiggins Depression (*DEP*) content scale.

Butcher et al. (1992) reported that the *A-anx* scale appears to measure general maladjustment as well as symptoms relating to depression and somatic complaints. Clinical correlates in the Archer and Gordon (1991b) study were derived from staff ratings on the Devereux Adolescent Behavior (DAB) Rating Scale, parental reports on the Child Behavior Checklist (CBCL), and presenting problems as indicated in the adolescent's psychiatric records. These authors found that high *A-anx* scores for adolescent girls were related to low endurance and fatigue, domination by peers, obsessional thought processes, anxiety, and timidity, whereas high scores for males were related to problems in concentration, the occurrence of suicidal thoughts, and sadness and depression. Arita and Baer (1998) explored the correlates of several MMPI-A Content scales in a sample of 62 adolescent inpatients and reported that the *A-anx* and *A-dep* scales tended to share similar correlates reflective of emotional distress, tension, and nervousness. Kopper, Osman, Osman, and Hoffman (1998) found scores from the *A-anx* scale associated with results from a self-report suicide probability scale in a sample of 143 adolescent inpatients. Veltri et al. (2009) reported *A-anx* scale elevations were related to suicidal ideation for boys and girls, and Handel et al. (2011) found higher *A-anx* scores associated with increased social and attentional problems across gender. The *A-anx* scale is one of only two Content scales for which Sherwood and her colleagues (1997) were unable to derive meaningful subscale components.

TABLE 6.3 Raw Score Intercorrelations of the Content and Basic Scales for Female Adolescents in the MMPI-A Normative Sample

Content Scales

	A-anx	A-obs	A-dep	A-hea	A-aln	A-biz	A-ang	A-cyn	A-con	A-lse	A-las	A-sod	A-fam	A-sch	A-trt
F_1	.36	.27	.50	.54	.59	.60	.29	.30	.54	.47	.37	.35	.55	.61	.54
F_2	.41	.32	.54	.55	.60	.63	.34	.31	.49	.54	.38	.46	.51	.56	.60
F	.42	.32	.55	.58	.64	.65	.34	.32	.54	.54	.40	.44	.56	.61	.61
L	-.19	-.30	-.14	.06	.01	-.02	-.31	-.19	-.25	-.12	-.10	.14	-.11	-.10	-.08
K	-.62	-.68	-.53	-.31	-.50	-.41	-.62	-.70	-.40	-.48	-.23	-.29	-.46	-.35	-.55
Hs	.62	.44	.59	.91	.48	.50	.33	.36	.33	.49	.29	.29	.40	.42	.46
D	.60	.33	.68	.51	.53	.34	.13	.22	.17	.57	.35	.47	.37	.31	.47
Hy	.33	.03	.34	.56	.15	.20	-.03	-.12	.03	.19	.14	-.02	.17	.16	.08
Pd	.59	.41	.68	.49	.59	.51	.39	.40	.50	.49	.31	.19	.68	.46	.51
Mf	.07	.05	.04	-.13	-.11	-.20	-.07	-.16	-.28	-.06	-.10	-.06	-.09	-.21	-.16
Pa	.56	.41	.63	.54	.55	.60	.28	.15	.38	.49	.23	.27	.42	.38	.47
Pt	.84	.78	.81	.58	.63	.62	.58	.57	.49	.73	.42	.39	.53	.50	.69
Sc	.76	.67	.79	.68	.71	.78	.54	.56	.60	.69	.44	.41	.66	.56	.74
Ma	.43	.48	.36	.36	.33	.52	.46	.51	.57	.26	.11	-.11	.47	.36	.36
Si	.54	.51	.59	.38	.60	.34	.31	.44	.24	.67	.47	.77	.37	.38	.62

TABLE 6.4 Raw Score Intercorrelations of the Content and Basic Scales for Male Adolescents in the MMPI-A Normative Sample

Content Scales

	A-anx	A-obs	A-dep	A-hea	A-aln	A-biz	A-ang	A-cyn	A-con	A-lse	A-las	A-sod	A-fam	A-sch	A-trt
F₁	.39	.21	.52	.63	.55	.64	.25	.11	.39	.47	.42	.34	.59	.64	.50
F₂	.42	.26	.53	.61	.56	.68	.24	.14	.35	.55	.45	.40	.56	.60	.58
F	.43	.25	.55	.65	.59	.70	.26	.13	.38	.54	.46	.40	.61	.65	.58
L	-.15	-.35	-.08	.28	.02	.06	-.33	-.39	-.29	-.02	.12	.14	-.01	.02	-.06
K	-.56	-.66	-.44	-.06	-.40	-.33	-.61	-.72	-.37	-.39	-.07	.22	-.33	-.26	-.44
Hs	.54	.27	.50	.90	.46	.47	.23	.09	.18	.44	.37	.35	.45	.40	.37
D	.50	.14	.54	.55	.43	.27	-.02	-.10	-.05	.45	.36	.46	.29	.24	.29
Hy	.21	-.15	.26	.63	.15	.16	-.14	-.39	-.09	.12	.24	.11	.20	.15	-.01
Pd	.54	.33	.64	.49	.57	.46	.33	.23	.43	.42	.38	.21	.67	.51	.43
Mf	.27	.14	.20	.11	.11	.04	.00	-.13	-.14	.16	.02	.20	.09	-.11	-.01
Pa	.53	.34	.62	.58	.56	.64	.24	.05	.25	.47	.35	.35	.50	.44	.45
Pt	.83	.76	.79	.48	.64	.60	.54	.50	.43	.69	.38	.46	.56	.52	.63
Sc	.74	.58	.79	.64	.73	.77	.49	.43	.50	.66	.46	.47	.72	.63	.69
Ma	.37	.50	.32	.18	.29	.44	.50	.54	.59	.25	-.09	.07	.46	.38	.37
Si	.58	.48	.58	.40	.61	.38	.26	.31	.13	.63	.42	.81	.39	.34	.57

TABLE 6.5 Raw Score Intercorrelations of the MMPI-A Content Scales and the MMPI Wiggins Content Scales for 58 Females in an Adolescent Inpatient Sample

MMPI-A Content Scales

	A-anx	A-obs	A-dep	A-hea	A-aln	A-biz	A-ang	A-cyn	A-con	A-lse	A-las	A-sod	A-fam	A-sch	A-trt
HEA	.54	.38	.44	.84	.42	.39	.15	.26	.33	.51	.23	.51	.17	.21	.44
DEP	.87	.81	.92	.61	.69	.43	.42	.53	.37	.85	.64	.54	.50	.47	.72
ORG	.77	.64	.60	.90	.50	.57	.38	.41	.44	.62	.35	.50	.29	.54	.53
FAM	.35	.44	.46	.22	.61	.28	.43	.46	.54	.44	.42	.11	.94	.35	.56
AUT	.42	.49	.38	.32	.45	.43	.50	.86	.70	.47	.39	.15	.47	.50	.57
FEM	-.10	-.11	-.11	.05	-.11	-.12	-.14	-.33	-.35	-.20	-.13	-.05	-.12	-.17	-.26
REL	.02	-.14	-.04	.18	-.08	.00	-.25	-.18	-.24	.02	-.18	.01	-.44	-.28	-.15
HOS	.54	.71	.45	.45	.44	.55	.83	.63	.72	.43	.41	.14	.52	.72	.58
MOR	.80	.74	.85	.53	.64	.35	.33	.54	.29	.88	.53	.58	.38	.36	.65
PHO	.57	.52	.38	.54	.35	.41	.32	.21	.29	.42	.15	.45	.23	.36	.32
PSY	.65	.58	.57	.62	.62	.86	.54	.53	.62	.56	.35	.34	.47	.59	.58
HYP	.34	.44	.16	.24	.15	.42	.65	.58	.58	.15	.14	-.13	.31	.50	.28
SOC	.50	.39	.55	.45	.46	.07	-.09	.22	-.02	.62	.36	.93	.08	.12	.46

Source: Archer (2005). Copyright © by Routledge. Reprinted with permission.

TABLE 6.6 Raw Score Intercorrelations of the MMPI-A Content Scales and the MMPI Wiggins Content Scales for 64 Males in an Adolescent Inpatient Sample

MMPI-A Content Scales

Wiggins Scales	A-anx	A-obs	A-dep	A-hea	A-aln	A-biz	A-ang	A-cyn	A-con	A-lse	A-las	A-sod	A-fam	A-sch	A-trt
HEA	.46	.39	.56	.86	.46	.42	.02	-.11	-.14	.42	.09	.41	-.09	.14	.30
DEP	.78	.73	.90	.68	.66	.55	.16	.19	-.03	.66	.23	.50	.05	.30	.59
ORG	.57	.53	.65	.90	.54	.51	.01	-.10	-.06	.54	.11	.55	-.09	.23	.42
FAM	.19	.25	.08	.02	.18	.13	.47	.31	.26	.10	.21	-.06	.82	.27	.19
AUT	.03	.24	-.06	-.28	.15	.09	.61	.88	.65	.12	.29	-.05	.38	.39	.31
FEM	.24	.12	.12	.24	.03	.22	-.04	-.19	-.01	.05	-.02	.15	-.00	.03	-.08
REL	-.03	-.19	-.00	.12	.11	.11	.08	-.07	.06	.08	-.24	.10	-.01	.06	.08
HOS	.34	.54	.18	.15	.27	.30	.79	.73	.59	.18	.27	.08	.45	.56	.42
MOR	.78	.83	.73	.55	.56	.47	.29	.39	-.02	.76	.20	.49	.02	.32	.59
PHO	.33	.33	.37	.62	.46	.55	.13	.00	.08	.32	.06	.47	-.12	.26	.36
PSY	.49	.61	.67	.63	.70	.89	.32	.29	.30	.64	.28	.59	.22	.47	.66
HYP	.38	.57	.04	.05	.14	.09	.72	.68	.40	.16	.06	-.04	.23	.34	.36
SOC	.39	.31	.41	.55	.47	.43	-.11	-.06	-.19	.46	.11	.86	-.04	.13	.43

Source: Archer (2005). Copyright © by Routledge. Reprinted with permission.

TABLE 6.7 Wiggins Content Scale Items Retained in the MMPI-A

Wiggins Content Scale	Items on MMPI	Number (and Percent) of Items Retained on MMPI-A	
Social Maladjustment (SOC)	27	22	(81.5%)
Depression (DEP)	33	31	(93.9%)
Feminine Interests (FEM)	30	16	(53.3%)
Poor Morale (MOR)	23	20	(87.0%)
Religious Fundamentalism (REL)	12	1	(8.3%)
Authority Conflict (AUT)	20	20	(100.0%)
Psychoticism (PSY)	48	40	(83.3%)
Organic Symptoms (ORG)	36	31	(86.1%)
Family Problems (FAM)	16	16	(100.0%)
Manifest Hostility (HOS)	27	18	(66.7%)
Phobias (PHO)	27	15	(55.6%)
Hypomania (HYP)	25	18	(72.0%)
Poor Health (HEA)	28	17	(60.7%)

The following descriptors are applicable to adolescents who produce high scores on the *A-anx* scale:

- Anxious, tense, nervous, and ruminative.
- Problems in concentration and attention.
- Low endurance and fatigability.
- Sadness and depression.
- Higher probability of suicidal thoughts and ideation.

Adolescent-Obsessiveness (A-obs) Scale

The *A-obs* scale consists of 15 items, 12 of which also appear on the MMPI-2 obsessiveness (*OBS*) scale and 13 items that appear on the original form of the MMPI. All of the items in the *A-obs* scale are scored in the *true* direction. The MMPI-A Obsessiveness scale contains items concerning ambivalence and difficulty in making decisions, excessive worry and rumination, and the occurrence of intrusive thoughts. Sherwood et al. (1997) did not report subscale components for the *A-obs* Content scale. Adolescents who score high on *A-obs* may also exhibit some compulsive behaviors. The *A-obs* scale is highly correlated with scale 7 of the basic profile, and negatively correlated with scale *K*.

Butcher et al. (1992) report that high *A-obs* scores in a clinical sample were related to anxious and dependent behaviors in boys and to suicidal ideations or gestures in girls. A clear correlate pattern was not identified in the Archer and Gordon (1991b) study. Veltri et al. (2009) observed that higher *A-obs* scale scores were associated with ratings of lower self-esteem for girls and Handel et al. (2011) reported that higher *A-obs* scores correlated with increased parental ratings of withdrawal and depression for girls. Content Component scales were not derived for the *A-obs* scale.

The following are characteristics or correlates associated with high *A-obs* scores:

- Excessive worry and rumination.
- Difficulty in making decisions.
- The occurrence of intrusive thoughts and problems in concentration.

Adolescent-Depression (A-dep) Scale

The *A-dep* scale consists of 26 items, of which 25 also appeared on the MMPI-2 Depression content scale. Further, 24 of the 26 items on the *A-dep* scale were derived from the original form of the MMPI. *A-dep* scale items appear to be related to depression and sadness, apathy, low energy, and poor morale. In the Archer and Gordon (1991b) inpatient sample, *A-dep* scores were highly correlated with scores from the Wiggins Depression (*DEP*) Content scale ($r = .92$ for females and $r = .90$ for males). *A-dep* scores were not highly correlated with scale 2, but were strongly associated with scores from Basic scales 7 and 8 (see Tables 6.3 and 6.4). Despite the relatively low-magnitude correlation between scale 2 and the *DEP* Content scale, research by Bence, Sabourin, Luty, and Thackrey (1995) has shown that both scales have approximately equal effectiveness in accurately identifying depressed patients in a sample of adult psychiatric inpatients. Archer et al. (1996) found that the MMPI-2 *DEP* Content scale added incrementally to information provided from Basic scale 2 in the prediction to scores on both self-report and clinician ratings of depression. Cashel, Rogers, Sewell, and Holliman (1998) examined MMPI-A Content scale correlates in clinical and non-clinical adolescent samples and reported that *A-dep* scores were positively correlated with several items from the Schedule of Affective Disorders and Schizophrenia for School Aged Children (K-SADS-III-R) reflective of depressive symptoms including depressed mood, guilt, and suicidal acts. Arita and Baer (1998) found the *A-dep* scale produced a correlation of $r = .58$ with Reynolds Adolescent Depression Inventory (RADS) in their investigation of adolescent inpatients. Veltri et al. (2009) found *A-dep* scores related to suicidal ideation for both genders, and Handel et al. (2011) found *A-dep* scores associated with anxiety, depression, affective problems, and internalizing for both boys and girls. Several of the items on the *A-dep* scale involve feelings of pessimism and hopelessness. Two *A-dep* scale items (177 and 283) directly relate to the occurrence of suicidal ideation.

Butcher et al. (1992) reported that high *A-dep* scores for adolescents in clinical settings were associated with a variety of behaviors and symptoms related to depression and the occurrence of suicidal ideation and gestures. Archer and Gordon (1991b) also found suicidal thoughts to be related to high *A-dep* scores for girls, whereas suicidal attempts were related to high *A-dep* scores for boys. Sherwood et al. (1997) identified four component scales for *A-dep* that were labeled Dysphoria (*A-dep$_1$*), Self-Depreciation (*A-dep$_2$*), Lack of Drive (*A-dep$_3$*), and Suicidal Ideation (*A-dep$_4$*).

The following characteristics are associated with high *A-dep* scores:

- Sadness, depression, and despondency.
- Fatigue and apathy.
- A pervasive sense of hopelessness that may include suicidal ideation.

Adolescent-Health Concerns (A-hea) Scale

The MMPI-A Health Concerns scale includes 37 items, of which 34 also appear on the MMPI-2 Health Concerns *(HEA)* scale. Thirty-four of the 37 items on the *A-hea* scale appeared on the original form of the MMPI. Twenty-three items on the *A-hea* scale also appear on scale *1* of the standard or Basic MMPI-A Clinical scales and scores from these two scales are highly correlated. The *A-hea* scale is one of only two MMPI-A Content scales that contain a majority of items keyed in the *false* direction. Adolescents who produce elevated scores on the *A-hea* Content scale are endorsing physical symptoms across a wide variety of areas including gastrointestinal, neurological, sensory, cardiovascular, and respiratory systems. These adolescents feel physically ill, and are worried about their health. In the Archer and Gordon (1991b) inpatient sample, *A-hea* scale scores were also highly correlated ($r = .90$ for males and females) with scores from the Wiggins Organic Symptoms *(ORG)* content scale.

Williams et al. (1992) found high *A-hea* scores to be related to somatic complaints for adolescents in their clinical sample, and to misbehavior, school problems, and poor academic performance for normal adolescents. Archer and Gordon (1991b) found high scores for females to be associated with the occurrence of suicidal thoughts, tiredness, and fatigue, whereas high-scoring boys were described as exhibiting poor reality testing, concentration difficulties, and somatic concerns. Veltri et al. (2009) did not report any meaningful correlates for the *A-hea* scale in their study, but Handel et al. (2011) found *A-hea* scores related to somatic complaints and somatic problems for girls. Future research should examine the extent to which poor physical health, including chronic medical conditions, affect *A-hea* scores. Sherwood et al. (1997) developed three component subscales for *A-hea* which were labeled Gastrointestinal Complaints (*A-hea$_1$*), Neurological Symptoms (*A-hea$_2$*), and General Health Concerns (*A-hea$_3$*).

The following descriptors are associated with elevated scores on *A-hea*:

- General physical concerns and complaints that may also include more specific gastrointestinal or neurological symptoms.
- Tiredness, weakness, and fatigue.

Adolescent-Alienation (A-aln) Scale

The MMPI-A Alienation scale is 20 items in length and does not directly correspond to any of the MMPI-2 Content scales. The *A-aln* scale is designed to identify adolescents who are interpersonally isolated and alienated, and feel pessimistic about social interactions. They tend not to believe that others understand or are sympathetic to them, and perceive their lives as being unfair or harsh. They may feel that they are unable to turn to, or depend on, anyone. These adolescents would be expected to have few or no close friends. The *A-aln* scale is most highly correlated with MMPI Basic scale *8* ($r = .71$ for females and $r = .73$ for males). Data from Archer and Gordon (1991b) indicate that this MMPI-A Content scale is most highly correlated with the Wiggins Depression (*DEP*) Content scale for females ($r = .69$) and with the Wiggins Psychoticism (*PSY*) scale for males ($r = .70$).

Williams et al. (1992) reported that the *A-aln* scale exhibited correlates in both the normative and clinical samples related to feeling emotionally distant from others. In the Archer and Gordon (1991b) clinical sample, high scores among girls were related to withdrawal, lying, and irritability, whereas high scores for boys were related to provocativeness, excessive use of fantasy, and the occurrence of hallucinations and suicidal thoughts. Kopper et al. (1998) reported that *A-aln* scale scores contributed significantly to adolescent inpatients' self-reports on a measure of suicide probability. Veltri et al. (2009) also found the *A-aln* scale related to histories of suicidal attempts or gestures for boys in a forensic sample. Handel et al. (2011) reported *A-aln* scale scores related to social problems and internalizing for girls, and anxiety and depression for adolescents across genders. Sherwood et al. (1997) provided three component subscales for *A-aln*: Misunderstood ($A\text{-}aln_1$), Social Isolation ($A\text{-}aln_2$), and Interpersonal Skepticism ($A\text{-}aln_3$).

The following are characteristics associated with high *A-aln* scores:

- Sense of interpersonal alienation, and frustration.
- Social withdrawal and isolation.

Adolescent-Bizarre Mentation (A-biz) Scale

The *A-biz* scale consists of 19 items, of which 17 also appear on the MMPI-2 Bizarre Mentation (*BIZ*) scale. Eleven of the 19 items on the *A-biz* scale also appear on the MMPI-A *F* scale. All but one of the *A-biz* scale items can be found in the original MMPI item pool. Adolescents who produce elevated scores on the *A-biz* scale are characterized by the occurrence of psychotic thought processes. They report strange and unusual experiences, which may include auditory, visual, or olfactory hallucinations. They may also have paranoid symptoms and delusions, including beliefs that they are being plotted against, or controlled by, others. *A-biz* scores are highly correlated with scales *F* and *8* from the basic

MMPI-A profile in the normative sample (see Tables 6.3 and 6.4), and with the Wiggins Psychoticism (*PSY*) scale in the Archer and Gordon (1991b) inpatient sample (see Tables 6.5 and 6.6). Williams et al. (1992) reported that the *A-biz* scale appeared to measure general maladjustment among normal adolescents, and was associated in their clinical sample with the occurrence of bizarre sensory experiences and psychotic symptoms. Archer and Gordon (1991b) found that high *A-biz* scores among female inpatients were related to hallucinations, poor emotional control, and poor reality testing, whereas high scores for males were associated with fighting, legal difficulties, the perpetration of sexual abuse, hallucinations, and poor reality testing. Veltri et al. (2009) reported that *A-biz* scale scores were related to self-mutilation for girls and a history of verbal threats for boys. Handel et al. (2011) found elevations on *A-biz* related to a history of thought problems and social problems for girls in a forensic setting. Sherwood and her colleagues identified Psychotic Symptomatology (*A-biz$_1$*) and Paranoid Ideation (*A-biz$_2$*) components for the *A-biz* Content scale.

The following characteristics are associated with elevated *A-biz* scale scores:

- Poor reality testing.
- Deficits in impulse control.
- Strange and unusual beliefs or thoughts.
- Presence of paranoid symptomatology, including hallucinations and delusions, and possible thought disorder or psychosis.

Adolescent-Anger (A-ang) Scale

The MMPI-A Anger scale consists of 17 items, of which 11 also appear on the MMPI-2 Anger (*ANG*) scale. Twelve of the *A-ang* items appeared on the original form of the MMPI. Clark (1994) examined the relationship between the MMPI-2 *ANG* scale and concurrent measures of anger and subjective distress in a sample of 97 men admitted to an inpatient chronic pain program. Results of this study indicated that the MMPI-2 *ANG* scale is a reliable index of the predisposition to the external expression of anger and this scale was found to be correlated $r = .71$ with the Spielberger (1988) trait measure of anger. Additionally, individuals who produced elevated (T $\geq$ 65) scores on the MMPI-2 anger scale could be described as displaying frequent and intense anger, feeling frustrated, being quick-tempered, and being impulsive and prone to interpersonal problems. Although the MMPI-2 *ANG* scale was found to be an effective measure of anger externalization, scores on this Content scale were not related to state experiences of anger or to patterns of inwardly directed anger.

Adolescents who score high on the MMPI-A *A-ang* scale may be described as irritable, grouchy, and impatient. Problems with anger may include the potential of physical assaultiveness, and four of the items on the *A-ang* scale (Items 34, 128, 445, and 458) specifically relate to the issue of physical aggression.

Williams et al. (1992) found that high *A-ang* scores among adolescents in clinical settings were related to histories of assaultive behaviors. Veltri et al. (2009) found *A-ang* scores related to aggressiveness, anger, assaultiveness and fighting, and Handel et al. (2011) reported higher *A-ang* scores associated with increased incidents of aggressiveness and conduct problems. Like the other MMPI-A scales related to externalizing behaviors, *A-ang* scores are negatively and highly correlated with scale *K* in the normative sample. In addition, the *A-ang* scale was highly correlated ($r = .79$ for boys and $r = .83$ for girls) with scores from the Wiggins Hostility (*HOS*) scale in the Archer and Gordon (1991b) inpatient sample. Additionally, these authors found high *A-ang* scores were associated with truancy, poor parental relationships, defiance and disobedience, anger, and assaultiveness for girls, and high heterosexual interest, drug abuse, hyperactivity, and threatened assaultiveness for boys. Toyer and Weed (1998) found *A-ang* scores positively correlated to counselor's ratings of anger in a sample of 50 court-adjudicated adolescents in outpatient treatment. Arita and Baer (1998) reported an intercorrelation of $r = .59$ between the *A-ang* scale and scores from the Externalizing scale on the Youth Self-Report version of the Child Behavior Checklist (YSR) and $r = .59$ intercorrelation between the *A-ang* and scores on the Trait form of the State-Trait Anger Expression Inventory (*STAXI-T*). Sherwood et al. (1997) developed two component subscales for *A-ang* which were identified as Explosive Behavior (A-ang_1) and Irritability (A-ang_2). The following features are associated with high *A-ang* scores:

- Anger and interpersonal hostility.
- Irritability, grouchiness, and impatience.
- Poor anger control and physical aggressiveness.

Adolescent-Cynicism (A-cyn) Scale

The *A-cyn* scale includes 22 items, 21 of which also appear on the MMPI-2 Cynicism (*CYN*) scale. All of the *A-cyn* items are scored in the *true* direction and appeared on the original form of the MMPI. Adolescents who produce elevations on this MMPI-A Content scale may be described as distrustful, cynical, and suspicious of the motives of others. They tend to believe that all individuals manipulate and use each other selfishly for personal gain. They assume that others behave in a manner that appears ethical or honest only because of the fear of being caught and punished for misbehavior. They expect others to lie, cheat, and steal in order to gain advantage. The *A-cyn* scale correlates highly, and negatively, with scale *K* of the MMPI-A Basic scale profile. Data from the Archer and Gordon (1991b) adolescent inpatient sample indicate that the *A-cyn* scale correlates highly ($r = .86$ for females and $r = .88$ for males) with the Wiggins Authority Problems (*AUT*) content scale.

Williams et al. (1992) reported few meaningful external correlates for this scale in their investigation of MMPI-A normative and clinical samples.

Archer and Gordon (1991b) found that high *A-cyn* scores among female adolescents were related to the occurrence of sexual abuse and poor parental relationships as primary presenting problems, and to staff ratings of these adolescents as resistant and displaying a negative attitude. The *A-cyn* scale produced few correlates for male inpatient adolescents. Those correlates that were obtained involved the increased occurrence of hallucinations and the excessive use of fantasy. Clark (1994) examined correlates of the MMPI-2 *CYN* Content scale in a sample of 97 male chronic pain patients. Results of this investigation provided few consistent descriptors associated with *CYN* scale elevations, and the authors concluded that caution should be employed in using the MMPI-2 *CYN* scale in clinical settings. More recently, Veltri et al. (2009) reported that boys with higher *A-cyn* scale scores were more likely to have a history of petty thievery, and Handel et al. (2011) found more elevated *A-cyn* scores were unrelated to any relevant correlates. The lack of consistency in clinical descriptors derived for the MMPI-A *CYN* scale also suggests caution in the use of this MMPI-A measure. The Sherwood et al. (1997) components for the *A-cyn* Content scale are Misanthropic Beliefs ($A\text{-}cyn_1$) and Interpersonal Suspiciousness ($A\text{-}cyn_2$).

Based on the item content of the *A-cyn* scale, the following descriptors may be associated with high scores on this measure:

- Guarded and suspicious of the motives of others.
- Unfriendly, manipulative, and hostile in relationships.

Adolescent-Conduct Problems (A-con) Scale

The MMPI-A Conduct Problems scale is composed of 23 items, of which 7 appear on the MMPI-2 Antisocial Practices (*ASP*) scale. Twelve of the 23 items on the *A-con* scale were derived from the item pool of the original MMPI. The *A-con* scale was developed to identify adolescents who report problem behaviors, including impulsivity, risk-taking behaviors, and antisocial behaviors. Sherwood and her colleagues have developed three discrete components for this content scale: Acting-Out Behaviors ($A\text{-}con_1$), Antisocial Attitudes ($A\text{-}con_2$), and Negative Peer Group Influences ($A\text{-}con_3$). Adolescents who produce elevations on this scale are likely to exhibit behaviors that may result in school suspensions and legal violations, and are more likely to receive conduct disorder diagnoses. In addition to behaviors and actions related to conduct problems, however, the *A-con* scale also measures attitudes and beliefs likely to be in conflict with societal norms and standards. In the MMPI-A normative sample, the *A-con* scale produced substantial correlations ($r > .50$) with scales 8 and 9 of the Basic scale profile for both genders, and was correlated ($r = .65$ for males and $r = .70$ for females) with the Wiggins Authority Problems (*AUT*) Content scale in the inpatient sample.

Williams et al. (1992) reported that high scores on *A-con* were associated with the occurrence of significant behavior problems. Archer and Gordon (1991b) found high *A-con* scores among males to be associated with presenting problems including theft, truancy, drug abuse, legal difficulties, alcohol abuse, and assaultive behaviors. Among females, high *A-con* scores were related to truancy, defiance and disobedience, anger, and running away from home. Arita and Baer (1998) reported *A-con* scores were correlated r = .57, r = .56 and r = .48 with the externalizing, delinquency, and aggressive scores, respectively, from the Youth Self-Report version of the Child Behavior Checklist (YSR). Veltri et al. (2009) found higher *A-con* scales related to substance abuse histories for boys and girls, and to oppositional behaviors and prior criminal charges for girls. Handel reported that *A-con* scores were related to rule-breaking and externalizing behaviors for both boys and girls in their forensic sample.

The following characteristics or correlates are associated with high *A-con* scores:

- Teenagers who are likely to be in trouble because of their behavior.
- Poor impulse control and antisocial behaviors.
- Attitudes and beliefs that conflict with societal norms and standards.
- Problems with authority figures.
- Increased likelihood of conduct disorder diagnoses.

Adolescent-Low Self-Esteem (A-lse) Scale

The *A-lse* scale consists of 18 items, all of which also appear on the MMPI-2 *LSE* Content scale. The *A-lse* scale attempts to identify adolescents who have low self-esteem and little self-confidence. Adolescents who score high on this Content scale often feel inadequate and useless, and not as capable and competent as others. They recognize many faults and flaws in themselves, both real and imagined, and feel unrespected or rejected by others. Among the Basic scales, *A-lse* produces the highest correlations with scales *7*, *8*, and *0* (see Tables 6.3 and 6.4). In addition, *A-lse* scores are highly correlated with scores from the Wiggins Poor Morale (*MOR*) scale (*r* = .76 for males and *r* = .88 for females). The Sherwood et al. (1997) component subscales for this content scale are Self-Doubt (*A-lse₁*) and Interpersonal Submissiveness (*A-lse₂*).

Williams et al. (1992) reported that high scores on the *A-lse* scale are associated with negative self-view and poor school performance. Among girls in their clinical sample, high scores on this scale were also associated with the occurrence of depression. In the Archer and Gordon (1991b) inpatient sample, high *A-lse* scores among girls were related to the occurrence of obsessive thoughts, social withdrawal, tiredness and fatigue, and suicidal thoughts. High scores among boys were related to suicidal thoughts, passivity, and self-blame or condemnation. Veltri et al. (2009) found higher *A-lse* scores related to lower clinical ratings of self-esteem for both boys in a forensic sample and girls in a clinical sample. Handel et al. (2011) reported an association between the *A-lse* scale and social problems, social withdrawal, and depression for boys and girls in their forensic sample.

The following descriptors or correlates are associated with elevated scores on *A-lse*:

- Poor self-esteem or self-confidence.
- Feelings of inadequacy and incompetency.
- Interpersonal passivity, discomfort, and withdrawal.

Adolescent-Low Aspirations (A-las) Scale

The MMPI-A Low Aspirations scale is composed of 16 items and does not have a direct counterpart among the MMPI-2 Content scales. The Sherwood et al. (1997) components for this content scale are Low Achievement Orientation (*A-las₁*) and Lack of Initiative (*A-las₂*). Like the *A-hea* scale, the majority of the items in the *A-las* content scale are scored in the *false* direction. Adolescents who score high on the *A-las* scale have few educational or life goals, and view themselves as unsuccessful. They do not apply themselves, tend to procrastinate, and give up quickly when faced with a frustrating or difficult challenge. The *A-las* scale does not produce any correlations exceeding .50 with the MMPI-A Basic scales, or with the Wiggins content scales (see Tables 6.3 through 6.6). Among Supplementary scales, the *A-las* scale was most highly associated with the Immaturity (*IMM*) scale, reflected in a correlational value of $r = .59$ for the normative sample.

Williams et al. (1992) found *A-las* scores were related to poor achievement in school activities and to conduct-disordered behaviors including running away and truancy. In the Archer and Gordon (1991b) inpatient sample, high *A-las* scores among boys were related to occurrence of arrests, legal difficulties, and suicidal threats. High scores for females were related to an inability to delay gratification, a defiant and resistant attitude, and frustration and anger in response to difficulties in learning or mastering new concepts and materials. Veltri found higher *A-las* scale scores unrelated to any relevant correlates for boys in a forensic setting or girls in an acute inpatient sample. Handel et al. (2011) found higher *A-las* scores related to higher scores on a measure of Attention-Deficit/Hyperactivity Disorder (ADHD) for boys and girls.

The following correlates are associated with elevated scores on the *A-las* scale:

- Poor academic achievement.
- Low frustration tolerance.
- Lack of initiative and direction.
- Persistent pattern of underachievement.

Adolescent-Social Discomfort (A-sod) Scale

The MMPI-A Social Discomfort scale consists of 24 items, of which 21 also appear on the MMPI-2 Social Discomfort scale. Sixteen of the items on the A-sod scale also appear on the MMPI-A Si Basic profile scale. Adolescents who produce elevated scores on the A-sod scale tend to be uncomfortable in social situations. They avoid social events, and find it difficult to interact with others. Sherwood et al. (1997) labeled the component dimensions of this Content scale Introversion (A-sod$_1$) and Shyness (A-sod$_2$). Among the basic MMPI-A scales, the A-sod is most highly correlated ($r > .75$) with the Si scale for both males and females (see Tables 6.3 and 6.4). The A-sod scale also produces a very high level of correlation ($r > .85$) with the Wiggins Social Maladjustment (SOC) scale, as shown in Tables 6.5 and 6.6.

Williams et al. (1992) found high A-sod scores to be associated with social withdrawal and discomfort for both boys and girls, and with depression and eating disorder problems for females. Archer and Gordon (1991b) found high A-sod scores among inpatient girls to be related to social withdrawal, apathy, fatigue, shyness, and the avoidance of competition with peers. High A-sod scores among boys were related to an increased frequency of provocative behaviors, anxiety and nervousness, and suicidal thoughts. Arita and Baer (1998) report A-sod scale scores were correlated (r = .63) with scores from the Social Introversion dimension of the Multiscore Depression Inventory (MDI) among adolescent inpatients. Veltri et al. (2009) reported higher A-sod scores related to depression and anxiety in his samples. Handel et al. (2011) found higher levels of withdrawal/depression among girls with elevated A-sod scores.

The following characteristics are associated with high A-sod scores:

- Social discomfort and withdrawal.
- Shyness and social introversion.

Adolescent-Family Problems (A-fam) Scale

The MMPI-A Family Problems scale includes 35 items, of which 15 also appear on the MMPI-2 Family Problems Content scale. Twenty-one of the items on the A-fam scale were derived from the original form of the MMPI. Adolescents producing elevations on the A-fam scale report the presence of substantial family conflict and discord. They are likely to have frequent quarrels with family members, and report little love or understanding within their families. They feel misunderstood and unjustly punished by family members, and may report being physically or emotionally abused. They may wish to run away or escape from their homes and families. Sherwood et al. (1997) divided the content of A-fam into two components, labeled Familial Discord (A-fam$_1$) and Familial Alienation (A-fam$_2$). Among the MMPI-A Basic scales, A-fam is most highly correlated ($r > .65$) with scores from scales Pd and Sc (see Tables 6.3 and 6.4).

Among the Wiggins content scales, *A-fam* scores are most highly correlated ($r > .80$) with the Wiggins Family Problems (*FAM*) scale (see Tables 6.5 and 6.6).

Williams et al. (1992) reported that high scores on the *A-fam* scale were associated with a variety of delinquent and neurotic symptoms and behaviors. Girls who produced high *A-fam* scores in the Archer and Gordon (1991b) inpatient sample were found to have more problems with anger, to be loud and boisterous, and to have a higher frequency of running away from home. Boys who scored high on this Content scale were more likely to engage in drug and/or alcohol abuse, to have anger control problems, and to have a history of physical abuse. In the research by Veltri and colleagues (2009), *A-fam* scale scores were related to anger and substance abuse histories for boys in a forensic setting, and a history of oppositional behavior and sexual abuse for girls in an acute inpatient setting. Handel et al. (2011) reported that *A-fam* scale scores were related to oppositional-defiant behaviors, conduct problems, and ADHD for boys and girls in their forensic sample.

The following characteristics are associated with high *A-fam* scores:

- Perception of family environment as unsupportive, hostile, unloving, or punitive.
- Increased probability of acting out, including running away from home.
- Resentment, anger, and hostility toward family members.

Adolescent-School Problems (A-sch) Scale

The MMPI-A School Problems scale consists of 20 items. This scale was created especially for the MMPI-A, and does not have a counterpart among the MMPI-2 scales. Only nine of the items that appear on the *A-sch* scale were derived from items appearing on the original instrument. Adolescents who score high on the *A-sch* scale do not like school, and are likely to encounter many behavioral and academic problems within the school setting. They may have developmental delays or learning disabilities, or may exhibit behavioral problems that have significantly interfered with academic achievement and their acquisition of academic skills. Sherwood et al. (1997) components for this content scale include School Conduct Problems (*A-sch₁*) and Negative Attitudes (*A-sch₂*). Among the MMPI-A Basic scales, *A-sch* scores are most highly correlated with scales F ($r > .60$) and Sc ($r > .55$). The *A-sch* score is also correlated with the Wiggins Hostility (*HOS*) scale ($r > .50$) and with the Immaturity (*IMM*) Supplementary scale ($r > .70$).

Williams et al. (1992) reported that high *A-sch* scores were related to the occurrence of academic and behavioral problems in the school environment and may also serve as a measure of general maladjustment. Archer and Gordon (1991b) found that high scores on this MMPI-A Content scale were related to the occurrence of academic decline and failure, truancy, and defiance among adolescent female inpatients. Among boys, high scores were associated with legal difficulties, drug abuse, fighting, and intense interest in the opposite sex. Toyer and Weed (1998) reported scores from the *A-sch* Content scales correlated with juvenile offender status as well as counselor's ratings of court-adjudicated adolescents' extent of difficulty in academic settings. Milne and Greenway (1999) investigated a sample of 170 adolescents and found elevations on *A-sch* related to lower scores on Wechsler Intelligence Scale for Children-III (WISC-III) Full Scale and Verbal IQ scores for boys, but this association was weaker for girls. Veltri et al. (2009) reported that higher *A-sch* scale scores were related to a history of substance abuse for boys, and a history of school suspension for girls. Handel et al. (2011) found that attention–deficit disorder, both inattentive and impulsive types, were related to higher *A-sch* scores for boys and girls in their forensic sample.

The following correlates or characteristics are associated with high *A-sch* scores:

- Negative attitude toward academic activities and achievement.
- Poor school performance, including behavioral and academic problems and deficits.
- Possibility of learning disabilities or significant developmental delays and learning problems.

Adolescent-Negative Treatment Indicators (A-trt) Scale

The MMPI-A Negative Treatment Indicator scale consists of 26 items, of which 21 also appeared on the MMPI-2 *TRT* scale. Only nine of the items in the *A-trt* scale are derived from the original MMPI instrument. Adolescents who produce elevations on the *A-trt* scale may present barriers to treatment stemming from apathy or despondency concerning their ability to change, or from suspiciousness and distrust of help offered by others (including mental health professionals). These adolescents may feel they are incapable of making significant changes in their lives, or that working with others in the change process is ineffective or a sign of weakness. The Sherwood et al. (1997) components for this Content scale are Low Motivation ($A\text{-}trt_1$) and Inability to Disclose ($A\text{-}trt_2$). The *A-trt* scale is most highly correlated ($r > .60$) with scales *Pt* and *Sc* among the MMPI-A Basic scales (see Tables 6.3 and 6.4). The *A-trt* scale is also highly correlated ($r > .60$) with the Immaturity (*IMM*) Supplementary scale, and the Wiggins Depression (*DEP*) and Psychoticism (*PSY*) Content scales.

In the Archer and Gordon (1991b) inpatient sample, high *A-trt* scores among boys were associated with interest in the opposite sex, poor sibling relationships, the excessive use of fantasy, and a tendency to physically threaten peers. Elevated *A-trt* scores for girls were associated with poor physical coordination and odd physical movements. Williams et al. (1992) failed to find a clear pattern of clinical correlates for the *A-trt* scale. Veltri et al. (2009) found *A-trt* scale scores related to suicidal attempts and gestures for boys in their forensic sample, and to suicidal ideation for girls in an acute inpatient setting. In the forensic sample investigated by Handel et al. (2011), *A-trt* scale scores were related to anxiety, depression and internalizing problems for girls.

Based on the content of the *A-trt* scale, the following are correlates likely to be associated with high scores:

- Presence of negative attitudes or expectations concerning mental health treatment.
- Pessimism concerning one's ability to change.
- The belief that talking about problems with others is not helpful or useful, or is a sign of weakness.

Supplementary Scales

The MMPI-A Supplementary scales consist of a set of six measures created by a variety of researchers. Three of the Supplementary scales were adopted from the original MMPI with relatively limited modification and were also included in the MMPI-2 (Butcher et al. 1989). These measures include Welsh's (1956) Anxiety and Repression scales, and the MacAndrew Alcoholism scale (MacAndrew, 1965), denoted the *MAC-R* in the MMPI-A. In addition, the Immaturity (*IMM*) scale, the Alcohol-Drug Problem Acknowledgment (*ACK*) scale, and the Alcohol-Drug Problem Proneness (*PRO*) scale are measures created especially for the MMPI-A.

Three general statements may be offered concerning the MMPI-A Supplementary scales:

1. The raw score totals for all Supplementary scales are converted to T-score values based on linear T-score transformation procedures. Identical to the MMPI-A Basic scales and Content scales, however, a gray or shaded zone denoting marginal-range elevations for Supplementary scales occurs between T-scores 60 through 65, inclusive.
2. None of the Supplementary scales may be scored within the first 350 items of the MMPI-A booklet. Each of the Supplementary scales require the administration of the full test booklet.
3. Supplementary scale results should be used to refine, but not replace, the interpretation of the MMPI-A Basic scales.

MMPI-A Supplemental Scales

The following section provides a brief overview of each of the MMPI-A Supplemental scales. Table 6.8 provides the intercorrelations of the Supplementary scales, and Tables 6.9 and 6.10 show the correlations of these measures with the MMPI-A Basic scales.

MacAndrew Alcoholism Scale—Revised (MAC-R)

The MacAndrew Alcoholism scale (*MAC*) was originally created by MacAndrew in 1965 by contrasting the item responses of 300 male alcoholics with those of 300 male psychiatric patients. Items selected for the *MAC* scale showed the greatest endorsement differences between these two groups (excluding two

TABLE 6.8 Raw Score Intercorrelations of the MMPI-A Supplementary Scales for Male and Female Adolescents in the MMPI-A Normative Sample

Females

	Scales	MAC-R	ACK	PRO	IMM	A	R
	MAC-R		.56	.45	.43	.22	−.38
M	ACK	.57		.57	.64	.38	−.12
a	PRO	.45	.60		.54	.30	−.07
l	IMM	.40	.62	.54		.53	.05
e	A	.23	.41	.33	.58		−.22
s	R	−.26	−.09	−.05	.05	−.24	

Source: Archer (1997b). Copyright © 1997 by Lawrence Erlbaum Associates, Inc. Reprinted with permission.

TABLE 6.9 Raw Score Intercorrelations of the MMPI-A Supplementary and Basic Scales for Female Adolescents in the MMPI-A Normative Sample

Scale	MAC-R	ACK	PRO	IMM	A	R
F_1	.49	.59	.45	.68	.34	.17
F_2	.46	.56	.35	.72	.40	.19
F	.50	.61	.41	.75	.40	.19
L	−.01	−.15	−.25	−.03	−.27	.39
K	−.22	−.30	−.22	−.43	−.73	.37
Hs	.26	.36	.29	.48	.54	.07
D	.02	.24	.22	.43	.54	.32
Hy	.05	.14	.20	.13	.16	.21
Pd	.43	.54	.53	.57	.55	−.02
Mf	−.32	−.23	−.13	−.35	.07	−.32
Pa	.35	.42	.30	.48	.54	.06
Pt	.26	.46	.36	.62	.90	−.17
Sc	.42	.58	.44	.73	.79	−.09
Ma	.52	.48	.41	.40	.43	−.39
Si	−.06	.20	.12	.52	.68	.18

Source: Archer (1997b). Copyright © 1997 by Lawrence Erlbaum Associates, Inc. Reprinted with permission.

TABLE 6.10 Raw Score Intercorrelations of the MMPI-A Supplementary and Basic
Scales for Male Adolescents in the MMPI-A Normative Sample

Scale	MAC-R	ACK	PRO	IMM	A	R
F_1	.35	.61	.47	.70	.29	.22
F_2	.33	.57	.40	.70	.34	.20
F	.36	.62	.45	.74	.34	.22
L	−.06	−.04	−.11	.07	−.30	.47
K	−.24	−.20	−.13	−.30	−.70	.52
Hs	.12	.33	.29	.48	.40	.23
D	−.17	.13	.14	.32	.36	.48
Hy	−.12	.14	.19	.15	−.02	.46
Pd	.33	.54	.55	.58	.46	.05
Mf	−.29	−.08	−.03	−.12	.23	.13
Pa	.27	.48	.33	.54	.46	.17
Pt	.22	.41	.35	.58	.88	−.16
Sc	.30	.58	.46	.74	.74	−.06
Ma	.54	.50	.42	.40	.43	−.47
Si	−.09	.14	.06	.47	.67	.20

Source: Archer (1997b). Copyright © 1997 by Lawrence Erlbaum Associates, Inc. Reprinted with permission.

items directly related to alcohol consumption). The final 49 items selected by these procedures correctly classified 81.5% of subjects in the cross-validation sample of male alcoholic and nonalcoholic psychiatric outpatients (MacAndrew, 1965). Based on their review of the MMPI literature in the substance abuse area, Sutker and Archer (1979) concluded that research findings on the *MAC* scale supported the view that it was "the most promising of current MMPI-derived alcoholism scales" (p. 127).

The *MAC* scale is the only MMPI special scale that has received substantial empirical investigation with adolescents (Archer, 1987b). This literature has shown *MAC* scale scores to be related to substance abuse among adolescents in public school settings, as well as in hospital and residential psychiatric and drug treatment programs. Recommended adolescent *MAC* raw score cutoff values across assessment settings have ranged from Wolfson and Erbaugh's (1984) cutoff of 24 for females and 26 for males to Archer's (1987b) recommended cutoff of 28 for both male and female adolescents. Findings by Gantner, Graham, and Archer (1992) indicated a raw score cutoff value of 28 for males and 27 for females provided maximum accurate classification of substance abusers from psychiatric inpatients, whereas values of 26 for males and 25 for females provided optimal discrimination of substance abusers from a sample of normal high school students. Further, as shown in Tables 6.11 and 6.12, findings by Archer and Klinefelter (1992) indicate that the probability of obtaining an elevated *MAC* scale score is associated with the type of basic scale MMPI codetype produced by an adolescent. Adolescents producing the

4-9/9-4 code, for example, were much more likely to produce elevated *MAC* scores, whereas adolescents producing the *2-3/3-2* code were more likely to produce lower range *MAC* scale scores. Greene (1994) also showed a strong relationship between adults, *MAC* scale elevations and MMPI codetype, subject gender, and treatment setting.

Similar to findings in adult populations, high *MAC* scores among adolescents appear to be related to the abuse of a variety of drugs in addition to alcohol. Andrucci, Archer, Pancoast, and Gordon (1989), for example, found high *MAC* scores related to abuse of amphetamines, barbiturates, cocaine, hallucinogens, and marijuana. In addition to indicating the possibility of substance abuse problems, elevated *MAC* scale scores have also been associated with a variety of personality characteristics. For example, Archer, Gordon et al. (1989) found high *MAC* adolescents to be described as assertive, independent, self-indulgent, undercontrolled, and much more likely to have an arrest record and to receive conduct disorder diagnoses. These findings are consistent with earlier reports by Rathus, Fox, and Ortins (1980), who found that *MAC* scale scores were related to delinquent behaviors, as well as results by Wisniewski, Glenwick, and Graham (1985), who found that high *MAC* scores in a high school sample were related to a higher number of disciplinary incidents and lower grade point averages. Basham (1992) examined a wide variety of MMPI scales as measures of acting out in a sample of 327 adolescent inpatients. He concluded that the *MAC* scale appears to measure a broad antisocial personality dimension rather than the presence of a specific alcohol or drug abuse problem. Svanum and Ehrmann (1992) found that adult alcoholics with high *MAC* scores were characterized by gregariousness, social drinking, belligerence and aggression while drinking, and a high incidence of alcohol-related legal problems. MacAndrew (1981) described individuals who produce elevations on *MAC* as pursuing a bold, impulsive lifestyle, with little concern for the consequences of behaviors.

The *MAC* scale has probably received extensive attention in the adolescent MMPI literature because of the importance many clinicians and researchers have placed on drug and alcohol problems within this age group. Although the *MAC* scale holds substantial potential as a useful screening device for substance abuse among adolescents, several cautions appear appropriate regarding its use. Archer (1987b), for example, observed that the findings in adult samples suggest that the *MAC* scale may have little diagnostic utility among Black respondents, and that substantial caution should be used when interpreting the *MAC* in non-White populations. According to Greene (2011), accuracy hit rates are probably too low to justify the use of the *MAC* as a screening device to detect substance abuse problems among patients in medical treatment settings. Wasyliw, Haywood, Grossman, and Cavanaugh (1993) reported findings that indicate that clinicians should be particularly cautious in interpreting the *MAC* scale when they suspect that respondents have attempted to minimize the report of psychopathology on

TABLE 6.11 MMPI Codetype Classification and MAC Scale Elevations at Two Criterion Levels for Male Adolescent Psychiatric Patients

Codetype	MAC Cutoff Scores				MAC	MAC SD
	<24	>24	<28	>28		
3	8 (47%)	9 (53%)	15 (88%)	2(12%)	23.7	4.7
4	4 (8%)	44 (92%)	17 (35%)	31 (65%)	28.8	4.0
5	10 (36%)	18 (64%)	20 (71%)	8 (29%)	24.7	4.0
9	3 (11%)	24 (89%)	8 (30%)	19 (70%)	29.3	4.6
13–31	10 (43%)	13 (57%)	15 (65%)	8 (35%)	24.3	5.9
14–41	1 (6%)	15 (94%)	5 (31%)	11 (69%)	29.3	4.2
15–51	1 (9%)	10 (91%)	6 (55%)	5 (45%)	27.7	4.9
17–71	0 (0%)	12 (100%)	9 (75%)	3 (25%)	26.4	2.4
18–81	0 (0%)	15 (100%)	6 (40%)	9 (60%)	29.4	3.7
23–32	9 (64%)	5 (36%)[*a]	13 (93%)	1 (7%)	20.6	5.4
24–42	7 (25%)	21 (75%)	20 (71%)	8 (29%)	25.3	4.0
25–52	11 (79%)	3 (21%)[*a]	12 (86%)	2 (14%)	21.6	4.5
34–43	3 (14%)	18 (86%)	9 (43%)	12 (57%)	26.9	4.3
35–53	2 (20%)	8 (80%)	5 (50%)	5 (50%)	27.4	3.6
45–54	9 (38%)	15 (62%)	15 (63%)	9 (37%)	25.3	5.0
46–64	1 (2%)	42 (98%)[*a]	9 (21%)	3 (79%)[*b]	30.1	3.6
47–74	0 (0%)	11 (100%)	2 (18%)	9 (82%)	30.1	3.0
48–84	3 (19%)	13 (81%)	9 (56%)	7 (44%)	27.4	4.3
49–94	1 (3%)	38 (97%)[*a]	8 (21%)	31 (79%)[*b]	31.5	4.2
56–65	3 (25%)	9 (75%)	7 (58%)	5 (42%)	25.6	5.1
67–76	2 (20%)	8 (80%)	5 (50%)	5 (50%)	27.4	4.9
68–86	5 (36%)	9 (64%)	8 (57%)	6 (43%)	26.3	5.4
69–96	1 (7%)	14 (93%)	3 (20%)	12 (80%)	31.5	5.9
78–87	3 (17%)	15 (83%)	6 (33%)	12 (67%)	28.8	5.0
No Code	70 (31%)	153 (69%)	141 (63%)	82 (37%)[*b]	26.1	4.5
Other Codes	32 (27%)	88 (73%)	64 (53%)	56 (47%)	26.8	5.4
Total	199 (24%)	630 (76%)	437 (53%)	392 (47%)	27.0	5.0

Source: Archer and Klinefelter (1992). Relationships Between MMPI Codetypes and MAC Scale Elevations in Adolescent Psychiatric Samples. *Journal of Personality Assessment*. Copyright © 1992 by Lawrence Erlbaum Associates, Inc. Reprinted with permission.

Notes

* $p < .002$

a Significant MAC elevation frequency difference found for codetype comparisons using MAC ≥24 criterion.

b Significant MAC elevation frequency difference found for codetype comparisons using MAC ≥28 criterion.

Values within parentheses indicate percentage of cases occurring at varying MAC scale values within specific codetypes.

TABLE 6.12 MMPI Codetype Classification and MAC Scale Elevations at Two Criterion Levels for Female Adolescent Psychiatric Patients

Codetype	MAC Cutoff Scores					
	<24	>24	<28	>28	MAC	MAC SD
4	8 (31%)	18 (69%)	17 (65%)	9 (35%)	25.5	4.4
9	6 (29%)	15 (71%)	18 (86%)	3 (14%)	24.6	3.5
12–21	14 (74%)	5 (26%)	15 (79%)	4 (21%)	22.9	4.5
13–31	7 (41%)	10 (59%)	12 (71%)	5 (19%)	24.1	4.2
18–81	7 (41%)	10 (59%)	11 (65%)	6 (35%)	24.9	5.1
23–32	12 (86%)	2 (14%)*[a]	14 (100%)	0 (0%)	19.3	3.6
24–42	15 (44%)	19 (56%)	28 (82%)	6 (18%)	23.3	4.6
46–64	11 (50%)	11 (50%)	14 (64%)	8 (36%)	25.3	4.8
48–84	8 (36%)	14 (64%)	15 (68%)	7 (32%)	25.0	4.7
49–94	3 (10%)	27 (90%)*[a]	11 (37%)	19 (63%)*[b]	8.3	3.5
69–96	0 (0%)	10 (100%)	3 (30%)	7 (70%)*[b]	30.2	4.0
78–87	3 (25%)	9 (75%)	9 (75%)	3 (25%)	24.8	3.3
89–98	0 (0%)	11 (100%)	2 (18%)	9 (82%)*[b]	30.1	2.8
No Code	65 (48%)	70 (52%)	13 (84%)	22 (16%)	23.1	4.4
Other Codes	69 (54%)	59 (46%)	105 (82%)	23 (18%)	23.2	4.7
Total	228 (44%)	290 (56%)	387 (75%)	131 (25%)	24.1	4.8

Source: Archer and Klinefelter (1992). Relationships Between MMPI Codetypes and MAC Scale Elevatiosn in Adolescent Psychiatricb Samples. *Journal of Personality Assessment.* Copyright © 1992 by Lawrence Erlbaum Associates, Inc. Reprinted with permission.

Notes

* $p < .004$

a Significant MAC elevation frequency difference found for codetype comparisons using MAC ≥24 criterion.

b Significant MAC elevation frequency difference found for codetype comparisons using MAC ≥28 criterion.

Values within parentheses indicate percentage of cases occurring at varying MAC scale values within specific codetypes.

the MMPI. Additionally, Gottesman and Prescott (1989) observed that lower range cutting scores, such as a value of 24 or above, which has frequently been employed for adults, would misclassify a high percentage of normal adolescents as a result of false positive errors. For example, the MAC-R scale mean value for adolescents in the MMPI-A sample was 21.07 for males and 19.73 for females (Butcher et al., 1992). Both Gottesman and Prescott (1989) and Greene (1988) noted the critical effects of substance abuse base rates on the clinical usefulness of the MAC scale. Many studies have examined the validity of the MAC scale based on equal, or nearly equal, samples of substance abuse and non-substance abuse groups. These studies have often yielded impressive rates of accurate classification of approximately 80% (e.g., MacAndrew, 1979). However, when hit rates are recalculated using more realistic estimates of the base rate of substance abuse, substantially less impressive accuracy is often obtained (e.g., Gantner et al., 1992; Gottesman & Prescott, 1989).

In the creation of the MMPI-A, a revised form of the *MAC* scale (i.e., the *MAC-R* scale) was developed. The MMPI-A *MAC-R* scale contains 49 items and is identical in length to the original *MAC* scale. Forty-five of the original *MAC* items were retained in the *MAC-R* scale, with four *MAC-R* items added. These latter items were used to replace the four items deleted from the original *MAC* scale in the formation of the MMPI-A.

There have been no studies on the comparability of the *MAC* and *MAC-R* scales for the MMPI-A. Research by Greene, Arredondo, and Davis (1990), however, indicates that the original *MAC* scale and the *MAC-R* scale of the MMPI-2 appear to produce comparable scores and may be used in a similar manner by clinicians. Gallucci (1997b) examined the contributions of the *MAC-R* to the identification of substance abuse patterns among 88 male and 92 female adolescents receiving substance abuse treatment. He reported that the *MAC-R* scale made the largest contribution to the correct classification of adolescents into varying categories of substance abusers (e.g., undercontrolled versus overcontrolled), although all three MMPI-A substance abuse supplementary scales make significant contributions to this classification task. Gallucci (1997a) apparently employed the same sample to evaluate scale correlates, and reported that the MMPI-A *MAC-R* and Alcohol/Drug Problem Proneness (*PRO*) scales produced similar patterns of correlates, with identical correlations of r = .31 with clinician's ratings of substance abuse. Veltri et al. (2009) investigated MMPI-A scale correlates in a sample of 157 boys from a forensic sample and 197 girls from an acute psychiatric inpatient setting. Results for both samples showed a significant correlation between *MAC-R* scale scores and history of substance abuse for boys (r = .33) and girls (r = .27). In general, it is expected that the following correlates would be related to raw score values of 28 or greater on the *MAC-R* scale of the MMPI-A:

- Increased likelihood of alcohol or drug abuse problems.
- Interpersonally assertive and dominant.
- Self-indulgent and egocentric.
- Unconventional and impulsive.
- Greater likelihood of conduct disorder diagnoses.
- Greater likelihood of legal involvement and violation of social norms.

In addition, individuals who produce low-range scores on the *MAC-R* might be expected to be dependent, conservative, indecisive, overcontrolled, and sensation-avoidant. As noted by MacAndrew (1981), individuals who abuse alcohol but produce low *MAC* scores (false negatives) are likely to be neurotic individuals who may use alcohol to self-medicate their affective distress.

The Alcohol/Drug Problem Acknowledgment (ACK) Scale

The Alcohol/Drug Problem Acknowledgment (*ACK*) scale was developed for the MMPI-A to assess an adolescent's willingness to acknowledge alcohol or drug use-related symptoms, attitudes, or beliefs (Butcher et al., 1992). The *ACK* scale consists of 13 items initially selected based on the rational judgment that item content was relevant to drug use, and further refined based on statistical criteria, including item correlations. The *ACK* scale is quite similar to the Addiction Acknowledgment Scale (*AAS*) created for the MMPI-2 (Weed, Butcher, McKenna, & Ben-Porath, 1992). Svanum, McGrew, and Ehrmann (1994) demonstrated the relative usefulness of the *AAS* as a direct measure of substance abuse, in contrast to more subtle measures such as the *MAC-R* scale, in detecting substance dependence in a sample of 308 college students. Choi, Kurtz, and Proctor (2012) recently found that while *MAC-R*, *PRO*, and *ACK* scale scores were each related to a substance abuse measure in a sample of 86 adolescents in a midwestern school, the former two scales were unable to account for additional variance in students' substance abuse reports beyond that accounted for solely by the *ACK* scale.

Elevations on the *ACK* scale indicate the extent to which an adolescent acknowledged or admitted alcohol and/or drug problems in their MMPI-A self-description. It should be noted, however, that not all items on the *ACK* scale directly involve an acknowledgment of drug use. Some items, for example items 81 and 249, deal with attitudes, beliefs, or behaviors that may be associated with drug use, but do not directly indicate the presence or absence of alcohol or drug use behaviors. For both boys and girls in the MMPI-A sample, the mean raw score for *ACK* was approximately 4, and a raw score total of 9 or greater converts to T-score values that exceed T = 70.

Several studies have evaluated the performance of the MMPI-A *ACK* scale. Gallucci (1997a) compared the correlates of the *ACK* scale with patterns for the MMPI-A *MAC-R* and *PRO* scales in a sample of adolescents receiving substance abuse treatment. This researcher found that the *ACK* scale produced a correlation value that was very similar to the *MAC-R* and *PRO* scales correlations with clinician's ratings of substance abuse, but appeared to be a more specific measure in the sense of generally producing lower correlations with non-substance abuse related criterion. Gallucci concluded, "These results were consistent with interpretation of the *ACK* scale as a somewhat specific measure of a young person's willingness to acknowledge problematic substance abuse" (p. 91). Toyer and Weed (1998) examined the MMPI-A substance abuse scales, as well as other selected scales, in their investigation of 50 court-adjudicated youths participating in outpatient counseling. The results of their study indicated that the *ACK* scale produced the highest correlation with counselor ratings of drug and alcohol use (r = .36) of any of the MMPI-A substance abuse scales. Micucci (2002) investigated the accuracy of the MMPI-A substance abuse scales in identifying substance abuse problems in a sample of 79 adolescent psychiatric inpatients. In this study, 89.9% of substance abuse cases were accurately identified by at least one of the three scales, with the overall accuracy of classification similar across genders and ethnicity, although there was a tendency for more false positive misclassifications to occur for males. *ACK, MAC-R,* and *PRO* were better at screening out cases of substance abuse (identifying for true negatives), than in accurately identifying adolescents who were using substances (identifying true negatives). The highest level of correct classification was achieved by identifying substance abuse using the criterion of T ≥ 60 or T ≥ 65 on the *ACK* scale. The former cutoff score achieved greater sensitivity, while the latter cutoff criterion achieved the highest degree of specificity. Tirrell, Archer, and Mason (2004) examined the concurrent validity of the MMPI-A substance abuse scales *MAC-R, ACK,* and *PRO* in distinguishing adolescents in groups of 100 substance abusers, 100 non-substance abusing psychiatric patients, and 100 adolescents selected from the MMPI-A normative sample. The overall findings clearly indicated that the *MAC-R, ACK,* and *PRO* scales generated the most impressive findings in the less challenging discrimination task of separating adolescent substance abusers from adolescents in the normative sample. Further, the *ACK* scale demonstrated the highest level of effectiveness in differentiating adolescent substance abusers from adolescent psychiatric patients, and was the single best predictor for this classification task. Veltri et al. (2009) reported correlations between substance abuse histories and *ACK* scale scores of r = .42 for boys and r = .44 for girls.

The Alcohol/Drug Problem Proneness (PRO) Scale

The Alcohol/Drug Problem Proneness (*PRO*) scale consists of 36 items. These items were empirically selected based on item endorsement differences found between adolescents in alcohol and drug treatment programs and adolescents receiving inpatient psychiatric services (Butcher et al., 1992). Thus, the scale construction method used for *PRO* is similar to that employed in the development of the *MAC* scale. Based on cross-validated research findings noted in the MMPI-A manual (Butcher et al., 1992), T-score values of 65 and greater are associated with an increased potential for the development of alcohol and drug problems. The 36 items in the *PRO* scale cover a wide variety of content, including familial characteristics, peer group features, antisocial behaviors and beliefs, and academic interests and behaviors. Veltri and his colleagues (2009) found significant correlations between the *PRO* scale and substance abuse history for both boys (r = .46) in a forensic sample and girls (r = .36) in an acute psychiatric inpatient setting.

The Immaturity (IMM) Scale

The Immaturity (*IMM*) scale was developed by Archer, Pancoast, and Gordon (1994) as a Supplementary scale for the MMPI-A. The *IMM* scale assesses psychological maturation during adolescence using Loevinger's (1976) concept of ego development as a conceptual focus. Items for the *IMM* scale were selected based on a multi-stage procedure involving both rational and statistical criteria. In the initial stage, MMPI-TX item correlations were computed with scores derived from the Holt (1980) Short Form adaptation of the Loevinger and Wessler (1970) Sentence Completion Test of ego development in a sample of 222 normal adolescents. Preliminary items were selected for the *IMM* scale based on the occurrence of correlation coefficients achieving a significance level of $\leq .01$. In the second stage of scale construction, raters independently evaluated the degree to which preliminary items were related to Loevinger's concept of ego development. Items were retained in the preliminary *IMM* scale if at least four of the six raters were in agreement on the appropriateness of the item to the ego development construct. In the third stage, preliminary *IMM* scale items were eliminated if the removal of the item increased the scale's internal reliability (alpha coefficient value) in either the normal sample of 222 adolescents or in a sample of 122 adolescent inpatients who had completed the MMPI-TX. Finally, each of the 704 items in the experimental MMPI-TX Form were examined in terms of their correlations with the *IMM* scale. New items were added to the *IMM* scale if items demonstrated both a conceptual and statistical relationship to the ego development construct.

The final form of the *IMM* scale consists of 43 items. The alpha coefficient value for the *IMM* scale in the MMPI-A normative sample was .83 for females and .80 for males. As expected, *IMM* mean raw score values were significantly higher for males than for females in both the clinical sample (18.69 vs. 14.88) and the MMPI-A normative sample (13.47 vs. 11.75). This gender-related difference in *IMM* mean scores is consistent with conclusions from a review (Cohn, 1991) of the results from 63 studies using the Sentence Completion Test. Cohn reported that females consistently showed higher developmental levels than males during adolescence.

The 43 items in the *IMM* scale concern aspects of personality including lack of self-confidence, externalization of blame, lack of insight and introspection, interpersonal and social discomfort and alienation, "living for the present" without concern for future consequences, the occurrence of hostile and anti-social attitudes, and egocentricity and self-centeredness. High scores on the *IMM* scale would be expected to be associated with impulsive adolescents who have a limited capacity for self-awareness. Their egocentricity is likely to impair their ability to engage in reciprocal and mutually satisfying interpersonal relationships, and their cognitive processes could be characterized as concrete and simplistic. Within Loevinger's model of ego development, individuals producing elevated *IMM* scores are likely to reflect a *preconformist* stage of development. Interpersonal relationships during the preconformist stage have been described as opportunistic, demanding, and exploitive (Loevinger, 1976).

Preliminary data on the *IMM* scale (Archer, Pancoast, & Gordon, 1994) from both normal and clinical samples indicated that adolescents who produced high scores on this measure had a higher incidence of school difficulties and problems. Research by Imhof and Archer (1997) examined the concurrent validity of the *IMM* scale in a residential treatment sample of 66 adolescents, ages 13 through 18, inclusive. In addition to the MMPI-A, participants were administered measures of intelligence, reading ability, and maturation. The results of this study provided support for the construct validity of the MMPI-A as a measure of maturational development. As predicted, individuals who scored higher on the *IMM* scale tended to produce lower full scale and verbal IQ scores and to exhibit lower levels of moral and ego development. Results from a multiple regression analysis indicated that a linear combination of three variables including identity development, reading ability, and moral development accounted for nearly one-half (46%) of the total variance in *IMM* scale raw scores. Zinn, McCumber, and Dahlstrom (1999) used 75 female and 76 male college undergraduates to cross-validate the MMPI-A *IMM* scale. In addition to the 43 items from the *IMM* scale, all these participants completed the Washington University Sentence Completion Test (WUSCT) developed by Loevinger and Wessler (1970) as a projective method of assessing ego development, and a brief biographical questionnaire. High interrater reliability (r = .80) was established for scoring the WUSCT. The distribution of *IMM* scale scores was used to partition adolescents into groups of low, medium, and high scores, and WUSCT scores were found to vary significantly between these categories. Zinn and her colleagues concluded that the MMPI-A *IMM* scale could be used as a reliable objective measure of Loevinger's concept of ego maturity. Veltri et al. (2009) reported an association between higher *IMM* scale scores and anger for boys in a forensic sample. Handel and his colleagues (2011) found *IMM* scale scores to be significantly related to social problems and rule-breaking behaviors for boys and girls in their forensic sample.

Based on the current literature, the following correlates appear applicable to adolescents who produce high *IMM* scores:

- Easily frustrated and quick to anger.
- Impatient, loud, and boisterous.
- Tend to tease or bully others.
- Not trustworthy or dependable.
- Defiant and resistant.
- Likely to have a history of academic and social difficulties.
- Likely to have lower verbal IQs and lower language ability.

Additionally, adolescents who produce low scores on the *IMM* scale are likely to be described as controlled, stable, patient, cooperative, and predictable.

Welsh's Anxiety (A) and Repression (R) Scales

As noted by Graham (2012), a large majority of the factor analytic studies on MMPI scale-level data has typically found two basic MMPI dimensions or factors accounting for a majority of basic scale score variance. The first factor has been assigned a variety of labels, including *general maladjustment* and *lack of ego resiliency* and the second factor has been referred to as *ego control* or *inhibition*. Welsh (1956) developed the Anxiety (*A*) and Repression (*R*) scales to assess the respondent's standing along these first and second dimensions, respectively.

The Anxiety scale was originally created as a 39-item scale keyed in such a manner that higher scores on the *A* scale were associated with a greater degree of psychopathology. High scores have been described as reflective of individuals who are maladjusted, anxious, depressed, pessimistic, inhibited, and uncomfortable (Graham, 2012). Although these adjectives are largely negative in tone, it has also been noted that high scores on the *A* scale are associated with substantial emotional distress that may serve as a motivator for positive change in the psychotherapeutic process. In contrast, low scores on the *A* scale have been related to a preference for activity, freedom from anxiety and discomfort, sociability, manipulativeness, and impulsivity (Graham, 2012). Archer, Gordon, et al. (1989) examined special scale correlates in a sample of 68 adolescent inpatients. These authors reported that the high-scoring *A* adolescent could be described as fearful, anxious, guilt-prone, overwhelmed, and self-critical. High-scoring *A* adolescents also tended to be viewed by both self (on other self-report instruments) and others, including family members and treatment staff, as significantly more maladjusted than other adolescent inpatients. MMPI scale *A* and basic scale *Pt* were highly correlated ($r = .90$) in this sample, and a higher incidence of presenting problems related to suicide attempts, thoughts, and ideations were related to elevations on the *A* scale. More recently, Veltri et al. (2009) reported boys producing high *A* scale scores were more anxious, depressed, and had lower self-esteems, while Handel et al. (2011) found high-scoring *A* girls to be anxious, depressed, and internalizing.

In the MMPI-A, Welsh's *A* scale has been reduced to 35 items. In general, the following correlates are associated with elevations on scale *A*:

- Tense and anxious.
- Fearful and ruminative.
- Maladjusted and ineffective.
- Self-critical and guilty.
- Overwhelmed.

The Repression scale originally consisted of 40 items developed by Welsh (1956) to assess the second dimension that emerges when the standard MMPI scales are subjected to factor analysis. Like the *A* scale, the *R* scale appears in the original version of the MMPI, the MMPI-2, and in the MMPI-A. In the MMPI-A, the *R* scale has been reduced to 33 items, all of which are scored in the *false* direction. In research by Archer, Gordon, et al. (1989), *R* scale scores were found to be negatively correlated with scale *9* and *MAC* scale values, and positively correlated with several scales, including *L*, *K*, and the neurotic triad (scales *Hs*, *D*, and *Hy*). This finding is consistent with expectations based on the loading patterns reported for the second factor of the MMPI. This factor typically shows positive loadings on the neurotic triad and a negative loading on scale *9* (Graham, 2000; Greene, 2000). Significant correlates for the high *R* scale adolescent in the Archer et al. study included the following:

- Overcontrolled.
- Shows little feeling.
- Inhibited and constricted.
- Pessimistic and defeated.

In contrast, adolescents who produced low scores on *R* were described as talkative, spontaneous, and optimistic. Archer (1987b) also noted, however, that low *R* scores among adolescent psychiatric patients are related to aggressiveness, impulsivity, argumentativeness, and a tendency to employ acting-out defense mechanisms. Veltri et al. (2009) reported that boys in a forensic sample producing high *R* scale scores experienced more anhedonia (i.e., an inability to experience pleasure), anxiety, and lower self-esteem. Handel et al. (2011) were unable to identify meaningful correlates for the *R* scale in their forensic sample.

The Harris–Lingoes and Si Subscales

As we have noted, the empirical keying method employed by Hathaway and McKinley resulted in the creation of basic scales that were heterogeneous in terms of content areas. In order to help clinicians to determine the content endorsement associated with MMPI basic scale elevations, Harris and Lingoes (1955) constructed subscales for six of the basic scales, using the following process:

> The items scored in each scale were examined, and those which seemed similar in content, or to reflect a single attitude or trait, were grouped into a subscale. In effect, the item correlations were estimated, purely subjectively. The items were grouped on the basis of these estimates, and then given a name which was thought to be descriptive of the inferred attitude underlying the sorting of the items in the scored direction.

(p. 1)

Harris and Lingoes used this method to develop 27 content subscales for six of the basic MMPI clinical scales, that is, *2, 3, 4, 6, 8,* and *9*. They did not attempt to restrict items to placement on only one subscale, and consequently there is substantial item overlap among the subscales and a high degree of subscale correlation.

The authors did not develop content subscales for scales *1* or *7* because they considered these measures to be homogeneous (Graham, 2012), and they did not create subscales for *5* or *0* because these scales are often viewed as "non-clinical" scales or involving dimensions separate or apart from the standard "clinical" scales. Caldwell (1988), Levitt (1989), and Levitt and Gotts (1995) reviewed the Harris–Lingoes subscales in their discussions of MMPI special scales, and a symposium was focused on these subscales (Colligan, 1988).

Relatively little research has been conducted on the Harris and Lingoes subscales in terms of the construct validity of these measures (Greene, 2011). Harris and Christiansen (1946) found significant differences on eight Harris–Lingoes subscales between patients judged successful versus unsuccessful in psychotherapy. Gocka and Holloway (1963) found few significant correlations between demographic variables and scores on the Harris–Lingoes subscales. Calvin (1975), however, empirically identified behavioral correlates for many of the Harris–Lingoes subscales, and these have been incorporated into the standard descriptions provided for these subscales in guides such as the Greene (2011) and Graham (2012) texts. Wrobel (1992) investigated the concurrent validity of the MMPI Harris–Lingoes subscales in terms of the ability of these measures to predict clinicians' ratings of 85 adult outpatients. Results supported the validity of the majority of Harris–Lingoes subscales, but caution was urged in the interpretive use of subscales *Hy1* (Denial of Social Anxiety), *Hy2* (Need for Affection), *Pd3* (Social Imperturbability), *Pa3* (Naivete), *and Ma2* (Psychomotor Acceleration). In relation to this latter caution, Krishnamurthy, Archer, and Huddleston (1995) noted that a special problem arises for the *Hy1* and *Pd3* subscales because these measures cannot produce clinical range elevations (T $\geq$ 65) on the MMPI-2. Further, MMPI-A T-score values cannot exceed 66 for *Hy1* and 67 for *Pd3* for adolescents of either gender. These limitations occur because these subscales are markedly short (six items), and mean raw score values are approximately 4 with a standard deviation of approximately 2. Thus, it can be readily seen that the linear T-score transformation procedure cannot produce elevated T-scores for these subscales for any obtained raw score. Krishnamurthy et al. (1995) concluded that these two Harris–Lingoes subscales should be deleted from standard use on both the MMPI-2 and MMPI-A because these measures cannot provide useful information and results are easily susceptible to misinterpretation.

Gallucci (1994) evaluated the validity of the Harris–Lingoes subscales in a sample of 177 adolescent inpatients using standardized criterion measures including therapist ratings of symptomatology. Findings indicated that the Harris–Lingoes subscales *Hy2* (Need for Affection), *Hy5* (Inhibition of Aggression) and *Pa3* (Naivete) function as inhibitory scales and that *Ma1* (Amorality) and *Ma3* (Imperturbability) serve as excitatory scales in this sample of adolescents. Pancoast and Archer (1988) showed that the standard adult norms produce marked elevations for normal adolescents on the Harris–Lingoes subscales, particularly for

Pd1 (Familial Discord), *Pa1* (Persecutory Ideas), several of the subscales related to scale *8*, and *Ma2* (Psychomotor Acceleration). These findings support the belief that adult norms would tend to produce very substantial distortions in the interpretation of adolescents' MMPI profiles. Colligan and Offord (1989) provided a set of adolescent norms for the Harris–Lingoes subscales derived from their contemporary adolescent sample collected with the original MMPI instrument. The *MMPI Adolescent Interpretive System*, developed by Archer (1987a), published by Psychological Assessment Resources, used these Harris–Lingoes subscale T-score values in providing computer-based test interpretation for the *original* form of the MMPI, and these subscales are also included in the MMPI-A versions of this computer program (Archer, 1995, 2003, 2013).

The Harris–Lingoes subscales have been carried over into testing materials and scoring programs for the MMPI-2 and the MMPI-A. This was possible because very few standard scale items from scales *2, 3, 4, 6, 8,* and *9* were deleted in the development of these instruments. A few Harris–Lingoes subscales have been slightly shortened in the revised instruments, however, because of item deletions. And, because Harris and Lingoes apparently included some subscale items that were not scored on the corresponding Basic scale (e.g., some items appear on *Pd* subscales that are not scored on the *Pd* scale), these items were deleted from membership in the MMPI-A and MMPI-2 Harris–Lingoes subscales. Finally, the Harris–Lingoes subscales were renumbered in the MMPI-A and in the MMPI-2 to eliminate the lettered subscripts employed by Harris and Lingoes to delineate several of their subscales. The revised numbering system is designed to simplify the method used to denote specific subscales. Adolescent norms for the MMPI-A Harris–Lingoes subscales, based on the 1,620 boys and girls in the normative sample, are available in the test manual for this instrument (Butcher et al., 1992). The MMPI-A profile form for the Harris–Lingoes *Si* subscales for boys is shown in Figure 6.2.

Unlike the MMPI-A scales previously reviewed, the Harris–Lingoes subscales are not recommended for routine use if hand-scoring procedures are used. This is because hand-scoring of the Harris–Lingoes subscales is quite time-consuming, and these data are primarily useful in supplementing Basic scale profiles under certain conditions (i.e., in selective cases). For example, Graham (2012) recommended the use of the Harris–Lingoes subscales if a subject receives an elevated score on a Clinical scale when that elevation was unexpected from the client's history and other information available or when the clinician is interpreting Basic scale elevations that occur within a marginally elevated range (corresponding to a T = 60 to 65 range on the MMPI-A). This latter recommendation implicitly recognizes that when Basic scale elevations are within normal limits, or markedly elevated, Harris–Lingoes values are relatively less important. Additionally, Friedman et al. (2001) raised several concerns and cautions regarding the use of the Harris–Lingoes subscales that appear to be well founded. First, they noted that Harris and Lingoes made

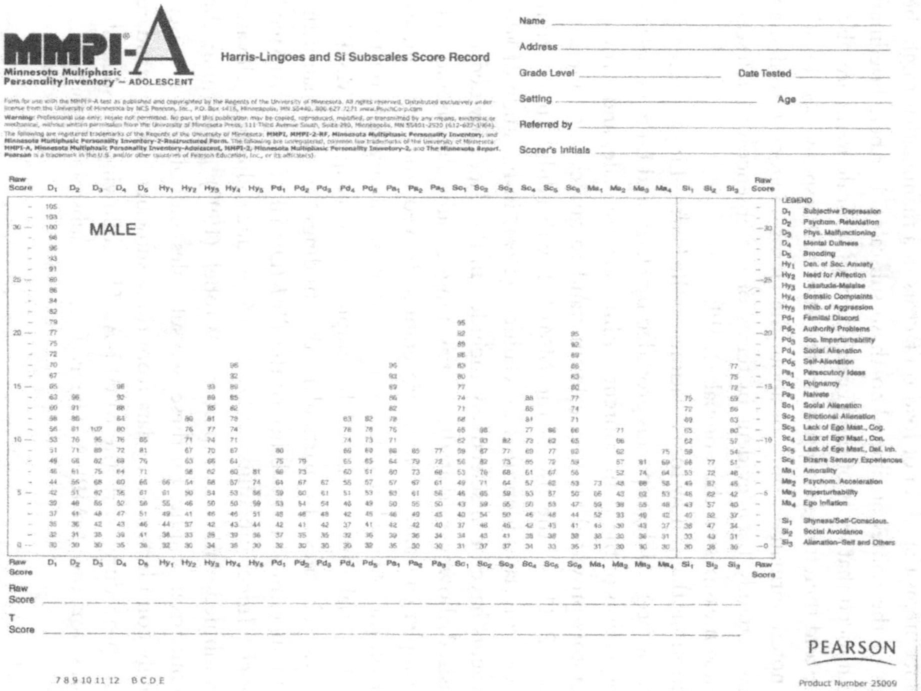

FIGURE 6.2 Profile for Harris–Lingoes and *Si* subscales (male).

Source: From the Minnesota Multiphasic Personality Inventory-Adolescent (MMPI®-A) Manual for Administration, Scoring, and Interpretation by Butcher, et al. Copyright © 1992 by the Regents of the University of Minnesota. Reproduced with the permission of the University of Minnesota Press. All rights reserved. "Minnesota Multiphasic Personality Inventory" and "MMPI" are trademarks owned by the Regents of the University of Minnesota.

no attempts to cross-validate item selection in their subscales, and the external validity data concerning these measures is quite limited. In this regard, Friedman et al. cited the results of the investigation by Miller and Streiner (1985), in which independent judges were unable to accurately group items into the rational categories employed by Harris and Lingoes for the majority of these subscales. Friedman et al. also reviewed the factor analytic results of Foerstner (1986), which showed that several of the Harris–Lingoes subscales contained items that did not load on factors in a manner that might be expected, given the names attributed to these subscales. Further, Friedman et al. (2001) noticed that most of the Harris–Lingoes subscale items are obvious in nature and therefore susceptible to the effects of response set. Finally, the authors noted normative concerns about the Harris–Lingoes subscales, an issue that has certainly been evident in terms of the absence of adolescent norms for these measures on the original MMPI.

The descriptions that follow for elevations on the Harris–Lingoes subscales are based on the original descriptions provided by Harris and Lingoes (1955), a rational inspection of the item content within each subscale, and a review of the descriptors provided for the scales in standard guides (e.g., Graham, 2012; Greene, 2011) to the use of the MMPI-2 with adults. In addition, Harris–Lingoes correlates identified by Gallucci (1994) in his study of adolescent inpatients have been selectively included in the data provided here. It is emphasized, however, that the Harris–Lingoes subscales should only be used to supplement and refine interpretation derived from the standard validity and clinical scales. Further, given the lack of validity data on these measures, substantial caution should be employed in using the MMPI-A Harris–Lingoes subscales. In particular, the findings by Krishnamurthy et al. (1995) concerning the inability of the $Hy1$ (Denial of Social Anxiety) and $Pd3$ (Social Imperturbability) subscales to produce clinically elevated T-scores, combined with the report by Wrobel (1992) concerning the absence of concurrent validity for these two subscales, indicate that test users should strongly consider omitting data from these subscales in their standard interpretation procedures with the MMPI-A. The following are suggested interpretations for the MMPI-A Harris–Lingoes subscales, grouped by parent scale.

Scale 2 (Depression) Subscales

Subjective Depression (D_1). High scores on the D_1 subscale may be associated with the following characteristics:

- Feelings of depression, unhappiness, and guilt.
- Lack of energy and interest in everyday activities.
- Deficits in concentration and attention.
- Self-critical tendencies.

Psychomotor Retardation (D₂). High scores on the D_2 subscale may be associated with:

- Lack of energy or inability to mobilize resources.
- Social withdrawal and social avoidance.
- Denial of hostile or aggressive impulses.

Physical Malfunctioning (D₃). High scores on the D_3 subscale may be associated with the following characteristics:

- Concerns and preoccupation with physical health.
- Reporting of a wide array of physical symptoms.

Mental Dullness (D₄). High scores on the D_4 subscale may be associated with the following characteristics:

- Complaints of difficulties with memory, concentration, or judgment.
- Lack of energy.
- Poor self-concept and feelings of inferiority.
- Difficulty in making decisions.

Brooding (D₅). High scores on the D_5 subscale may be associated with the following characteristics:

- Lack of energy, apathy, and lethargy.
- Excessive sensitivity to criticism.
- Feelings of despondency and sadness.

Scale 3 (Hysteria) Subscales

Denial of Social Anxiety (Hy₁). Higher scores on the Hy_1 subscale may be associated with the following characteristics:

- Social extroversion.
- Ease in talking to, and dealing with, others.

Need for Affection (Hy₂). High scores on the Hy_2 subscale may be associated with the following characteristics:

- Strong needs for attention and affection.
- Optimistic and trusting in relationships.
- Denial of cynical, hostile, or negative feelings about others.

Lassitude-Malaise (Hy₃). High scores on the Hy_3 subscale may be associated with the following characteristics:

- Unhappiness and discomfort.
- Fatigue, physical problems, and the perception of poor physical health.

- Sadness and despondency.
- Poor appetite and sleep disturbance.

Somatic Complaints (Hy_4). High scores on the Hy_4 subscale may be associated with the following characteristics:

- Multiple somatic complaints and concerns.
- Head or chest pains.
- Fainting, dizziness, and problems with balance.
- Nausea, vomiting, and gastrointestinal disturbances.

Inhibition of Aggression (Hy_5). High scores on the Hy_5 subscale may be associated with the following characteristics:

- Denial of hostile or aggressive impulses.
- Perfectionistic tendencies.
- Self-perception as decisive.
- Self-perception as socially sensitive.

Scale 4 (Psychopathic Deviate) Subscales

Familial Discord (Pd_1). High scores on the Pd_1 subscale may be associated with the following characteristics:

- View of home and family as unpleasant, hostile, or rejecting.
- View of home situation as lacking in love.
- The occurrence of frequent quarrels and conflict within the family.
- Views family members as hypercritical and controlling.

Authority Problems (Pd_2). High scores on the Pd_2 subscale may be associated with the following characteristics:

- History of legal violations and antisocial behaviors.
- History of conflicts with individuals in authority.
- Resentful of societal standards, customs, or norms.

Social Imperturbability (Pd_3). Higher scores on the Pd_3 subscale may be associated with the following characteristics:

- Denial of social anxiety and dependency needs.
- Social extroversion and social confidence.
- Tendency to hold strong opinions that are vigorously defended.

Social Alienation (Pd_4). High scores on the Pd_4 subscale may be associated with the following characteristics:

- Feeling misunderstood, alienated, and isolated.
- Feelings of loneliness, unhappiness, and estrangement from others.

- Tendency to blame others for problems or conflicts.
- Feelings of despondency and sadness.

Self-Alienation (*Pd₅*). High scores on the Pd_5 subscale may be associated with the following characteristics:

- Emotional discomfort and unhappiness.
- Problems in concentration and attention.
- Feelings of guilt, regret, and remorse.
- Possibility of excessive alcohol use.

Scale 6 (Paranoia) Subscales

Persecutory Ideas (*Pa₁*). High scores on the Pa_1 subscale may be associated with the following characteristics:

- A sense of being treated unfairly by others.
- Externalization of blame for problems and frustrations.
- Use of projection.
- Possible presence of persecutory ideas and delusions of persecution.

Poignancy (*Pa₂*). High scores on the Pa_2 subscale may be associated with the following characteristics:

- View of self as sensitive, high-strung, and easily hurt.
- Belief that one feels emotions more intensely than do others.
- Loneliness, sadness, and a sense of being misunderstood.
- Self-perception of uniqueness or specialness.

Naivete (*Pa₃*). High scores on the Pa_3 subscale may be associated with the following characteristics:

- Naively trusting and optimistic.
- Denial of hostile or cynical feelings or attitudes.
- Presentation of high moral or ethical standards.
- Unlikely to act impulsively.

Scale 8 (Schizophrenia) Subscales

Social Alienation (*Sc₁*). High scores on the Sc_1 subscale may be associated with the following characteristics:

- Lack of rapport with others.
- Avoidance of social situations and withdrawal from relationships.
- Sense of being misunderstood, unfairly criticized, or unjustly punished by others.
- Hostility or anger toward family members.

Emotional Alienation (Sc₂). High scores on the Sc_2 subscale may be associated with the following characteristics:

- Feelings of self-criticalness, despondency, depression, and despair.
- Possibility of suicidal ideation.
- View of life as difficult or hopeless.
- Possibility of sadistic or masochistic experiences.

Lack of Ego Mastery—Cognitive (Sc₃). High scores on the Sc_3 subscale may be associated with the following characteristics:

- Admission of strange thought processes.
- Feelings of unreality.
- Problems in concentration and attention.

Lack of Ego Mastery—Conative (Sc₄). High scores on the Sc_4 subscale may be associated with the following characteristics:

- Feelings of psychological weakness and vulnerability.
- Problems in concentration and attention.
- Lack of energy and psychological inertia.
- Guilt, despondency, depression, and possible suicidal ideation.

Lack of Ego Mastery—Defective Inhibition (Sc₅). High scores on the Sc_5 subscale may be associated with the following characteristics:

- Loss of control over emotions and impulses.
- Restlessness, irritability, and hyperactivity.
- Episodes of uncontrollable laughing or crying.
- Possible dissociative experiences or symptoms.

Bizarre Sensory Experiences (Sc₆). High scores on the Sc_6 subscale may be associated with the following characteristics:

- Strange or unusual sensory experiences.
- Loss of emotional control.
- The occurrence of a variety of neurological symptoms including paralysis, loss of balance, or involuntary muscular movements.

Scale 9 (Hypomania) Subscales

Amorality (Ma₁). High scores on the Ma_1 subscale may be associated with the following characteristics:

- A tendency to perceive others as motivated by selfishness and self-gain.
- Endorsement of antisocial or asocial attitudes, beliefs, or behaviors.
- Drug abuse.

Psychomotor Acceleration (Ma_2).   High scores on the Ma_2 subscale may be associated with the following characteristics:

- Acceleration of thought or speech.
- Tension, restlessness, and hyperactivity.
- Need to seek out excitement and stimulation.
- Attraction to sensation-seeking and risk-taking behaviors.

Imperturbability (Ma_3).   High scores on the Ma_3 subscale may be associated with the following characteristics:

- Denial of social anxiety.
- Comfort and confidence in social situations.
- Freedom or independence from the influence of the opinions of others.
- Tendency to seek out excitement.

Ego Inflation (Ma_4).   High scores on the Ma_4 subscale may be associated with the following characteristics:

- Feelings of self-importance, possibly including grandiosity.
- Resentfulness of perceived demands from, or interference by, others.

Si *Subscales*

As previously noted, Harris and Lingoes did not attempt to develop subscales for the MMPI basic scales *1, 5, 7*, and *0*. Graham, Schroeder, and Lilly (1971) performed factor analyses of scales *5* and *0* based on the item-level responses of adults in normal and psychiatric settings. Serkownek (1975) utilized the findings from the Graham et al. factor analyses to develop subscales for scales *5* and *0*. The Serkownek subscales received relatively limited clinical attention with adolescents on the original form of the MMPI, and may not be applicable to the MMPI-A because of the extensive item deletions that occurred for scales *5* and *0*.

Ben-Porath, Hostetler et al. (1989) developed *Si* scale subscales for the MMPI-2 based on their analyses of the responses of normal college men and women. After creating preliminary scales based on item-level factor analysis, three subscales were developed using procedures to maximize internal consistency (alpha coefficient values) while producing scales that were composed of non-overlapping or mutually exclusive items. Sieber and Meyer (1992) examined the relationship of the *Si* subscales to a variety of self-report measures believed to be differentially related to these three subscales in a sample of 410 college students. The results of this study provided evidence of the concurrent validity of the *Si* subscales and supported the use of these scales with the MMPI-2. The *Si* subscales developed by Ben-Porath et al. for the MMPI-2 were carried over to the MMPI-A without modification and are grouped with the Harris–Lingoes subscales on a single profile sheet.

Si_1 has been labeled *Shyness/Self-Consciousness* and the following characteristics may be associated with elevations on the Si_1 subscale:

- Shy around others and easily embarrassed.
- Ill at ease in social situations.
- Uncomfortable in new situations.

Ben-Porath, Hostetler, et al. (1989) labeled Si_2 as *Social Avoidance*. The following characteristics or features are associated with elevations on this subscale:

- Dislike or avoidance of social activities.
- Avoidance of contact or involvement with others.

The Si_3 subscale was labeled *Alienation—Self and Others*. This Si subscale appears to involve psychiatric symptomatology that interferes with the ability to adaptively engage with, or relate to, others. The following are characteristics or features that may be associated with elevations on Si_3:

- Low self-esteem and self-concept.
- Self-critical and lack of confidence in judgment.
- Nervous, fearful, and indecisive.
- Suspicious or fearful of others.

Thus far in this chapter we have dealt with a variety of scales and subscales which are designed to augment the interpretation of the MMPI-A Basic scales (e.g., the Content and Supplementary scales), or were developed as a means of refining or "breaking out" components of other scales (e.g., Content Component scales and the Harris–Lingoes and Si subscales). We will now turn our attention to MMPI-A special scales which were created to provide a broader or macro view of the individuals' psychological functioning. These MMPI-A scales are the Personality Psychopathology Five (PSY-5) scales.

The Personality Psychopathology Five (PSY-5) Scales

The Personality Psychopathology Five (PSY-5; Harkness & McNulty, 1994) is a descriptive, dimensional model of personality initially designed to complement categorical personality disorder diagnosis. It is one of a number of personality models based on a five-factor conceptual system of hierarchical personality traits. The PSY-5 model was originally applied to the MMPI-2 by Harkness, McNulty, and Ben-Porath (1995) in their development of the PSY-5 scales for this instrument, and the findings on the MMPI-2 PSY-5 scale were summarized by Harkness, McNulty, Ben-Porath, and Graham (2002). Harkness, Finn, McNulty, and Shields (2012) summarized the literature on the PSY-5 scales related to the MMPI-2,

MMPI-A and MMPI-2-RF. As will be discussed in Chapter 7, the PSY-5 scales have also been adapted in a revised form for the MMPI-A-RF. The MMPI-A profile from the Supplementary and PSY-5 scales for girls is shown in Figure 6.3.

McNulty, Harkness, Ben-Porath, and Williams (1997) examined the MMPI-2 PSY-5 scales and selected 104 items that also appeared in the MMPI-A test booklet. Rational item selection was used to identify additional items from questions uniquely found on the MMPI-A and preliminary scales were refined using statistical methods designed to increase internal consistency based on the MMPI-A normative sample and the clinical sample reported in the MMPI-A manual (Butcher et al., 1992). The resulting MMPI-A PSY-5 scales were identified as Aggressiveness (*AGGR*), Psychoticism (*PSYC*), Constraint (*CONS*), Negative Emotionality/ Neuroticism (*NEGE*), and Positive Emotionality/Extroversion (*EXTR*). The Constraint and Positive Emotionality/Extroversion scale were later reversed and changed to Disconstraint (*DISC*) and Introversion/Low Positive Emotionality (*INTR*), respectively, to facilitate scoring and interpretation. The median coefficient alpha for the five scales was .76 in both the clinical and normative sample. In addition, data collected from a record review form, the Child Behavior Checklist (CBCL), and the Devereux Adolescent Behavior Rating Scale (DAB) were utilized to explore the correlate patterns for each of these five dimensions. The item composition of the MMPI-A based PSY-5 scales is shown in Table 6.13. Harkness et al. (1995) note that the PSY-5 scales differ from other MMPI scales in their emphasis on specific personality traits or dispositional differences, rather than on major psychopathological dimensions. The data from several MMPI-A investigations of these scales suggest the following correlate patterns for each of the PSY-5 scales:

The following characteristics may be associated with elevations on the Aggressiveness (AGGR) scale:

- Poor temper control.
- Assaultive or aggressive.
- More likely to exhibit externalizing and acting-out behaviors.

The following characteristics may be associated with elevations on the Psychoticism (PSYC) scale:

- More likely to exhibit psychotic-like behaviors.
- More likely to appear anxious and obsessive.

The following characteristics or features may be associated with elevations on the Disconstraint (DISC) (originally named Constraint) scale:

- More likely to exhibit externalizing behaviors.
- More likely to engage in acting out and drug use.
- More likely to exhibit delinquent behavior.

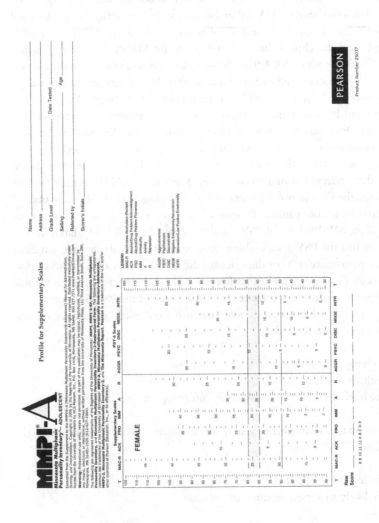

FIGURE 6.3 Profile for Supplementary and PSY-5 scales (female).

TABLE 6.13 Item Composition of the MMPI-A Based PSY-5 Scales

Scale	Items
Aggressiveness (AGGR)	24, 34, **47**, **81**, **128**, 200, 201, 282, **303**, **325**, **334**, **354**, (355), 367, 378, **382**, 453, 458, 461, (465)
Psychoticism (PSYC)	12, **22**, 29, **39**, **45**, **92**, **95**, **132**, **136**, **225**, **250**, **286**, **295**, 296, **299**, **315**, **332**, **337**, (**387**), **417**, **439**
Disconstraint (DISC) (originally named Constraint)	**32**, 69, **80**, (**96**), **99**, **101**, **117**, (**120**), 144, **197**, **234**, (**246**), (**249**), **323**, **338**, **361**, **380**, **389**, 440, 456, (**457**), (460), 462,
Negative Emotionality/ Neuroticism (NEGE)	**49**, (**60**), **78**, **89**, **111**, (**134**), **139**, **159**, **185**, (**209**), **271**, **281**, **285**, **357**, 364, **368**, (**375**), **383**, **392**, **394**, 412, (**424**)
Introversion/Low Positive Emotionality (INTR) (originally named Positive Emotionality/ Extraversion)	(**9**), (**46**), (**58**), (**71**), (**74**), (**82**), (**91**), (**105**), (**125**), (**170**), (**179**), (**180**), (**228**), (262), (**289**), (**292**), (**298**), (**319**), (**322**), (**329**), (**331**), (**335**), (436), (**447**), (450), 463, 473, (476)

Source: Copyright © 1997 by the American Psychological Association. Adapted with permission from McNulty, Harkness, Ben-Porath and Williams (1997). *Assessing the Personality Psychopathology Five (PSY-5) in adolescents: New MMPI-A Scales*. Psychological Assessment.

Note
Items in parentheses are scored if False; all others are scored if True. Items in boldface type also appear on the corresponding MMPI-2-based PSY-5 scale (see Table E-1 in Butcher et al., 1992, for item number conversions).

The following characteristics or features may be associated with elevations on the Negative Emotionality/Neuroticism (NEGE) scale:

• Anxious, tense, worried.
• Guilt and remorse.
• Excessive reliance or dependency on adults.

The following characteristics may be associated with elevations on the Introversion (INTR) scale, originally named Positive Emotionality/Extroversion:

• Social isolation.
• Interpersonally uncommunicative and withdrawn.

Veltri and his colleagues (2009) examined the empirical correlates for a variety of MMPI-A scales including the PSY-5 scales in a sample of 157 boys from a forensic setting and 197 girls from an acute psychiatric inpatient setting. These authors found that internalizing variables such as anhedonia, depression, psychomotor retardation, and suicidal ideation were significantly related to INTR scale scores, while NEGE scores were related to fatigue, anxiety, and suicidal ideation.

Externalizing variables showed a pattern of significant correlations with AGGR scores including anger, history of fighting, and oppositional behavior. Further, DISC scale scores were related to a variety of impulsive and disinhibited behaviors including a history of substance abuse, school suspensions, criminal charges, and running away. Finally, scores on the PSYC scale were related to the presence of auditory hallucinations.

Veltri et al. (2014) examined the relationship between the MMPI-A PSY-5 scale scores and violent and non-violent behaviors among 260 adolescent boys and girls in a forensic setting. Results indicated, consistent with expectations, that elevations on the Disconstraint (DISC) scale were associated with non-violent delinquency, whereas Aggressiveness (AGGR) was characterized by the use of instrumental aggression and violent forms of delinquency. The authors concluded that their findings held implications for informing the manner in which clinicians interpreted the MMPI-A PSY-5 scales. For example, clinicians evaluating an adolescent with elevated scores on DISC but normal-range scores on the AGGR scale might infer that the adolescent likely has a history of engaging in non-violent delinquent behaviors and has a lower likelihood for engaging in violent behaviors in the future. In contrast, an adolescent producing elevations on both the DISC and AGGR scales is more likely to have a history of violent acts and a higher risk for committing violent acts in the future.

Bolinskey, Arnau, Archer, and Handel (2004) examined the MMPI-A PSY-5 scales in a sample of 545 adolescents receiving inpatient psychiatric treatment. These researchers employed item-level PCA to determine the internal structure of each of the PSY-5 scales and to aid in the creation of facet subscales for each of the PSY-5 scales. Results indicated that the MMPI-A PSY-5 scales, with the exception of the Negative Emotionality/Neuroticism scale, could be meaningfully subdivided into two components and Table 6.14 shows the item composition and reliability of the PSY-5 domain and facet scores from this study. Overall, their results supported the construct validity of the MMPI-A PSY-5 scales and provided a promising set of facet subscales. The authors noted that future research will be needed to establish the external correlate patterns found for the facet subscales, as well as to demonstrate the overall applicability of the PSY-5 constructs to the assessment of adolescents in light of the emphasis by Harkness & McNulty (1994) on personality disorder symptomatology in the original development of these scales.

Stokes, Pogge, Sarnicola, and McGrath (2009) explored the usefulness of the Bolinskey et al. (2004) MMPI-A PSY-5 facet scales in an adolescent inpatient psychiatric sample of 662 adolescents. Correlational analyses were used to examine the relationship between the PSY-5 facet scales and therapist ratings, chart-review variables, and self-report measures. The authors concluded that their findings provided support for the validity of the MMPI-A PSY-5 facet scales. The facet scales generally demonstrated acceptable levels of internal

TABLE 6.14 Item Composition and Reliability of MMPI-A PSY-5 Domain and Facet Scores

Facet	Items	Alpha
AGGR		**.79**
Hostility	24, 34, 81, 128, 201, 282, 303, 354, (355), 367, .76 453, 458, 461, 465	.76
Grandiosity/Indignation	47, 200, 325, 334, 378, 382	.57
DISC		**.80**
Delinquent Behaviors and Attitudes	32, 80, (96), 101, 144, 197, 234, (246), (249), 323, 338, 361, 380, 440, (460), 467	.77
Norm Violation	69, 99, 117, (120), 389, 456, (457), 462	.57
INTR		**.83**
Low Drive/ Expectations	(9), (58), (71), (74), (91), (105), (170), (179), (228), (329), (436), (447), (450), 473	.77
Low Sociability	(46), (82), (125), (180), (262), (289), (292), (298), (319), (322), (331), (335), 463, (476)	.72
PSYC		**.81**
Psychotic Beliefs/ Experiences	12, 22, 39, 95, 132, 136, 250, 299, 315, 332, 337, (387), 439	.78
Odd Mentation	29, 45, 92, 296, 417	.59
NEGE*		**.78**

Source: Bolinskey et al. (2004). Copyright © Sage Publications. Reprinted with permission of the author.
Notes
AGGR = Aggressiveness; DISC = Disconstraint, INTR = Introversion/Low Positive Emotionality. PSYC = Psychoticism; NEGE = Negative Emotionality/Neuroticism.
Analyses indicated a single factor for NEGE; thus, no facet scales were constructed for this PSY-5 scale. Items in parentheses are scored in the False direction.

consistency and were related in predictable and meaningful ways to self-report and symptom ratings. For example, externalizing symptoms were related to the Hostility and Delinquent Attitudes facet scales, internalizing symptoms were most closely related to the presence of High Neuroticism facet scale and the Low-Drive/Expectations facet scales, and bizarre features and psychotic symptoms were found to be most strongly associated with the Psychotic Experiences and Odd Mentations facet scales.

In conclusion, the findings on the MMPI-A PSY-5 scales appear to be quite encouraging both in terms of the reliability of these scales and the external correlate patterns produced by the PSY-5 scales. Additional research will be necessary to fully evaluate the extent to which PSY-5 facet scales for the MMPI-A can provide reliable and accurate information for test users in the interpretation of adolescent profiles.

7

OVERVIEW OF THE MMPI-A-RF

The MMPI-A-RF is a new instrument for the assessment of psychopathology among adolescents that is heavily influenced by the structure and underlying concepts involved in the MMPI-2-RF. However, the development of the MMPI-A-RF also placed an emphasis on creating scales uniquely sensitive to adolescent developmental issues (e.g., Negative Peer Influences) and adolescent problem areas (e.g., Negative School Attitudes). Further, even though many scales share the same name or label on the MMPI-A-RF and the MMPI-2-RF, it would be erroneous to assume that these scales were identical. Many of these scales with shared names across the two tests differ substantially in terms of their item composition.

While the MMPI-A-RF may be viewed as an adaptation of the MMPI-2-RF for adolescent respondents, the MMPI-A-RF also has strong relationships to the MMPI-A. Table 7.1 shows the intercorrelations between the MMPI-A-RF Validity scales and the Validity scales of the MMPI-A. This table reflects, for example, strong relationships ($r \geq .80$) between measures of underreporting or defensiveness (e.g., K and K-r) as well as strong relationships ($r = .86$) between measures of overreporting (F and F-r). Table 7.2 illustrates the relationships between each of the MMPI-A Clinical and Content scales and their three highest correlations among the MMPI-A-RF Substantive scales in large samples of outpatient boys and girls. In general, most of these relationships reflect anticipated or expected correlations between MMPI-A scales and their counterparts on the MMPI-A-RF. For example, Basic scale Hs is correlated $r = .93$ with $RC1$, MMPI-A Content Scale A-biz is correlated $r = .80$ with $RC8$, and Content Scale A-Fam is correlated $r = .90$ with the MMPI-A-RF Family Problems (FML) Scale. Similarly, White and Krishnamurthy (2014) have reported a

TABLE 7.1 MMPI-A/MMPI-A-RF Validity Scale Correlations for Boys and Girls in the MMPI-A-RF Normative Sample

MMPI-A Scale	MMPI-A-RF Scale					
	VRIN-r	TRIN-r	CRIN	F-r	L-r	K-r
VRIN	.68	.14	.74	.64	.42	.10
TRIN	.13	.58	.18	.27	−.02	−.22
F_1	.56	.24	.63	.79	.34	−.08
F_2	.56	.29	.64	.82	.32	−.14
F	.59	.29	.68	.86	.35	−.12
L	.27	−.13	.31	.24	.80	.42
K	.02	−.29	.04	−.10	.33	.81

Source: Adapted from the MMPI-A-RF Manual with permission. Minnesota Multiphasic Personality Inventory-Adolescent-Restructured Form (MMPI®-A-RF) Manual for Administration, Scoring, and Interpretation by Butcher, et al. Copyright © 1992 by the Regents of the University of Minnesota. MMPI-A-RF Manual for Administration, Scoring, and Interpretation by Archer et al. Copyright © 2016 by the Regents of the University of Minnesota. Reproduced with the permission of the University of Minnesota Press. All rights reserved. "Minnesota Multiphasic Personality Inventory" and "MMPI" are trademarks owned by the Regents of the University of Minnesota.

correlation of r = .90 between *Hs − RC1* in their sample of high school girls, and an r = .80 value in the same sample between MMPI-A scale *L* and MMPI-A-RF scale *L-r*. However, it can also be noted in the MMPI-A-RF Manual (Archer et al., 2016a) that the MMPI-A Basic Scale *Sc* does not produce its highest correlations with the MMPI-A-RF *RC8* scale, and MMPI-A Basic Scale *Hy* does not produce a strong association with *RC3*. These latter findings underscore that the MMPI-A-RF bears some significant differences from the MMPI-A, and should be thought of as frequently overlapping, but distinctly different tests in many important respects.

MMPI-A-RF Validity Scales

Chapter 3 provides a description of each of the MMPI-A Validity scales related to defensiveness or underreporting (*L-r* and *K-r*), overreporting (*F-r*), and inconsistency (*VRIN-r*, *TRIN-r*, and *CRIN*). Chapter 3 also contains information concerning the interpretation of each of these Validity scales. Table 7.3 provides information on reliability, expressed in test-retest data, Cronbach's alpha coefficient internal consistency, and standard error of measurement results for each of the Validity scales in the normative sample and in a variety of other settings. As shown in this table, test-retest and internal consistency reliability data for measures of underreporting and overreporting are generally in the moderate range. In contrast, and as expected, measures of response consistency generally produce much lower reliability results, particularly on measures of internal consistency

TABLE 7.2 Three Most Highly Correlated MMPI-A-RF Substantive Scales With Each MMPI-A Clinical and Content Scale

MMPI-A Scale	Outpatient Boys (n = 6,851)			Outpatient Girls (n = 4,848)		
Hs	RC1 (.93)	NUC (.72)	MLS (.71)	MLS (.75)	RC1 (.94)	NUC (.74)
D	EID (.71)	MLS (.71)	RCd (.70)	MLS (.75)	EID (.77)	RCd (.75)
Hy	MLS (.61)	RC1 (.59)	NUC (.50)	MLS (.67)	RC1 (.68)	HPC (.56)
Pd	FML (.64)	RCd (.60)	RC4 (.59)	RCd (.63)	FML (.64)	RC6 (.61)
Mf	EID (–.43)	NEGE-r (.42)	SFD (.41)	STW (.25)	SFD (.26)	AGG (–.23)
Pa	THD (.73)	PSYC-r (.70)	RC6 (.69)	RC6 (.70)	THD (.73)	PSYC-r (.69)
Pt	EID (.91)	RCd (.88)	NEGE-r (.83)	RCd (.87)	EID (.91)	RC7 (.82)
Sc	EID (.83)	RCd (.83)	F-a (.74)	RCd (.81)	EID (.81)	F-a (.79)
Ma	RC9 (.67)	BXD (.65)	DISC-r (.55)	BXD (.62)	RC9 (.68)	AGG (.55)
Si	SHY (.81)	INTR-r (.78)	EID (.73)	INTR-r (.79)	SHY (.81)	EID (.72)
A-anx	EID (.89)	NEGE-r (.88)	RCd (.84)	NEGE-r (.87)	EID (.88)	RCd (.83)
A-obs	NEGE-r (.83)	RC7 (.80)	EID (.79)	RC7 (.79)	NEGE-r (.81)	EID (.78)
A-dep	RCd (.93)	EID (.91)	SFD (.77)	EID (.91)	RCd (.93)	SFD (.77)
A-hea	RC1 (.92)	NUC (.76)	F-a (.71)	NUC (.77)	RC1 (.94)	F-a (.74)
A-biz	PSYC-r (.84)	RC8 (.80)	THD (.78)	RC8 (.81)	PSYC-r (.84)	THD (.78)
A-ang	ANP (.85)	AGGR-r (.85)	AGG (.75)	AGGR-r (.86)	ANP (.86)	AGG (.75)
A-cyn	RC3 (.89)	K-r (–.58)	RC6 (.55)	AGGR-r (.59)	RC3 (.89)	THD (.58)
A-aln	EID (.75)	RCd (.74)	THD (.66)	RCd (.73)	EID (.73)	THD (.67)
A-con	BXD (.77)	DISC-r (.77)	ASA (.76)	DISC-r (.79)	ASA (.79)	BXD (.78)
A-lse	EID (.84)	RCd (.82)	SFD (.80)	RCd (.82)	EID (.84)	SFD (.80)
A-las	NFC (.56)	EID (.52)	HLP (.52)	HLP (.56)	NFC (.59)	EID (.56)
A-sod	INTR-r (.91)	SAV (.86)	SHY (.74)	SAV (.87)	INTR-r (.91)	SHY (.75)
A-fam	FML (.90)	AGGR-r (.57)	RCd (.57)	FML (.89)	FML (.89)	RC6 (.54)
A-sch	NSA (.82)	RC4 (.59)	DISC-r (.59)	RC4 (.59)	NSA (.82)	DISC-r (.58)
A-trt	HLP (.83)	RCd (.77)	EID (.77)	EID (.78)	HLP (.84)	EID (.78)

TABLE 7.3 Reliability and Standard Errors of Measurement for the MMPI-A-RF Validity Scales

	Test-Retest	Internal Consistency (Alpha)										Standard Error of Measurement (SEM)			
	Normative Sample Subset	Normative Sample		Outpatients		Inpatients		Correctional		School		Normative (Test-Retest)	Normative (Alpha)		Median Clinical (Alpha)
	Boys and Girls (154)	Boys (805)	Girls (805)	Boys (6,851)	Girls (4,848)	Boys (241)	Girls (178)	Boys (1,362)	Girls (394)	Boys (832)	Girls (422)	Boys and Girls (154)	Boys (805)	Girls (805)	Boys and Girls (15,128)
VRIN-r	.78	.45	.37	.27	.15	.25	.18	.31	.30	.23	.17	4	8	7	7
TRIN-r	.60	.34	.24	.16	.10	.30	.09	.20	.08	.15	.04	4	8	8	8
CRIN	.76	.60	.52	.42	.30	.43	.31	.46	.39	.39	.31	4	7	6	6
F-a	.51	.74	.71	.76	.75	.77	.70	.76	.75	.75	.75	6	5	5	6
L-r	.62	.53	.55	.53	.47	.43	.50	.54	.49	.53	.42	6	7	6	7
K-r	.74	.58	.60	.68	.66	.59	.50	.62	.65	.70	.68	6	6	6	6

Source: Adapted with permission from the MMPI-A-RF Manual. Adapted from the MMPI-A-RF Administration, Scoring, Interpretation and Technical Manual by Archer et al. Copyright © 2016 by the Regents of the University of Minnesota. Reproduced with the permission of the University of Minnesota Press. All rights reserved. "Minnesota Multiphasic Personality Inventory" and "MMPI" are trademarks owned by the Regents of the University of Minnesota.

Note

Numbers within parentheses specify sample size.

M M P I A RF™

Minnesota Multiphasic
Personality Inventory-Adolescent
Restructured Form™

Name _____

ID Number _____

Gender _____   Date Tested _____

Education _____   Age _____   Scorer's Initials _____

Profile for Validity Scales

T Score ____ ____ ____ ____ ____ ____ ____

Raw
Score ____ ____ ____ ____ ____ ____ ____

T Score ____ ____ ____ ____ ____ ____ ____

Cannot
Say (Raw) _____

MMPI-A-RF T scores are nongendered.

VRIN-r Variable Response Inconsistency   F-r Infrequent Responses
TRIN-r True Response Inconsistency   L-r Uncommon Virtues
CRIN   Combined Response Inconsistency   K-r Adjustment Validity

Hand-Scoring Directions for the MMPI-A-RF VRIN-r, TRIN-r, and CRIN Scales

See the VRIN-r and TRIN-r answer keys for steps 1 and 2.

3. In the blank spaces below, enter the number of item pairs that have both responses blackened from each of the VRIN-r and TRIN-r answer keys. Follow the directions below for calculating the raw score for VRIN-r, TRIN-r, and CRIN. To obtain T scores, record the raw scores in the spaces provided beneath the grid on the other side of this form. Plot the raw score for each scale on the graph and record the corresponding T score in the space provided.

VRIN-r

Number of item
pairs blackened

VRIN-r Key 1: _____

+

VRIN-r Key 2: _____

+

VRIN-r Key 3: _____

+

VRIN-r Key 4: _____

= [_____]

Maximum
raw score = 21

Add the numbers above to obtain the VRIN-r raw score.

TRIN-r

Number of item   Number of item
pairs blackened   pairs blackened

TRIN-r Key 1: _____   —   TRIN-r Key 2: _____ = _____ + 5 points = [_____]
                           (minus)

Maximum
raw score = 13
Minimum
raw score = 0

Subtract the score for TRIN-r Key 2 from the score for TRIN-r Key 1. Then add 5 points to obtain the TRIN-r raw score.

CRIN

Number of item pairs blackened	Number of item pairs blackened	Number of item pairs blackened	Number of item pairs blackened	Number of item pairs blackened	Number of item pairs blackened	
VRIN-r Key 1: _____	+ VRIN-r Key 2: _____	+ VRIN-r Key 3: _____	+ VRIN-r Key 4: _____	+ TRIN-r Key 1: _____	+ TRIN-r: Key 2: _____	= [_____]

Maximum
raw score = 34

Add the numbers above to obtain the CRIN raw score.

FIGURE 7.1   MMPI-A-RF Validity scale profile sheet.

Source: From the MMPI-A-RF Administration, Scoring, Interpretation and Technical Manual by Archer et al. Copyright © 2016 by the Regents of the University of Minnesota. Reproduced with the permission of the University of Minnesota Press. All rights reserved. "Minnesota Multiphasic Personality Inventory" and "MMPI" are trademarks owned by the Regents of the University of Minnesota.

reflected in alpha coefficients. Figure 7.1 shows the MMPI-A-RF Validity scale profile sheet.

Higher-Order (*H-O*) Scales

As previously noted, the MMPI-2-RF development process was used as a template for MMPI-A-RF scale development. Accordingly, the MMPI-A-RF employed a three-tiered structure representing different levels of breadth versus specificity. The three Higher-Order scales define the highest and broadest level of this hierarchy, the RC scales occupy the middle level, and the Specific Problems scales were developed to provide the most narrowband width at the base of the hierarchy.

The MMPI-A-RF Higher-Order scales were created to measure broadband constructs comparable to the Higher-Order scales found in the MMPI-2-RF. In order to achieve this goal, a PCA of scale RC level data was conducted and the resulting three-factor model provided the core components for each of the Higher-Order scales. The first component, Emotional/Internalizing Dysfunction (*EID*) was characterized by high loadings on measure of affective distress including *RCd*, *RC1*, *RC2* and *RC7*. The second component, Thought Dysfunction (*THD*) was largely defined by high loadings on *RC3*, *RC6* and *RC8*. Finally, the third component, labeled Behavioral/Externalizing Dysfunction (*BXD*) was characterized by high loadings on *RC4* and *RC9*. Figure 7.2 presents the H-O and RC scale profile sheet for the MMPI-A-RF. Table 7.4 also provides the reliability and standard error of measurement data for the Higher-Order scales, as well as comparable reliability results for each of the RC scales.

As shown in this table, internal reliability as measured by test-retest data and alpha coefficient internal consistency is moderately high for each of the Higher-Order scales, and the standard error of measurement for these scales generally ranges between 4 and 6 T-score points. Each of the Higher-Order scales are described below.

Emotional/Internalizing Dysfunction (EID) Scale

The *EID* is a 26-item scale developed to assess a broad range of emotional distress and internalizing problems. Consistent with a factor structure associated with MMPI-A Basic Scales 2 and 7, scores on *EID* provide an overall measure of emotional dysfunction and difficulty.

The following is a summary of descriptors for elevated *EID* scale scores (T ≥ 60):

- The presence of negative emotional experiences including depression, anxiety, helplessness and pessimism.
- The presence of significant emotional distress which, at higher ranges, may be perceived as debilitating.

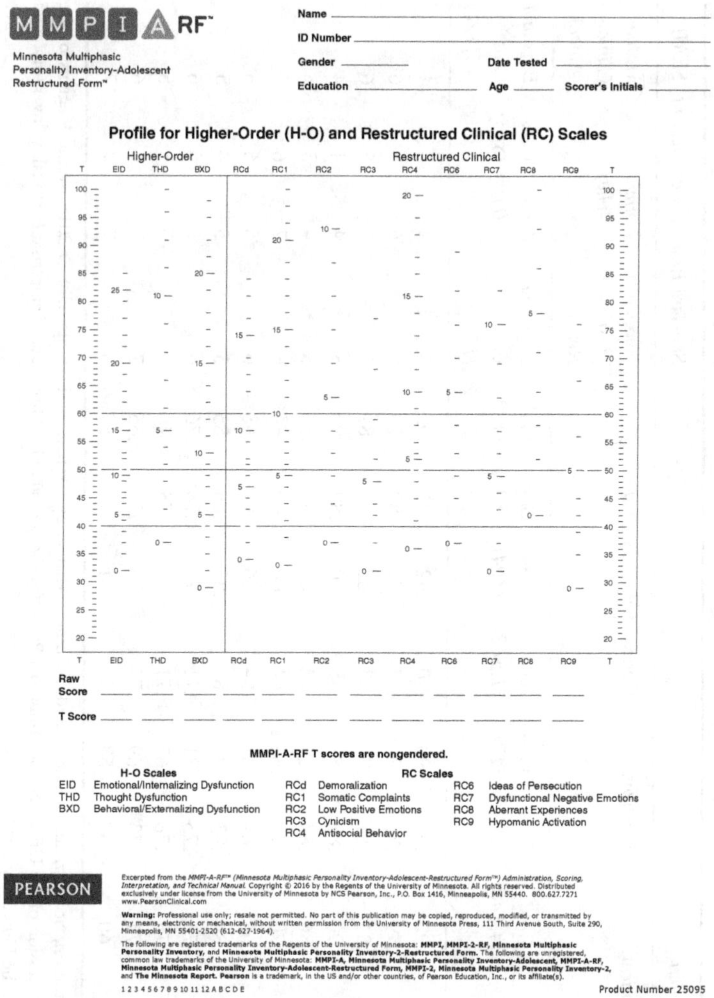

MMPI A RF™

Minnesota Multiphasic
Personality Inventory-Adolescent
Restructured Form™

Name _____

ID Number _____

Gender _____   Date Tested _____

Education _____   Age _____ Scorer's Initials _____

Profile for Higher-Order (H-O) and Restructured Clinical (RC) Scales

	Higher-Order					Restructured Clinical					

MMPI-A-RF T scores are nongendered.

H-O Scales		RC Scales	
EID	Emotional/Internalizing Dysfunction	RCd	Demoralization
THD	Thought Dysfunction	RC1	Somatic Complaints
BXD	Behavioral/Externalizing Dysfunction	RC2	Low Positive Emotions
		RC3	Cynicism
		RC4	Antisocial Behavior
		RC6	Ideas of Persecution
		RC7	Dysfunctional Negative Emotions
		RC8	Aberrant Experiences
		RC9	Hypomanic Activation

FIGURE 7.2 MMPI-A-RF Higher-Order (*H-O*) and Restructured Clinical (*RC*) scale profile sheet.

Source: From the MMPI-A-RF Administration, Scoring, Interpretation and Technical Manual by Archer et al. Copyright © 2016 by the Regents of the University of Minnesota. Reproduced with permission of the University of Minnesota Press. All rights reserved. "Minnesota Multiphasic Personality Inventory" and "MMPI" are trademarks owned by the Regents of the University of Minnesota.

TABLE 7.4 Reliability and Standard Errors of Measurement for the MMPI-A-RF Higher-Order (*H-O*) and Restructured Clinical (*RC*) Scales

| | Test-Retest | Internal Consistency (Alpha) | | | | | | | | | | Standard Error of Measurement (SEM) | | | | |
| | Normative Sample Subset | Normative Sample | | Outpatients | | Inpatients | | Correctional | | School | | Normative (Test-Retest) | Normative (Alpha) | | Median Clinical (Alpha) |
	Boys and Girls (154)	Boys (805)	Girls (805)	Boys (6,851)	Girls (4,848)	Boys (241)	Girls (178)	Boys (1,362)	Girls (394)	Boys (832)	Girls (422)	Boys and Girls (154)	Boys (805)	Girls (805)	Boys and Girls (15,128)
EID	.85	.84	.86	.92	.92	.92	.90	.90	.92	.91	.92	5	4	4	4
THD	.64	.70	.70	.77	.79	.78	.76	.77	.79	.80	.79	6	6	5	6
BXD	.71	.74	.72	.79	.81	.81	.82	.83	.82	.83	.81	5	5	5	6
RCd	.82	.80	.83	.89	.90	.88	.87	.88	.90	.89	.90	5	4	4	4
RC1	.78	.77	.78	.83	.86	.83	.84	.82	.86	.82	.86	5	4	5	5
RC2	.65	.60	.53	.68	.70	.72	.66	.64	.66	.69	.74	6	7	6	7
RC3	.60	.60	.65	.65	.66	.64	.61	.64	.66	.67	.68	6	6	6	6
RC4	.66	.80	.77	.83	.84	.83	.85	.85	.83	.86	.83	5	5	4	5
RC6	.58	.64	.66	.74	.76	.73	.71	.71	.74	.78	.76	6	6	5	6
RC7	.74	.63	.66	.75	.75	.78	.63	.71	.74	.75	.76	6	5	5	5
RC8	.56	.59	.55	.70	.71	.73	.69	.75	.78	.70	.65	7	7	6	6
RC9	.71	.45	.52	.57	.60	.58	.58	.59	.61	.55	.59	6	7	7	7

Source: Adapted from the MMPI-A-RF Administration, Scoring, Interpretation and Technical Manual by Archer, et al. Copyright © 2016 by the Regents of the University of Minnesota. Reproduced with the permission of the University of Minnesota Press. All rights reserved. "Minnesota Multiphasic Personality Inventory" and "MMPI" are trademarks owned by the Regents of the University of Minnesota.

Thought Dysfunction (THD) Scale

The *THD* scale is a 14-item measure of thought dysfunction. Individuals who produce elevated scores on this scale may be characterized by the presence of paranoid ideation, delusions, and auditory and visual hallucinations.

The following is a summary of descriptors for adolescents who produce high *THD* scale scores (T ≥ 60):

- May be reporting a broad range of symptoms or difficulties associated with disordered thinking including paranoid delusions and audio and visual hallucinations.
- At higher ranges, elevations on this scale may indicate the adolescent requires an evaluation for the use of antipsychotic medication or possible inpatient treatment for THD.

Behavioral/Externalizing Dysfunction (BXD) Scale

This 24-item scale was developed to assess a broad range of behavioral problems. The *BXD* scale provides an index of conduct-disordered behavior consistent with the *4-9/9-4* codetype on the MMPI-A. Adolescents who produce elevations on the *BXD* scale may exhibit a variety of conduct-disordered behaviors including thrill-seeking and risk-taking behaviors such as alcohol and drug abuse.

The following is a summary of descriptors for adolescents with elevated *BXD* scores (T ≥ 60):

- Likely to exhibit behavioral disconstraint.
- Significant history of externalizing and acting-out behaviors.
- Alcohol and substance abuse.
- Conduct-disordered and impulsive behaviors.

Restructured Clinical (RC) Scales

The first step in developing the MMPI-A-RF RC scales was to map MMPI-2-RF items for each RC scale onto the corresponding MMPI-A-RF RC scales. These preliminary MMPI-A-RF scales served as the seed scales for further development. These initial seed scales were then further refined by the use of rational review of item content combined with the results of statistical analysis such as alpha coefficients. In the next step, the seed scale items for *RCd* were combined with each preliminary MMPI-A-RF RC scale items and a series of exploratory factor analyses were conducted across several scale development samples. The goal of these analyses was to identify items that served as markers for the core or seed construct, separate from the *RCd* factor. Preliminary RC scale items were required to correlate most highly with their target scale in contrast to the other RC scales. The results of these analyses additionally indicated that an *RCd* scale could be identified for adolescents which was distinct from other RC scale constructs, and comparable to the role of the *RCd* scale within the MMPI-2-RF. In the final stages of MMPI-A-RF RC scale development, all of the seed scales were correlated with each remaining item in the 478 items of the MMPI-A to identify additional potential items which could be added to each of the RC scales to optimize convergent and discriminant validity correlations. The result of this process was the development of a set of MMPI-A-RF RC scales which overlap considerably with their MMPI-2-RF counterparts, but often include items specific to the MMPI-A item pool. MMPI-A-RF RC scales typically do not include all of the RC scale items found in their MMPI-2-RF counterparts.

Demoralization (RCd) Scale

The *RCd* scale is an 18-item measure of demoralization, defined as a dimension of unhappiness, poor morale, and high levels of life dissatisfaction. Additional scales related to *RCd* include Helplessness/Hopelessness (*HLP*), Self-Doubt (*SFD*), Inefficacy (*NFC*), and Obsessions/Compulsions (*OCS*).

The following is a summary of characteristics of adolescents who produce elevated scores on the *RCd* scale (T ≥ 60):

- Feels sad and depressed.
- Experiences low self-esteem.
- Problems in concentration and attention.
- Maintains low self-esteem.
- Low energy and fatigue.

Somatic Complaints (RC1) Scale

The *RC1* scale consists of 23 items presenting a wide array of somatic complaints including head pain, neurological symptoms, and gastrointestinal problems. An adolescent's actual health status, particularly the presence of chronic health conditions, may influence his or her results on the *RC1* scale. More modest elevations on *RC1* may reflect primarily the adolescent's physical health problems, but marked elevations typically include a complaint of psychological preoccupation with diffuse health concerns. Interpretation of elevations on *RC1* are often facilitated by consideration of scores on the Malaise (*MLS*), Gastrointestinal Complaints (*GIC*), Head Pain Complaints (*HPC*), Neurological Complaints (*NUC*), and Cognitive Complaints (*COG*) scales.

The following is a summary of characteristics of adolescents who produce elevated scores on *RC1* (T ≥ 60):

- Multiple and varied somatic complaints.
- Diffuse head pain and neurological complaints.
- Gastrointestinal symptoms.
- Problems in concentration and attention.
- Low energy and fatigue.

Low Positive Emotions (RC2) Scale

RC2 is a 10-item scale measuring a lack of positive emotional experiences, one of the primary components of depression. Adolescents who produce elevations on this scale typically report feeling unsuccessful, hopeless and ineffective.

The following is a summary of characteristics of adolescents who produce elevated scores on *RC2* (T ≥ 60):

- Reports low self-esteem.
- Fatigue and psychomotor retardation.
- Social withdrawal and introversion.
- Self-critical and self-punishing.

Cynicism (RC3) Scale

The *RC3* scale consists of nine items that describe adolescents who maintain a negative and cynical view of interpersonal relationships. Adolescents who produce elevations on this scale view the behavior of others as driven primarily by self-interest and a desire to manipulate others.

The following is a summary of characteristics of adolescents who produce elevated scores on *RC3* (T ≥ 60):

- Views others as motivated solely by self-interest.
- Cynical attitudes may interfere with the development of a therapeutic relationship.
- Is mistrustful in interpersonal relationships.

Antisocial Behavior (RC4) Scale

RC4 consists of 20 items presenting various aspects of antisocial and conduct-disordered behaviors. In interpreting elevations on *RC4* consideration should also be given to scores on the Negative School Attitudes (*NSA*), Antisocial Attitudes (*ASA*), Conduct Problems (*CNP*), Substance Abuse (*SUB*), and Negative Peer Influence (*NPI*).

The following is a summary of characteristics of adolescents who produce elevated scores on *RC4* (T ≥ 60):

- History of conduct-disordered behaviors.
- Abuse of alcohol or drugs.
- Affiliation with negative peer group.
- School disciplinary problems including school suspensions.
- Problems at home including running away.

Ideas of Persecution (RC6) Scale

RC6 is a nine-item scale presenting a variety of persecutory beliefs. These beliefs range from a sense of being treated unfairly by others to the occurrence of paranoid delusions and beliefs. *RC6* is one of the six MMPI-A-RF scales that contain critical response items content, but the interpretation of scores on *RC6* is not linked to any SP scale. As will be noted later in this chapter, items endorsed in the keyed direction in any of the six critical scales *(RC6, RC8, AGG, AXY, HLP* and *SUB)* are reported in the MMPI-A-RF Score Report if the scale T-score is ≥ 60 for a given scale.

The following is a summary of characteristics of adolescents who produce elevated scores on *RC6* (T ≥ 60):

- Feelings of being mistreated by others.
- Interpersonal suspiciousness and distrust.
- Aggressive behaviors including fighting.
- Oppositional behaviors.
- History of school truancy and suspensions.
- Possible presence of persecutory ideas and beliefs.
- Possible hallucinations and psychotic symptoms.

Dysfunctional Negative Emotions (RC7) Scale

RC7 is an 11-item scale measuring various aspects of negative emotional experiences. These experiences include anxiety, irritability, impatience, and apprehensiveness. Interpretation of elevated scores on *RC7* is facilitated by consideration of scores on the following SP scales: Obsessions/Compulsion (*OCS*), Stress/Worry (*STW*), Anxiety (*ANX*), Behavior-Restricting Fears (*BRF*), and Specific Fears (*SPF*).

The following is a summary of characteristics of adolescents who produce elevated scores on *RC7* (T ≥ 60):

- Reports anxiety which may include specific fears.
- Low self-esteem.
- Problems in concentration and attention.
- Irritability and impatience.

Aberrant Experiences (RC8)

RC8 is an eight-item scale related to the experience of unusual thoughts and perceptions. Adolescents who produce higher elevations on *RC8* may experience delusions as well as auditory and visual hallucinations. RC8 is one of the six MMPI-A-RF scales for which items endorsed in the keyed direction are reported on the MMPI-A-RF Score Report if the T-score for that scale is ≥ 60.

The following is a summary of characteristics of adolescents who produce elevated scores on *RC8* (T ≥ 60):

- Reports unusual thought processes.
- Engages in frequent daydreaming.
- May experience visual and/or audio hallucinations.

May experience delusional thinking and poor reality testing adolescents who produce elevations on this scale may require an evaluation for possible use of antipsychotic medications and their psychotic symptoms may serve as their primary intervention target.

Hypomanic Activation (RC9) Scale

The *RC9* scale consists of eight items which involve behaviors and attitudes related to hypomanic activation. *RC9* contains items which include a strong need for excitement and stimulation, high levels of psychomotor energy, racing thoughts, and periods of sleeplessness. Adolescents who produce elevated scores on this scale may be described as risk-taking and thrill-seeking.

The following is a summary of characteristics of adolescents who produce elevated scores on *RC9* (T ≥ 60):

- Heightened level of activation.
- History of conduct-disordered behaviors.
- Has many and varied interests.
- Heightened probability of history of aggressive behaviors.
- Evaluate for potential referral for mood-stabilizing medications.

Specific Problems Scales

The Specific Problems (SP) scales were developed as the third tier of MMPI-A-RF scales. The SP scales are characterized by a relatively narrow focus on specific areas of psychological functioning. The SP scales were developed to assess important characteristics associated with one of the RC scales or other clinically relevant areas of psychological functioning. The interpretation of SP scales is not limited, however, to facilitating the interpretation of the RC scales and SP scales may be interpreted regardless of the score on an associated RC scale. The SP scales were organized into four groups: Somatic/Cognitive scales, Internalizing scales, Externalizing scales, and Interpersonal scales.

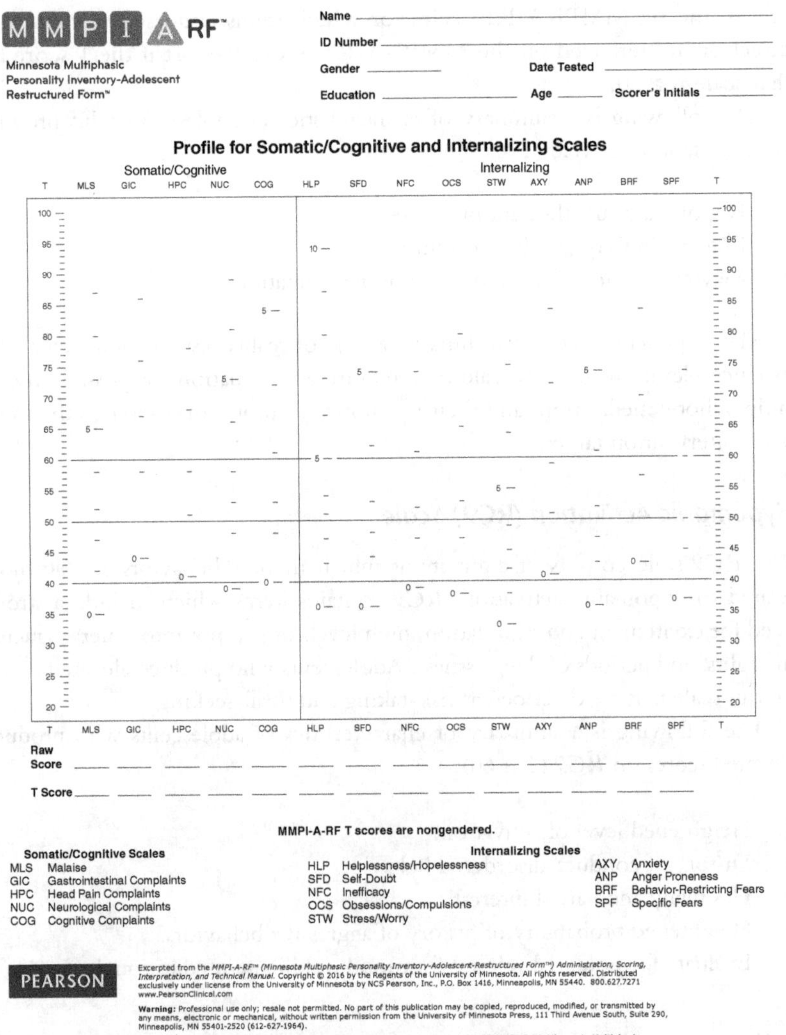
MMPI-A-RF™
Minnesota Multiphasic Personality Inventory-Adolescent Restructured Form™

Name ______
ID Number ______
Gender ______ Date Tested ______
Education ______ Age ______ Scorer's Initials ______

MMPI-A-RF T scores are nongendered.

Somatic/Cognitive Scales
MLS Malaise
GIC Gastrointestinal Complaints
HPC Head Pain Complaints
NUC Neurological Complaints
COG Cognitive Complaints

Internalizing Scales
HLP Helplessness/Hopelessness
SFD Self-Doubt
NFC Inefficacy
OCS Obsessions/Compulsions
STW Stress/Worry
AXY Anxiety
ANP Anger Proneness
BRF Behavior-Restricting Fears
SPF Specific Fears

FIGURE 7.3 MMPI-A-RF Somatic/Cognitive and Internalizing scales profile sheet.

Source: From the MMPI-A-RF Administration, Scoring, Interpretation and Technical Manual by Archer et al. Copyright © 2016 by the Regents of the University of Minnesota. Reproduced with the permission of the University of Minnesota Press. All rights reserved. "Minnesota Multiphasic Personality Inventory" and "MMPI" are trademarks owned by the Regents of the University of Minnesota.

Somatic/Cognitive Scales

The Somatic/Cognitive scales, as shown in Figure 7.3, are grouped with the Internalizing scales on the profile sheets of the MMPI-A-RF.

The Somatic/Cognitive scales have in common a shared emphasis on providing information concerning the adolescent's perception of his or her medical condition and health functioning. For this reason, accurate interpretation of scores for the Somatic/Cognitive scales requires that the test interpreter be aware of the adolescent's actual history of physical problems and health issues. Table 7.5 provides reliability and standard error of measurement data for the MMPI-A-RF Somatic/Cognitive scales. As shown in this table, internal consistency as reflected in Cronbach's alpha coefficient values range from $r = .53$ to $r = .80$ for these scales, and standard error of measurement values range from 5 to 7 T-score points. The following is a discussion of each of the Somatic/Cognitive scales.

Malaise (MLS) Scale

The *MLS* scale consists of eight items related to a general sense of poor physical health including fatigue and lack of energy. Elevated scores on this scale reflect a self-presentation that involves poor general health and physical debilitation. Adolescents who produce elevations on this scale typically have vague non-specific concerns about their health functioning. The following are descriptors associated with adolescents who produce elevated scores on the MLS scale (T ≥ 60):

- Generalized sense of poor physical health.
- Weakness and fatigue.
- Low energy.
- Poor concentration.
- Sleeplessness.

Gastrointestinal Complaints (GIC) Scale

The *GIC* scale consists of four items which involve gastrointestinal complaints including stomach discomfort and pain, nausea and vomiting. The following are descriptors associated with adolescents who produce elevated scores on the *GIC* scale (T ≥ 60):

- Reports gastrointestinal complaints and discomfort.
- Reports nausea and stomach upset.
- Reports vomiting.

Head Pain Complaints (HPC) Scale

The *HPC* scale is composed of four items involving headache and head pain. Consistent with the interpretation of all of these somatic scales, interpretation

TABLE 7.5 Reliability and Standard Errors of Measurement for the MMPI-A-RF Somatic/Cognitive Scales

| | Test-Retest | Internal Consistency (Alpha) | | | | | | | | | | Standard Error of Measurement (SEM) | | | |
| | Normative Sample Subset | Normative Sample | | Outpatients | | Inpatients | | Correctional | | School | | Normative (Test-Retest) | Normative (Alpha) | | Median Clinical (Alpha) |
	Boys and Girls (154)	Boys (805)	Girls (805)	Boys (6,851)	Girls (4,848)	Boys (241)	Girls (178)	Boys (1,362)	Girls (394)	Boys (832)	Girls (422)	Boys and Girls (154)	Boys (805)	Girls (805)	Boys and Girls (15,128)
MLS	.72	.54	.53	.65	.69	.60	.60	.57	.64	.65	.71	6	7	7	7
GIC	.65	.59	.69	.72	.78	.69	.78	.69	.75	.73	.80	6	5	6	6
HPC	.68	.51	.59	.60	.69	.61	.59	.60	.65	.59	.66	6	6	7	7
NUC	.58	.59	.54	.62	.67	.67	.67	.62	.68	.62	.67	6	7	7	7
COG	.65	.55	.61	.70	.74	.73	.73	.68	.75	.69	.75	6	6	6	7

Note
Numbers within parentheses specify sample size.

of the *HPC* scale requires knowledge of the adolescent's actual medical condition that may influence his or her responses to the *HPC* scale. The following are descriptors associated with adolescents who produce elevated scores on the *HPC* scale (T ≥ 60):

- Head pain and discomfort.
- Multiple somatic complaints.
- Problems in concentration.

Neurological Complaints (NUC) Scale

The *NUC* scale consists of seven items describing a variety of neurological problems including involuntary muscle movements, dizziness, numbness and weakness. Accurate interpretation of the *NUC* scale may require a neuropsychological or neurological evaluation to rule out a variety of medical conditions which may produce elevations on the *NUC* scale.

The following are descriptors associated with adolescents who score high on the *NUC* scale (T ≥ 60):

- Vague neurological complaints.
- Problems with concentration.
- Muscle weakness, and lack of control over movement.
- Areas of numbness or loss of sensation.
- Periods of dizziness.

Cognitive Complaints (COG) Scale

The *COG* scale consists of five items that cover a variety of cognitive difficulties including problems in concentration, memory problems, and cognitive confusion. Elevations on the *COG* scale may be related to a variety of conditions including ADHD.

The following are descriptors associated with adolescents who produce elevations on the *COG* scale (T ≥ 60):

- Diffuse pattern of cognitive difficulties including memory problems and lack of concentration.
- Attention problems.
- Problems in concentration.
- Academic deficits and learning problems.
- Slow speech quality.

Adolescents with elevated *COG* scale scores may require evaluations for ADHD and other neurodevelopmental disorders.

Internalizing Scales

The reliability estimates for each of the nine Internalizing scales of the MMPI-A-RF are shown in Table 7.6. Three of these scales assist in the assessment of various forms of demoralization. These scales include Helplessness/Hopelessness (*HLP*), Self-Doubt (*SFD*), and Inefficacy (*NFC*). The remaining internalizing scales measure aspects of Dysfunctional Negative Emotions and include Obsessions/Compulsions (*OCS*), Stress/Worry (*STW*), Anxiety (*AXY*), Anger Proneness (*ANP*), Behavior-Restricting Fears (*BRF*), and Specific Fears (*SPF*) scales. We will begin with a review of the three scales related to demoralization.

Helplessness/Hopelessness (HLP) Scale

The *HLP* scale consists of 10 items reflecting a general sense of pessimism and hopelessness. Adolescents who produce elevated scores on the *HLP* scale generally feel that they are unlikely to succeed in life and that they experience a variety of negative emotions. As one of the six MMPI-A-RF Critical scales, items endorsed in the critical direction will be provided in the MMPI-A-RF Score Report for adolescents whose T-score is ≥ 60 on this scale.

The following are descriptors associated with adolescents who produce elevations on the *HLP* scale (T ≥ 60):

- Feelings of hopelessness and helplessness.
- Suicidal ideation.
- Experiences low self-esteem.
- Presence of depression-related disorders.

Self-Doubt (SFD) Scale

The *SFD* scale consists of five items reflecting low self-esteem and poor self-confidence. Adolescents who produce elevations on this scale report strong feelings for self-doubt and inferiority. They are self-critical and have feelings of uselessness.

The following are descriptors associated with adolescents who produce elevations on the *SFD* scale (T ≥ 60):

- Poor self-esteem.
- Feelings of self-doubt and low self-confidence.
- Self-disparagement.

Inefficacy (NFC) Scale

The *NFC* scale is composed of four items endorsed by adolescents who feel ineffective and useless.

TABLE 7.6 Reliability and Standard Errors of Measurement for the MMPI-A-RF Internalizing Scales

	Test-Retest	Internal Consistency (Alpha)										Standard Error of Measurement (SEM)			
	Normative Sample Subset	Normative Sample		Outpatients		Inpatients		Correctional		School		Normative (Test-Retest)	Normative (Alpha)		Median Clinical (Alpha)
	Boys and Girls (154)	Boys (805)	Girls (805)	Boys (6,851)	Girls (4,848)	Boys (241)	Girls (178)	Boys (1,362)	Girls (394)	Boys (832)	Girls (422)	Boys and Girls (154)	Boys (805)	Girls (805)	Boys and Girls (15,128)
HLP	.62	.59	.61	.74	.78	.74	.76	.71	.76	.75	.80	6	6	6	7
SFD	.73	.56	.60	.75	.77	.73	.68	.70	.78	.74	.77	6	6	6	6
NFC	.64	.52	.53	.65	.65	.67	.62	.65	.65	.65	.66	6	7	7	7
OCS	.56	.39	.45	.53	.51	.58	.51	.56	.62	.54	.49	7	8	8	7
STW	.67	.54	.58	.71	.70	.68	.61	.66	.70	.71	.74	6	6	7	6
AXY	.61	.37	.44	.59	.64	.60	.64	.63	.58	.64	.59	7	8	8	8
ANP	.63	.57	.52	.67	.67	.64	.66	.66	.66	.67	.71	6	7	7	7
BRF	.24	.43	.38	.37	.37	.35	.50	.40	.44	.44	.41	8	8	8	8
SPF	.67	.39	.39	.31	.38	.28	.32	.39	.39	.29	.42	5	7	8	7

Source: Adapted from the MMPI-A-RF Administration, Scoring, Interpretation and Technical Manual by Archer et al. Copyright © 2016 by the Regents of the University of Minnesota. Reproduced with the permission of the University of Minnesota Press. All rights reserved. "Minnesota Multiphasic Personality Inventory" and "MMPI" are trademarks owned by the Regents of the University of Minnesota.

Note
Numbers within parentheses specify sample size.

The following are descriptors associated with adolescents who produce elevated scores on the *NFC* scale:

- Feelings of self-doubt and poor self-esteem.
- Self-defeating and self-degrading beliefs.
- Socially passive and introverted.
- Experiences sad and depressed mood.

The following are MMPI-A-RF Internalizing scales that measure varying aspects of dysfunction or negative emotion. In addition, all SP scales may serve to assess relatively distinctive aspects of psychological functioning.

Obsessions/Compulsions (OCS) Scale

The *OCS* scale consists of four items describing various obsessive and compulsive behaviors. These may include obsessive behaviors such as ruminating over unpleasant thoughts or experiences, and compulsive activities, e.g., stepping over sidewalk cracks, or repetitive counting behaviors.

The following are descriptors associated with adolescents who produce elevations on the *OCS* scale (T ≥ 60):

- Preoccupation with orderliness and rigid organization.
- Is anxious and ruminative.
- At higher ranges, may engage in obsessive thoughts and/or compulsive behaviors.

Stress/Worry (STW) Scale

The *STW* scale consists of seven items reflecting various aspects of stress and apprehensiveness. Adolescents who produce elevated scores on the *STW* scale report a variety of stress-related symptoms including sleep complaints, problems in concentration, and a tendency to over-respond to stress.

The following are descriptors associated with adolescents who produce elevations on the *STW* scale (T ≥ 60):

- Complaints of stress and worry.
- Anxious and apprehensive.
- Complaints of sleeplessness.
- Problems in concentration.

Anxiety (AXY) Scale

The *AXY* scale consists of four items describing a variety of anxiety symptoms. These symptoms include feelings of dread and uneasiness, nightmares, and pervasive feelings of anxiety. As one of the six MMPI-A-RF scales designed as having crucial responses, *AXY* items endorsed in the critical direction will be displayed on the MMPI-A-RF Score Report if this scale produces a T ≥ 60.

The following are descriptors associated with adolescents who produce elevated scores in the *AXY* scale (T ≥ 60):

- Feelings of anxiety and apprehensiveness.
- Problems in concentration.
- Multiple fears.
- Frequent nightmares.

Anger Proneness (ANP) Scale

The *ANP* scale consists of five items related to the experience and expression of anger. Adolescents who produce elevations on this scale report a high level of anger problems including irritability and impatience.

Following are descriptors associated with adolescents who produce elevated scores on the *ANP* scale (T ≥ 60):

- Frequent anger and irritability.
- Aggressive behaviors including verbal threats and fighting.
- Oppositional behavior.
- Conduct-disordered behavior.

Behavior-Restricting Fears (BRF) Scale

The *BRF* scale is a three-item scale presenting levels of fearfulness and anxiety that serve to interfere with and restrict normal activities. Adolescents who produce elevations on this score are generally anxious and fearful and may also have symptoms related to agoraphobia.

The following are descriptors associated with adolescents who produce elevations on the *BRF* scale (T ≥ 60):

- Depression and anxiety.
- Procrastination and difficulty completing projects.
- Possible agoraphobic behaviors.

Specific Fears (SPF) Scale

The *SPF* scale consists of four items which present several areas of specific fears. These areas include the fear of blood, snakes, and high places, and concerns and apprehensiveness about exposure to disease. Adolescents who produce elevations on this scale have reported a higher-than-average number of specific fears.

The following are descriptors associated with adolescents who score high on the *SPF* scale (T ≥ 60):

- Multiple fears and phobias.
- Possibility of the presence of a phobic disorder.

Externalizing Scales

There are six Externalizing scales on the MMPI-A-RF which measure facets or aspects of antisocial behavior (*RC4*) and hypomanic activation (*RC9*). The facet scales for *RC4* include Negative School Attitudes (*NSA*), Antisocial Attitudes (*ASA*), Conduct Problems (*CNP*), and Substance Abuse (*SUB*), and Negative Peer Influence (*NPI*). The Facet scale for *RC9* is Aggression (*AGG*). Similar to all SP scales, the Externalizing Scales not only help to identify specific facets of *RC4* and *RC9*, but are also interpretable even when the associated RC scales are not clinically elevated. For example, if *RC9* fell within a normal range, elevated scores on *AGG* would still be interpretable. Table 7.7 provides reliability and standard error of measurement data for the externalizing scales and Figure 7.4 presents the profile sheet for the MMPI-A-RF Externalizing and Interpersonal scales.

Negative School Attitudes (NSA) Scale

The *NSA* scale consists of six items reflecting negative attitudes or beliefs regarding school. Adolescents who produce elevations on this scale believe that school is boring, a waste of time, and dislike engaging in school activities.

The following are descriptors associated with adolescents who produce elevations on the *NSA* scale (T ≥ 60):

- Poor study habits.
- Frequent academic problems.
- Negative school attitudes.
- Difficulty in motivating to engage in school activities.
- Rule-breaking or oppositional behavior.

Antisocial Attitudes (ASA) Scale

The *ASA* scale consists of six items reflecting a variety of antisocial beliefs and attitudes. Adolescents who produce elevations on this scale engage in rule-bending and rule-breaking behaviors and report a variety of antisocial attitudes.

The following are descriptors associated with adolescents who produce elevations on the *ASA* scale (T ≥ 60):

TABLE 7.7 Reliability and Standard Errors of Measurement for the MMPI-A-RF Externalizing Scales

	Test-Retest	Internal Consistency (Alpha)										Standard Error of Measurement (SEM)			
	Normative Sample Subset	Normative Sample		Outpatients		Inpatients		Correctional		School		Normative (Test-Retest)	Normative (Alpha)		Median Clinical (Alpha)
	Boys and Girls (154)	Boys (805)	Girls (805)	Boys (6,851)	Girls (4,848)	Boys (241)	Girls (178)	Boys (1,362)	Girls (394)	Boys (832)	Girls (422)	Boys and Girls (154)	Boys (805)	Girls (805)	Boys and Girls (15,128)
NSA	.55	.54	.55	.73	.74	.78	.65	.74	.77	.74	.72	7	7	7	7
ASA	.56	.52	.47	.64	.64	.64	.63	.63	.66	.65	.58	6	7	7	7
CNP	.71	.62	.52	.69	.73	.61	.69	.64	.61	.71	.73	5	7	6	7
SUB	.46	.53	.56	.64	.67	.76	.78	.75	.76	.67	.68	7	7	7	6
NPI	.55	.37	.29	.43	.41	.42	.50	.48	.45	.46	.41	6	10	10	11
AGG	.55	.55	.55	.69	.73	.72	.71	.71	.77	.72	.72	6	7	6	6

Source: Adapted from the MMPI-A-RF Administration, Scoring, Interpretation and Technical Manual by Archer et al. Copyright © 2016 by the Regents of the University of Minnesota. Reproduced with the permission of the University of Minnesota Press. All rights reserved. "Minnesota Multiphasic Personality Inventory" and "MMPI" are trademarks owned by the Regents of the University of Minnesota.

Note
Numbers within parentheses specify sample size.

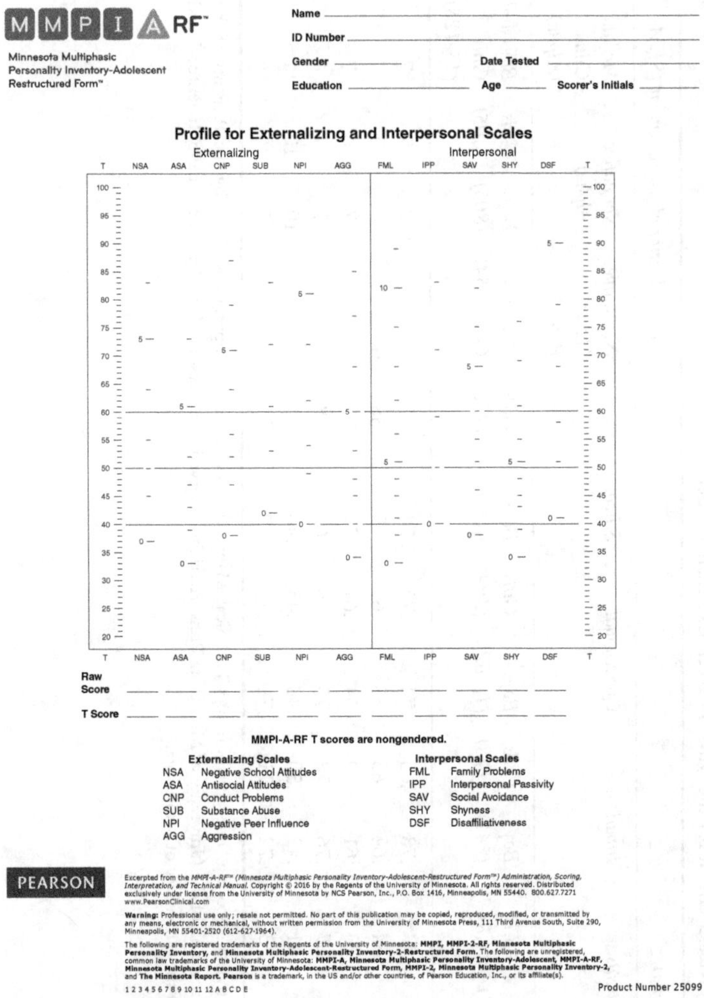

MMPI A RF™

Minnesota Multiphasic Personality Inventory-Adolescent Restructured Form™

Name ____

ID Number ____

Gender ____ Date Tested ____

Education ____ Age ____ Scorer's Initials ____

Profile for Externalizing and Interpersonal Scales

Externalizing: T NSA ASA CNP SUB NPI AGG

Interpersonal: FML IPP SAV SHY DSF T

Raw Score ____

T Score ____

MMPI-A-RF T scores are nongendered.

Externalizing Scales		Interpersonal Scales	
NSA	Negative School Attitudes	FML	Family Problems
ASA	Antisocial Attitudes	IPP	Interpersonal Passivity
CNP	Conduct Problems	SAV	Social Avoidance
SUB	Substance Abuse	SHY	Shyness
NPI	Negative Peer Influence	DSF	Disaffiliativeness
AGG	Aggression		

PEARSON

1 2 3 4 5 6 7 8 9 10 11 12 A B C D E

Product Number 25099

FIGURE 7.4 MMPI-A-RF Externalizing and Interpersonal scale profile sheet.

Source: From the MMPI-A-RF Administration, Scoring, Interpretation and Technical Manual by Archer et al. Copyright © 2016 by the Regents of the University of Minnesota. Reproduced with the permission of the University of Minnesota Press. All rights reserved. "Minnesota Multiphasic Personality Inventory" and "MMPI" are trademarks owned by the Regents of the University of Minnesota.

- History of school suspensions and disciplinary actions.
- Conduct problems and oppositional behaviors.
- Association with a negative peer group.

Conduct Problems (CNP) Scale

The *CNP* scale consists of seven items reflecting a variety of conduct disorder behaviors. Adolescents who produce elevations on the *CNP* scale report significant behavioral and academic problems in school, and problem behaviors at home which may include delinquent behaviors and running away from home.

The following are descriptors associated with adolescents who produce elevations on the *CNP* scale (T ≥ 60):

- Exhibits a broad range of conduct problems and rule-breaking behaviors.
- History of school suspensions.
- Legal violations including placement in juvenile detention.
- Poor academic achievement and performance, including school truancy.

Substance Abuse (SUB) Scale

The *SUB* scale consists of four items related to the abuse of drugs or alcohol. Adolescents who produce elevations on this scale have reported the problematic use of alcohol or drugs. Since *SUB* is one of the six MMPI-A-RF scales designated as having crucial responses, specific substance abuse items endorsed in the critical direction may be identified through review of the MMPI-A-RF Score Report if the T-score on *SUB* is ≥ 60.

The following are descriptors associated with adolescents who produce elevations on the *SUB* scale (T ≥ 60):

- Abuse of alcohol or drugs.
- Association with a negative peer group.
- History of legal charges and/or running away from home.
- Engages in rule-breaking behavior.

Negative Peer Influence (NPI) Scale

The *NPI* scale consists of five items associated with affiliation with a negative peer group. Adolescents who produce elevations on this scale have a history of conduct-disordered behaviors resulting from, or supported through, their affiliation with a negative peer group.

The following are descriptors associated with adolescents who produce elevations on the *NPI* scale (T ≥ 60):

- Oppositional and rule-breaking behavior.
- History of truancy and school suspension.
- Abuse of drugs and alcohol.

Aggression (AGG) Scale

The *AGG* scale consists of eight items associated with problems in physically aggressive behavior. Adolescents who produce marked elevations on this scale may employ physically aggressive and violent behavior as a means of intimidating and controlling others. If the adolescent's T-score on *AGG* is ≥ 60, each scale item endorsed in the critical direction will be found on the MMPI-A-RF Score Report.

The following are descriptors associated with adolescents who produce elevations on the *AGG* scale (T ≥ 60):

- Engages in aggressive behavior.
- Engages in violent behaviors including fighting.
- History of oppositional and rule-breaking behavior.
- History of school suspension.
- Possible placement in detention or on probation.
- History of problems with anger management and anger control.
- Engages in verbally threatening behavior.

Interpersonal Scales

The MMPI-A-RF contains a group of scales related to assessment of interpersonal functioning, which include Family Problems (*FML*), Interpersonal Passivity (*IPP*), Social Avoidance (*SAV*), Shyness (*SHY*), and Disaffiliativeness (*DSF*). Table 7.8 provides information on the internal reliability and standard error of measurement of the Interpersonal scales.

Family Problems (FML) Scale

The *FML* scale consists of eleven items describing an adolescent's attitudes and experiences in relation to his or her family members. The content of the *FML* scale includes negative family experiences, wanting to leave home, frequent conflicts with family members, and an adolescent's perception of lack of parental support.

The following are descriptors associated with adolescents who produce elevations on the *FML* scale (T ≥ 60):

- Conflictual family relationships.
- Reports lack of family support and understanding.
- Resents or blames family members for his or her difficulties.
- Family life is characterized by discord and disharmony.
- Problems with authority figures.
- History of running away from home.

TABLE 7.8 Reliability and Standard Errors of Measurement for the MMPI-A-RF Interpersonal Scales

| | Test-Retest | Internal Consistency (Alpha) | | | | | | | | | | Standard Error of Measurement (SEM) | | | |
| | Normative Sample Subset | Normative Sample | | Outpatients | | Inpatients | | Correctional | | School | | Normative (Test-Retest) | Normative (Alpha) | | Median Clinical (Alpha) |
	Boys and Girls (154)	Boys (805)	Girls (805)	Boys (6,851)	Girls (4,848)	Boys (241)	Girls (178)	Boys (1,362)	Girls (394)	Boys (832)	Girls (422)	Boys and Girls (154)	Boys (805)	Girls (805)	Boys and Girls (15,128)
FML	.71	.63	.67	.73	.76	.75	.71	.71	.76	.75	.77	6	6	6	6
IPP	.52	.36	.30	.46	.50	.55	.45	.37	.41	.37	.51	7	8	8	8
SAV	.66	.65	.61	.77	.81	.76	.84	.68	.74	.78	.82	6	6	6	6
SHY	.70	.68	.73	.77	.80	.79	.78	.76	.79	.76	.79	6	5	5	5
DSF	.38	.43	.45	.52	.53	.56	.51	.53	.60	.52	.52	7	8	7	7

Source: Adapted from the MMPI-A-RF Administration, Scoring, Interpretation and Technical Manual by Archer et al. Copyright © 2016 by the Regents of the University of Minnesota. Reproduced with the permission of the University of Minnesota Press. All rights reserved. "Minnesota Multiphasic Personality Inventory" and "MMPI" are trademarks owned by the Regents of the University of Minnesota.

Note

Numbers within parentheses specify sample size.

Interpersonal Passivity (IPP) Scale

The *IPP* scale consists of four items including the belief that one is easily downed in an argument, inadequate to serve as a group leader, or reluctant or unable to effectively assert their opinion.

The following are descriptors associated with adolescents who produce elevations on the *IPP* scale (T ≥ 60):

- Socially introverted and interpersonally passive.
- Low self-esteem.
- Unassertive.
- Easily dominated by others.

Social Avoidance (SAV) Scale

The *SAV* scale consists of seven items that deal with various aspects of social avoidance. Adolescents who score in moderate ranges (T-scores of 60 to 79) report the avoidance of some social situations and events, but a marked elevation on this scale (T ≥ 80) is associated with pervasive social avoidance and social withdrawal.

The following are descriptors associated with adolescents who produce elevations on the *SAV* scale (T ≥ 60):

- Few or no friends.
- Social Isolation and introversion.
- Uncomfortable around members of the opposite sex.

Shyness (SHY) Scale

The *SHY* scale consists of nine items describing various aspects of social shyness. Adolescents who produce elevated scores on this scale are introverted, lack confidence in social situations, and are bashful and easily embarrassed.

The following are descriptors associated with adolescents who produce elevations on the *SHY* scale (T ≥ 60):

- Introverted and socially isolated.
- Easily embarrassed and bashful.
- Feels socially inferior.
- Interpersonally anxious.

Disaffiliativeness (DSF) Scale

The *DSF* scale presents five items related to a preference for solitary and socially isolated activities. Adolescents who produce moderate elevations (T-score of

60 to 79) on this scale report some dislike of being around others, while adolescents producing marked (T ≥ 80) elevations strongly prefer solitary activities and activities that avoid social involvement.

The following are descriptors associated with adolescents who produce elevations on the *DSF* scale (T ≥ 60):

- Socially withdrawn.
- Few or no friends.
- Difficulty in trusting others.
- Uncomfortable in dealing with emotions around others.
- Disaffiliativeness may interfere with establishment of a therapeutic relationship.

Personality Psychopathology Five (PSY-5) Scales

The MMPI-A PSY-5 scales are a revision of the PSY-5 scales developed by Harkness, McNulty, and Ben-Porath (1995) for the MMPI-2, and by McNulty, Harkness, Ben-Porath, and Williams (1997) for the MMPI-A. All of these sets of PSY-5 scales were based on Harkness and McNulty's (1994) dimensional model of personality psychopathology, with the caution that this model of underlying personality traits may be expected to deal with characteristics which are less stable during adolescence than for adults. Table 7.9 provides reliability and standard error of measurement data for the MMPI-A-RF Personality Psychopathology Five (*PSY-5*) scales. These data indicate generally high alpha coefficient values for the PSY-5 scales ranging from r = .70 for inpatient girls on the *NEGE-r* scale to r = .84 for inpatient girls and for boys in correctional settings on the *DISC-r* scale. Further, standard error of measurement ranges from 5 to 8 T-score points across the MMPI-A-RF PSY-5 scales.

McNulty and Harkness developed the MMPI-A-RF revisions of the PSY-5 scales using a modern method of scale construction involving rational item selection, refinement of scale item membership through use of alpha coefficient internal reliabilities, and optimization of scale composition by examining preliminary scale correlations with relevant external criteria. Specifically, McNulty and Harkness employed several raters to review all 241 items of the MMPI-A to identify those items that could be uniquely assigned to the PSY-5 constructs. Those items were initially included on revised scales based on the unanimous agreement among the raters, or if an item had been among the 66 MMPI-A-RF items that appeared on one of the MMPI-A PSY-5 scales. Internal analyses were conducted in a variety of samples, separately by gender. These processes eventually produced a group of five PSY scales composed of 73 items of which none appeared on more than one of the PSY-5 scales (i.e., non-overlapping scale membership).

Figure 7.5 presents the MMPI-A-RF profile sheet for the PSY-5 scales.

TABLE 7.9 Reliability and Standard Errors of Measurement for the MMPI-A-RF Personality Psychopathology Five (PSY-5) Scales

	Test-Retest	Internal Consistency (Alpha)										Standard Error of Measurement (SEM)			
	Normative Sample Subset	Normative Sample		Outpatients		Inpatients		Correctional		School		Normative (Test-Retest)	Normative (Alpha)		Median Clinical (Alpha)
	Boys and Girls (154)	Boys (805)	Girls (805)	Boys (6,851)	Girls (4,848)	Boys (241)	Girls (178)	Boys (1,362)	Girls (394)	Boys (832)	Girls (422)	Boys and Girls (154)	Boys (805)	Girls (805)	Boys and Girls (15,128)
AGGR-r	.64	.57	.58	.72	.74	.75	.72	.75	.77	.74	.76	6	8	7	7
PSYC-r	.64	.69	.65	.74	.74	.79	.75	.77	.78	.76	.73	7	6	6	6
DISC-r	.71	.77	.73	.81	.83	.83	.84	.84	.83	.85	.83	5	5	5	5
NEGE-r	.72	.64	.67	.80	.79	.80	.70	.77	.79	.80	.83	6	5	6	5
INTR-r	.70	.70	.70	.81	.83	.81	.81	.76	.79	.81	.85	6	6	5	6

Source: Adapted from the MMPI-A-RF Administration, Scoring, Interpretation and Technical Manual by Archer et al. Copyright © 2016 by the Regents of the University of Minnesota. Reproduced with the permission of the University of Minnesota Press. All rights reserved. "Minnesota Multiphasic Personality Inventory" and "MMPI" are trademarks owned by the Regents of the University of Minnesota.

Note

Numbers within parentheses specify sample size.

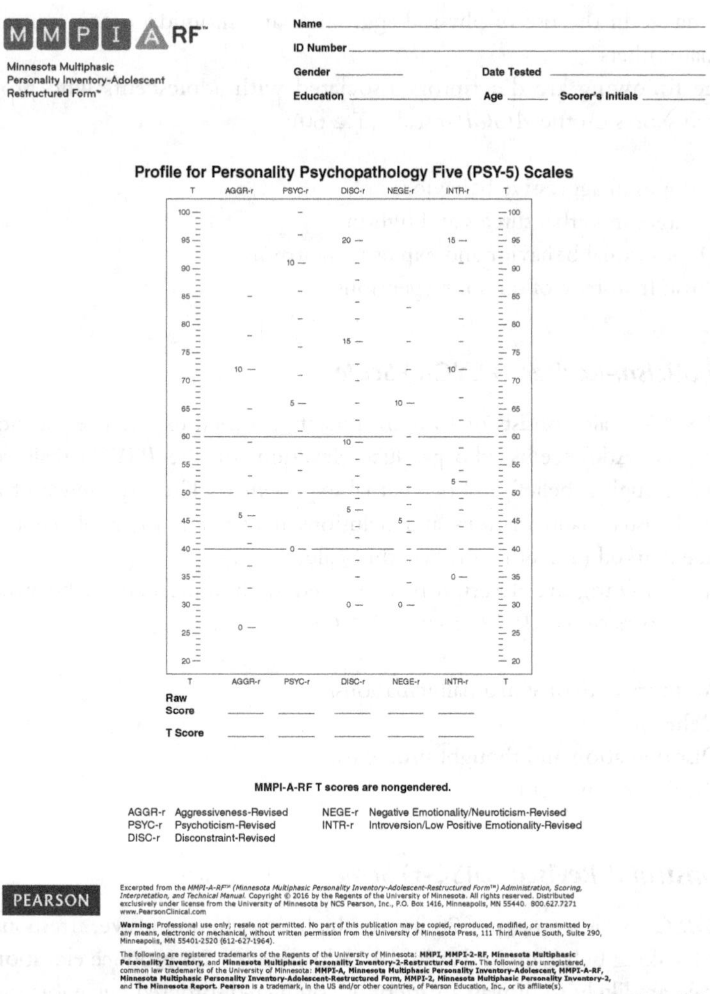

FIGURE 7.5 MMPI-A-RF Personality Psychopathology Five (PSY-5) scale profile sheet.

Source: From the MMPI-A-RF Administration, Scoring, Interpretation and Technical Manual by Archer et al. Copyright © 2016 by the Regents of the University of Minnesota. Reproduced with the permission of the University of Minnesota Press. All rights reserved. "Minnesota Multiphasic Personality Inventory" and "MMPI" are trademarks owned by the Regents of the University of Minnesota.

Aggressiveness-Revised (AGGR-r) Scale

The *AGGR-r* scale consists of 12 items describing various aspects of instrumental aggression, i.e., aggressive behavior used by an adolescent to achieve goals or accomplish objectives. Adolescents who produce elevated scores on the *AGGR-r* scale engage in the use of physical aggression and intimidation to control and dominate others.

The following are descriptors associated with adolescents who produce elevated scores on the *AGGR-r* scale (T ≥ 60):

- Engages in aggressive behavior.
- Engages in verbal threats and fighting.
- Oppositional behavior and explosive tantrums.
- Possible history of school suspensions.

Psychoticism-Revised (PSYC-r) Scale

The *PSYC-r* scale consists of 13 items reflecting varied experiences of thought disturbance. Adolescents who produce elevations on the *PSYC-r* scale report unusual thoughts, beliefs and perceptual experiences. The experience of auditory and visual hallucinations and delusions may occur for adolescents who produce marked (T ≥ 80) scores on this scale.

The following are descriptors associated with adolescents who produce elevated scores on the *PSYC-r* scale (T ≥ 60).

- Auditory and/or visual hallucinations.
- Delusions.
- Disorientation and thought problems.
- Psychotic symptoms.

Disconstraint-Revised (DISC-r) Scale

The *DISC-r* scale consists of 20 items which describe impulsive, irresponsible, and risk-taking behaviors and attitudes. Adolescents who produce elevations on this scale are likely to display a variety of conduct-disordered behaviors including abuse of drugs and alcohol.

The following are descriptors associated with adolescents who produce elevated scores on the *DISC-r* scale (T ≥ 60):

- The occurrence of criminal charges and possible placement in juvenile detention.
- History of school suspension and school problems.
- Drug and alcohol abuse.
- Running away from home.
- Rule-breaking and oppositional behavior.
- Fighting and aggressive behavior.
- Conduct-disordered behaviors.

Negative Emotionality/Neuroticism-Revised (NEGE-r) Scale

The *NEGE-r* scale consists of 13 items which describe a wide array of negative emotional experiences. Adolescents who produce an elevation on this scale are anxious, worried, nervous and over-responsive to stress.

The following are descriptors associated with adolescents who produce elevations on the *NEGE-r* scale (T ≥ 60):

- Problems with anxiety and depression.
- Problems with concentration.
- Feeling that something dreadful is about to happen.
- Possible suicidal ideation.
- Emotional discomfort that may serve as a motivating factor to engage in treatment.

Introversion/Low Positive Emotionality-Revised (INTR-r) Scale

The *INTR-r* scale consists of 15 items involving a lack of positive emotional experiences and social introversion. Adolescents who produce elevations on the *INTR-r* scale report anhedonia, social isolation and introversion.

The following are descriptors associated with adolescents who produce elevations on the *INTR-r* scale (T ≥ 60):

- Anhedonia.
- Sad/depressed affect.
- Low self-esteem.
- Social isolation.
- Fatigue and low energy.

Normative Issues

A major aspect of the development of the MMPI-A was the collection of an adolescent-specific normative sample across eight geographic locations in the United States. An important question in the development of the MMPI-A-RF concerned the extent to which the MMPI-A norms, collected in the late 1980s, could be extended to serve as the normative sample for the MMPI-A-RF. The central questioning regarding the appropriateness of the MMPI-A normative sample with the MMPI-A-RF centered on the extent to which important and substantive changes in adolescent response patterns may have occurred over the past decades. To evaluate this issue, the results of 11 studies reporting MMPI-A findings for non-clinical samples, conducted between 1995 and 2012, were reviewed to provide empirical data on this important issue. All of these studies provided information concerning means and standard deviations for the MMPI-A Basic Clinical scales for boys and girls in non-clinical samples. Four of these studies also provided data on additional MMPI-A scales, and two of these investigations (Carlson, 2001; Newton, 2008) also included mean and standard deviation data for all 69 MMPI-A scales.

The central focus of several of these studies was on the identification of response styles such as random responding or under- or overreporting by administering the MMPI-A to non-clinical samples under standard instructions and under instructions encouraging participants to simulate one or more response styles (i.e., Baer, Ballenger, Berry, & Wetter, 1997; Bagdade, 2004; Conkey, 2000; Stein, Graham, & Williams, 1995). Results of these studies consistently showed mean T-score values on MMPI-A Validity and Clinical scales ranging from the mid to high 40s, to the lower 50s. Three additional investigations reported MMPI-A scale scores from samples of academically gifted adolescents (Cross et al. 2004; Cross et al. 2008; Newton, 2008). Participants across these studies consistently showed mean T-score values ranging from the mid-40s to the low 50s. Two additional studies used non-clinical samples to contrast MMPI-A scores produced under computer test administrations versus traditional paper-and-pencil test administration (Carlson, 2001; Hays, 2003). These studies consistently showed T-scores ranging from the high 40s to the low 50s, with standard deviations of approximately 10 T-score points. These studies also showed general equivalence between test results achieved through computer administration versus standard administration. Finally, an investigation by Henry (1999) examined MMPI-A scores produced by a non-clinical sample of African-American adolescents and Yavari (2012) reported T-score means for a sample of high school students in the study of self-descriptive correlates of the K scale. The results of both of these latter investigations also demonstrated a pattern of Basic scale mean T-score values around 50 and standard deviation units around 10.

Collectively, these studies include data from 1,899 adolescents in studies conducted over the past 20 years. Table 7.10 shows the MMPI-A Basic scale means and standard deviations for the combined results of these 11 studies. As shown in this table, the overall Basic scale means for the combined studies are consistently within 3 T-score points of 50 across all scales, and standard deviations range from 8.43 on the F scale to 11.61 on the Si scale. Thus, these studies show no evidence of systematic changes in adolescent response patterns over the last two decades and support the adequacy of the MMPI-A normative sample in providing an accurate normative expectation for contemporary adolescents.

MMPI-A-RF Normative Sample

The MMPI-A-RF normative sample is a subset of the MMPI-A normative sample. The MMPI-A normative data were collected in junior high and

TABLE 7.10 MMPI-A Basic Scale Means and Standard Deviations for the Combined Results of 11 Studies Including Non-Clinical Sample Conducted From 1995 Through 2012

| T-Score | MMPI-A Scales | | | | | | | | | | | | |
| | Validity | | | Clinical | | | | | | | | | |
	L	F	K	Hs	D	Hy	Pd	Mf	Pa	Pt	Sc	Ma	Si
Mean	51.04	48.03	50.91	48.22	49.81	49.95	48.62	51.40	48.37	47.33	47.85	50.21	47.29
SD	9.27	8.43	9.13	9.92	10.22	9.36	9.06	9.91	9.35	10.46	10.07	10.64	11.61

Note

The combined sample size for Validity scales *L* and *K* is 1,087 and for scale *F* the sample is based on 1,193 adolescents. For all of the Basic Clinical Scales, the combined sample size is 1,899 adolescents.

high schools in California, Minnesota, New York, North Carolina, Ohio, Pennsylvania, Virginia and Washington State (Bucher et al., 1992). Since the intention of the MMPI-A-RF developers was to create a set of non-gendered norms for this instrument, it was deemed desirable to have an equal number of boys and girls in the MMPI-A-RF normative sample. The MMPI-A normative sample consisted of 805 boys and 815 girls. In developing the MMPI-A-RF normative sample, the normative sample of 805 boys was retained, and a subset of 805 girls was randomly selected from the 815 girls in the MMPI-A normative sample. The data for boys and girls were then combined into the MMPI-A-RF normative sample for a total sample of 1,610 adolescents. The age distributions for the MMPI-A-RF normative sample is shown in Table 7.11. Table 7.12 provides the grade level for the MMPI-A-RF normative sample of 1,610 adolescents. As shown in this table, relatively few adolescents are included at the seventh- or eighth-grade levels.

White and Krishnamurthy (2015) conducted a preliminary evaluation of the item endorsement frequencies for the 241 MMPI-A-RF items, as obtained through MMPI-A administration in clinical (R = 108) and non-clinical (R = 114) samples of adolescents. MMPI-A-RF item endorsement frequencies were examined for all items in terms of differences between clinical and high school student samples, evaluated separately by gender. Consistent with expectations, the majority of boys and girls in clinical samples showed higher item endorsement frequencies in the expected direction than their high school counterparts.

Like the MMPI-2-RF, the MMPI-A-RF uses non-gendered norms. As discussed by Ben-Porath and Tellegen (2008/2011), the use of gender-specific norms is typically based on the assumption that group differences in test

TABLE 7.11 Age Distribution of MMPI-A-RF Normative Sample

Age	Total N	Boys	Girls	%
14	366	193	173	22.7
15	438	207	231	27.2
16	427	228	199	26.5
17	292	135	157	18.1
18	87	42	45	5.4
Total	1610	805	805	100

Source: Adapted from the MMPI-A-RF Administration, Scoring, Interpretation and Technical Manual by Archer et al. Copyright © 2016 by the Regents of the University of Minnesota. Reproduced with the permission of the University of Minnesota Press. All rights reserved. "Minnesota Multiphasic Personality Inventory" and "MMPI" are trademarks owned by the Regents of the University of Minnesota.

Note
The mean age for the total sample is 15.56 (*SD* = 1.18).

TABLE 7.12 Grade Level of MMPI-A-RF Normative Sample

Grade	Total N	Boys	Girls	%
7	8	5	3	0.5
8	121	57	64	7.5
9	415	212	203	25.8
10	470	238	232	29.2
11	385	206	179	23.9
12	210	87	123	13
None Reported	1	0	1	0.1
Total	1610	805	805	100

Source: From the MMPI-A-RF Administration, Scoring, Interpretation and Technical Manual by Archer, et al. Copyright © 2016 by the Regents of the University of Minnesota. Reproduced with the permission of the University of Minnesota Press. All rights reserved. "Minnesota Multiphasic Personality Inventory" and "MMPI" are trademarks owned by the Regents of the University of Minnesota.

raw scores related to gender are not relevant to the constructs that are being assessed. Thus, for example, some may assume that gender differences observed between boys and girls in raw score distributions on a depression scale are not related to meaningful gender differences in the experience or expression of depression, and therefore these gender group differences should be eliminated by transforming test raw scores into standardized scores separately for boys and girls. Ben-Porath and Tellegen noted that the initial impetus for exploring the development of non-gendered norms occurred for the MMPI-2 as a result of the Federal Civil Rights Act of 1991 which prohibited consideration of gender-specific norms in employment settings. While the MMPI-A-RF would not be expected to be utilized in pre-employment screenings, the use of non-gendered norms was deemed appropriate because meaningful gender differences may occur in the experience or expression of various forms of psychopathology that would be masked by the use of gender-specific norms. Gender differences are better reflected through the use of non-gendered norms (e.g., Reynolds & Kamphaus, 2002) and an additional advantage of the use of non-gendered norms is that the scale scores for both boys and girls are calculated using the same conversion standard.

Uniform T-score Transformation

The adult norms developed by Hathaway and McKinley (1942) for the original form of the MMPI were based on linear transformation procedures that converted raw scores to T-score values. The MMPI-A-RF retains the use of linear T-scores for the Validity scales (i.e., TRIN-r, VRIN-r, F-r, L-r and K-r). However, researchers have long noted a problem that is associated with the use of linear T-score values for the Clinical scales of the original MMPI.

This problem is that identical T-score values do not represent the same percentile equivalents across the standard MMPI scales when derived using linear T-scores. This phenomenon occurs because MMPI scale raw score distributions are not normally distributed, and the degree to which they vary from the normal distribution fluctuates from scale to scale. Thus, using linear T-score conversion procedures, a T-score value of 70 on one scale may not represent a percentile value equivalent to that represented by a T-score value of 70 on another MMPI clinical scale. This discrepancy resulted in difficulties when directly comparing T-score values across MMPI scales. These difficulties were first discussed in detail by Colligan et al. (1983).

In developing the MMPI-2, uniform T-score transformation procedures were used in order to provide equivalent T-score values across the Clinical and Content scales (Tellegen & Ben-Porath, 1992). This same approach was used in the development of the MMPI-A-RF uniform T-scores. Uniform T-score values, for example, were developed for the RC scales by examining a distribution of scales and deriving a composite or average distribution of raw scores adjusting the distribution of each individual RC scale to maximize its match with the composite RC scale distribution. The purpose of developing a composite or uniform distribution was to allow the assignment of a T-score conversion value to each scale such that a given T-score value would convert to an equivalent percentile value across each of the scales.

Because uniform T-scores represent composite linear T-scores, this procedure serves to produce equivalent percentile values across scales for a given T-score. This procedure, however, also maintains the underlying skew in the distribution of scores from these measures. Thus, uniform T-scores are generally similar to values that would be obtained from linear T-scores (Edwards, Morrison, and Weissman, 1993b). Uniform T-scores do not have major effects on the underlying distribution of raw scores and do not serve to "normalize" the underlying raw score distribution. This is important in that the true distribution of scores on MMPI scales may not, in fact, follow the normal distribution curve, and therefore a normalization procedure may actually serve to distort T-score values by artificially lowering those that occur in the higher range (Tellegen & Ben-Porath, 1992).

Table 7.13 shows the percentile values for uniform T-scores for MMPI-A-RF scales at given T-score values. As shown in this table, uniform T-scores do not correct or normalize the underlying raw score distribution. For example, a T-score value of 50 does not equal a percentile value of 50, but rather a percentile equivalent value of 55. The uniform T-score procedure makes relatively small adjustments in individual scale raw score distributions achieved by creating a composite or overall distribution across the affected scales. These adjustments produce comparable percentile equivalents to be assigned to a T-score value so that a given T-score value will yield more equivalent percentile range across scale. For example, a T-score value of 60

TABLE 7.13 Percentile Equivalents for MMPI-A-RF Uniform T-Scores

Uniform T-Score	Equivalent Percentile
30	< 1
35	4
40	15
45	34
50	55
55	73
60	85
65	92
70	96
75	98
80	> 99

Source: From the MMPI-A-RF Administration, Scoring, Interpretation and Technical Manual by Archer, et al. Copyright © 2016 by the Regents of the University of Minnesota. Reproduced with the permission of the University of Minnesota Press. All rights reserved. "Minnesota Multiphasic Personality Inventory" and "MMPI" are trademarks owned by the Regents of the University of Minnesota.

would produce an equivalent percentile ranking at the 85th percentile across a variety of MMPI-A-RF scales.

In summary, the MMPI-A-RF has employed a set of norms which are very similar to the MMPI-A in terms of the normative sample and the use of uniform T-score transformation procedures. However, the use of non-gendered norms with the MMPI-A-RF represents a point of departure from the MMPI-A. A second major departure from the MMPI-A is the reduction of the demarcation point to define clinical range elevations to T ≥ 60 on the MMPI-A-RF.

The T ≥ 60 Definition of MMPI-A-RF Clinical Range Elevations

Normal-range mean profiles for adolescents in clinical samples were frequently obtained with the original version of the MMPI using the traditional T-score criteria of 70 or greater to define clinical range symptomatology. As previously noted, Ehrenworth and Archer (1985) recommended the use of a T-score value of 65 (rather than 70) for defining clinical range elevations for adolescents on the original instrument. In developing the MMPI-A, the criteria for clinical range profiles was reduced so that a T-score ≥ 65 determine clinical range elevations, while T-scores between 60 and 65 constitute a marginal range of elevations in which adolescents might be expected to show some, but not necessarily all, of the clinical correlates or traits associated with a higher range elevation for these MMPI-A scales. However, studies following the release of the MMPI-A conducted in samples of adolescents in clinical settings showed evidence of a significant problem with the occurrence of false-negative profiles, that is, adolescents who produced normal-range scores while in treatment in outpatient or inpatient psychiatric settings.

The MMPI-A-RF has eliminated the transitional or marginally elevated range or zone used on the MMPI-A, and redefined clinical range elevations as any T-score ≥ 60 on a clinical or substantive scale. Classification accuracy in identifying adolescents as normal versus psychologically impaired always represents a tradeoff or balance between the types of errors created by moving the T-score criteria upward or downward. For example, reducing the T-score criteria to T ≥ 60 to reduce the frequency of false-negative misclassifications of adolescents in clinical samples must result in an increase in the rate of false-positive misidentification of normal adolescents. Further, the relative cost of this tradeoff will always be related to the actual occurrence of psychopathology in a given population, that is, the actual base rate of psychopathology in a given sample or setting. Given the extensive literature indicating that the MMPI-A tended to produce relatively low scores for adolescents in clinical samples, the T-score criteria of 60 or greater to define clinical range psychopathology constitutes a logical step in attempting to address this issue. Future research studies in this area will shed light on the extent to which this modification successfully increased the overall accurate identification or hit rate outcomes for this test instrument.

Critical Responses and Critical Items

The MMPI-A-RF Score Report, available from Pearson, provides raw and T-score values for all MMPI-A-RF scales, the percentage of items answered on each scale, a list of unscorable items, and a list of items with critical content. One source of critical content derives from the concept of critical responses used on the MMPI-2-RF. Specifically, in parallel to the MMPI-2-RF, there are six critical scales on the MMPI-A-RF which include Aggression (*AGG*), Anxiety (*AXY*), Helplessness/Hopelessness (*HLP*), Ideas of Persecution (*RC6*), Aberrant Experiences (*RC8*), and Substance Abuse (*SUB*). Items endorsed in the keyed direction on each of these scales are reported in the MMPI-A-RF Score Report as Critical Responses. Thus, it is possible to evaluate, for example, the types of persecutory ideation associated with elevations on *RC6* by reviewing the actual item endorsement for this scale. In addition, the MMPI-A-RF also includes a set of critical items which were derived from the Forbey and Ben-Porath (1998) Critical Item list for the MMPI-A. The Forbey and Ben-Porath Critical Item List development process, based on a combination of empirical and rational steps, is described in the MMPI-A Manual Supplement (Ben-Porath et al. 2006). The final list of critical items developed for the MMPI-A by Forbey and Ben-Porath reflected 81 items sorted into 15 content-based categories.

TABLE 7.14 Forbey and Ben-Porath MMPI-A-RF Critical Item List

Content Area	# of Items
Aggression	2
Anxiety	4
Cognitive Problems	2
Conduct Problems	7
Depression/Suicidal Ideation	7
Eating Problems	2
Family Problems	2
Hallucinatory Experiences	3
Paranoid Ideation	6
School Problems	4
Self-Denigration	2
Somatic Complaints	6
Substance Use/Abuse	5
Unusual Thinking	1
Total Items	53

Source: From the MMPI-A-RF Administration, Scoring, Interpretation and Technical Manual by Archer et al. Copyright © 2016 by the Regents of the University of Minnesota. Reproduced with the permission of the University of Minnesota Press. All rights reserved. "Minnesota Multiphasic Personality Inventory" and "MMPI" are trademarks owned by the Regents of the University of Minnesota.

The MMPI-A Critical Item list was reviewed by Archer et al. (2016a) in terms of items which survived into the 241 item pool of the MMPI-A-RF. The resulting MMPI-A-RF Critical Item list, shown in Table 7.14 consists of 53 items grouped into 14 content categories.

Interpretations of individual items of the MMPI-A-RF results are generally not recommended because of reliability and validity issues associated with single-item responses. However, critical item review may give a clinician a sense of the nature and severity of problems that an adolescent has reported. For example, review of items in the Depression/Suicidal Ideation content area will reveal the extent to which an adolescent has endorsed items suggestive of suicidal ideation. Further, critical item review provides a solid basis for the clinician to explore important content areas with the adolescent during the process of test feedback and to initiate a therapeutic discussion of the adolescent's problem areas.

An Interpretive Strategy for the MMPI-A-RF

The interpretive process for the MMPI-A-RF will be illustrated in greater detail in Chapter 8. Interpretation of MMPI-A-RF results begins with a consideration of protocol validity, starting with the issue of whether the adolescent has provided enough responses, as reflected in the *CNS* score, in order to interpret test results. If a sufficient number of responses have occurred (less than 10 item omissions), the protocol may be evaluated in terms of consistency (scores on *VRIN-r*, *TRIN-r*, and *CRIN*) and in terms of response accuracy reflected in scales of underreporting (i.e., *L-r* and *K-r*) and overreporting (*F-r*). Interpretation of substantive scale scores can only be undertaken after potential threats to the validity of the test protocol have been ruled out using the validity scale interpretation model provided by Roger Greene (2011) as discussed in Chapter 6.

The interpretation of the Substantive scales follows a process that may be organized into four sequential stages: a review of the Higher-Order (H-O) scales, the Restructured Clinical (RC) scales, the Specific Problems (SP) scales and, finally, the Personality Psychopathology-5 (PSY-5) scales. As previously noted, the H-O scales represent the broadest constructs, the RC scales represent mid-level constructs, and the SP scales represent the most narrow-focused constructs designed to measure or augment facets of the RC scales. Thus, a clinical range elevation on the Emotional Dysfunction (*EID*) scale would lead to refinement of the description of the adolescent through examination of *RC2* and *RC7* at the mid-level, as well as SP scales in the Internalizing group such as Anxiety (*AXY*), Stress/Worry (*STW*), Anger Proneness (*ANP*), and Behavior-Restricting Fears (*BRF*). In contrast, a clinical range elevation on the Behavioral Dysfunction (*BXD*) H-O scale would lead to a mid-level examination of T-score values on *RC4* and *RC9*, and externalizing SP scales such as Aggression (*AGG*), Substance Abuse (*SUB*), and Conduct Disorder (*CNP*) and the Disconstraint (*DISC*-r) PSY-5 scale, at the third and most narrow review level. Finally, a clinical range elevation on the H-O Thought Dysfunction (*THD*) scale would lead to focused evaluation of the adolescent's scores on Ideas of Persecution (*RC6*) and Aberrant Experiences (*RC8*) on the RC scale or mid-level, and Psychoticism-Revised (*PSYC-r*) on the PSY-5 scales. In summary, the interpretive process consistently moves from the broadest scales at the H-O level, to the mid-range scales at the RC level, to the more specific facet scales at the SP and PSY-5 level. Finally, at the item level, the responses to the six critical scales are reviewed as provided in the extended score reports for the MMPI-A-RF, and the critical items across 14 content areas are also examined to provide an insight into the specific nature and characteristics of the psychopathology being reported by the adolescent.

Salient Differences Between the MMPI-A and MMPI-A-RF

The MMPI-A-RF is a new instrument designed to help in the identification and description of psychopathology among adolescents. Table 7.15 provides a summary of some of the important differences between the MMPI-A-RF and the MMPI-A.

TABLE 7.15 Salient Differences Between the MMPI-A and the MMPI-A-RF

Variable	MMPI-A	MMPI-A-RF
Year of Publication	1992	2016
Primary Influence	MMPI-2	MMPI-2-RF
Number of Items	478	241
Scale Structure	Extensive item overlap across scales	Non-overlapping items within hierarchical scale structure
Norms	Gender Specific	Non-gendered
T-Score criterion for clinical elevation	T ≥ 65	T ≥ 60

As noted in Table 7.15, the MMPI-A was a downward age extension of the MMPI-2 specifically designed for use with adolescents. In contrast, the MMPI-A-RF was designed and developed to serve as a downward age extension of the MMPI-2-RF for adolescents ages 14 through 18, heavily informed by the psychometric approach utilized in the development of this latter instrument by Tellegen and Ben-Porath. The MMPI-A-RF is not simply a revision of the MMPI-A, but represents a notable departure from its predecessor, in a manner that is similar to the change represented by the MMPI-2-RF in contrast to the MMPI-2. The MMPI-A-RF, at 241 items, is roughly half the item length of the 478-item MMPI-A. Test length is a critical issue in evaluating many adolescents who may not have an adequate attention span to successfully complete the 478 items of the MMPI-A. The development of the MMPI-A-RF may prove particularly instrumental in increasing the use of personality assessment measures in educational and forensic/criminal justice settings in which evaluation time constraints may be a crucial factor in limiting the use of the MMPI-A.

The MMPI-A, similar to the original MMPI, exhibits extensive item overlap across scales, contributing to higher than expected correlations between scales measuring unrelated constructs. The MMPI-A-RF developers sought to reduce scale intercorrelations, and hence potentially increased scale discriminant validity, by reducing the influence of the pervasive demoralization factor within scales and by eliminating item overlap between scales within each of the hierarchical levels (i.e., H-O, RC, and SP scales) of the MMPI-A-RF. While the two instruments share a largely overlapping normative sample, the MMPI-A-RF uses non-gendered norms in the transformation of raw scores to T-scores, in contrast to the gender-specific T-score transformation procedure developed for the MMPI-A. Finally, the T-score criteria used for defining clinical range elevations on the MMPI-A-RF is T ≥ 60, which may be contrasted with the T-score criteria of T ≥ 65 employed with the MMPI-A.

It is anticipated that support for administration and scoring for both the MMPI-A and the MMPI-A-RF will be available from the University of Minnesota Press and Pearson Assessments for the foreseeable future. Given the accelerated rate of accumulation of MMPI-A research over the past 20 years, when compared with the adolescent research done with the original form of the MMPI during the initial 40 years of use of that instrument, it is anticipated that the MMPI-A-RF will generate a substantial research literature over the next decade. The accumulation of this MMPI-A-RF research will be greatly aided by the fact that the MMPI-A-RF may be scored based on results obtained through the administration of the MMPI-A. Thus, currently existing MMPI-A datasets can be readily rescored using the items and scale structure of the MMPI-A-RF to provide important empirical information concerning the usefulness of this new test instrument.

The research literature on the MMPI-A-RF will undoubtedly show areas of advantage for this instrument (relative to the MMPI-A) in some specific assessment tasks with adolescents, and areas of limitations for the MMPI-A-RF in addressing other types of assessment issues or areas. It is likely that the ultimate evaluation of the MMPI-A-RF will be based on a scale-by-scale analysis of the instrument, rather than broad generalizations concerning the overall utility of the test instrument. The publication of the MMPI-A-RF offers test users a valuable alternative instrument to the MMPI-A, particularly in situations in which the 241-item length of the MMPI-A-RF serves as an important factor in successful test administration.

The reduction in test length provided by the MMPI-A-RF, however, was not the primary objective of the development of this test. The central objective in the development of the MMPI-A-RF was to improve on the discriminate validity achievable by the MMPI-A by reducing the ubiquitous and confounding influence of the demoralization factor commonly found in most personality inventories. Archer (2006) and Friedman et al. (2015), for example, noted that the extensive item overlap that occurs across the MMPI Basic scales (including the MMPI-A Basic scales) is attributable to the criterion keying method of item selection employed by Hathaway and McKinley (1943) for scale development, the degree of symptom overlap among psychiatric disorders, and the pervasive influence of shared first-factor variance, a factor labeled by Tellegen as Demoralization. While scales heavily influenced by the Demoralization factor might be expected to show strong evidence of convergent validity (i.e., high correlations with predicted external criteria), such scales typically suffer from relatively poor specificity or discriminate validity (i.e., the ability to discriminate between various forms of psychopathology). The MMPI-A-RF seeks to reduce the redundancy found among MMPI-A scales by isolating the demoralization factor and reducing its influence on the "seed" or "core" components of MMPI-A-RF scales. This process, if successful, should result in shorter scales (in contrast to

MMPI-A counterparts) with comparable convergent validity but improved discriminative ability. The MMPI-A-RF Manual (Archer, Handel, Ben-Porath, & Tellegen, 2016b) provides over 17,000 correlations between MMPI-A-RF scale scores and external criteria in a variety of adolescent samples. These data provide an important initial step in evaluating the MMPI-A-RF. Future research will further establish the extent to which the MMPI-A-RF has achieved the important objectives of maintaining convergent validity while demonstrating improvements in discriminant validity.

8

INTERPRETIVE STRATEGIES FOR THE MMPI-A AND MMPI-A-RF

The MMPI-A or MMPI-A-RF, used in conjunction with data from other psychometric sources, psychosocial assessment results, and clinical interview findings, provide a rich source of information concerning a variety of respondent characteristics. Test findings from the MMPI-A or MMPI-A-RF include data concerning profile validity and the adolescent's test-taking attitude. Validity findings also encompass the degree to which the adolescent's responses were consistent and accurate, both of which serve as essential components to establish the protocol validity. Test profiles also provide information concerning the presence or absence of psychiatric symptoms along a number of dimensions of psychopathology, including the nature, type and extent of symptomatology. Further, inspection of the adolescent's MMPI-A or MMPI-A-RF results allow for an overall estimate of the adolescent's adjustment level as well as providing information concerning the adolescent's characteristic defense mechanisms, and the relative effectiveness of these defenses in protecting the adolescent from consciously perceived emotional distress. The psychologist should also be able to form useful opinions concerning the adolescent's typical interpersonal relationships, including such issues as interpersonal dominance versus submissiveness, as well as the tendency to become actively engaged with others versus socially withdrawn and isolated.

The use of the MMPI-A or MMPI-A-RF will also typically yield valuable diagnostic impressions and hypotheses concerning the most effective modes of treatment for the adolescent patient. It is important to stress, however, that all test instruments are most productively used to generate a variety of diagnostic possibilities, rather than exclusive single diagnoses. Research has shown that MMPI-derived diagnoses and clinician-derived diagnoses differ frequently in clinical studies of adult psychiatric patients (Graham, 2012) and adolescent patients (Archer & Gordon, 1988). Research (e.g., Pancoast, Archer, & Gordon, 1988) has also indicated that simple systems designed to derive diagnosis from the MMPI appear to perform as well as more complex diagnostic classification systems developed for the MMPI such as those by Goldberg (1965, 1972) and by Meehl and Dahlstrom (1960). Perhaps the most important data yielded from the MMPI-A or MMPI-A-RF involves providing clinicians with information concerning treatment considerations and options. These data typically include information concerning the adolescent's level of motivation to engage in psychotherapy and openness to the therapeutic process. The clinician may also be able to derive information concerning the types of therapy, or combination of therapies, most likely to be effective with the adolescent (e.g., supportive psychotherapies, insight-oriented psychotherapies, cognitive-behavioral psychotherapies, or psychopharmacological interventions). Test results may also allow for inferences concerning the modalities of treatment most likely to be indicated, including individual, family, and group psychotherapies.

Common Steps in Test Interpretation

There are significant areas of overlap in the initial steps in the interpretation process between the MMPI-A and MMPI-A-RF, and we will deal with these common steps first in this chapter before we discuss interpretive guidance unique to either the MMPI-A or MMPI-A-RF.

The ability to derive meaningful and useful information from the MMPI-A or MMPI-A-RF is a function of the overall interpretive process utilized with this instrument. Table 8.1 summarizes a useful common interpretive approach for both instruments.

The first two common steps in interpreting both the MMPI-A and/or MMPI-A-RF emphasize the importance of consideration of the setting in which the test is administered, and the evaluation of history and background information available for the adolescent. Interpretive hypotheses generated from MMPI-A or MMPI-A-RF findings should be carefully coordinated with what is known about the adolescent from extra-test sources. It is possible to interpret a test profile in a "blind" fashion without consideration of the patient's background and history or features of the administration setting. Indeed, these latter sources of information are often not utilized in computerized interpretations of objective personality assessment instruments. Nevertheless, demographic, psychosocial, educational, medical and psychiatric history information generally increase the accuracy and utility of inferences derived from the MMPI-A and MMPI-A-RF.

The third step shown in Table 8.1 concerns the evaluation of the technical validity of the MMPI-A or MMPI-A-RF profile. Validity assessment approaches for the MMPI-A and MMPI-A-RF were presented in detail in

TABLE 8.1 Common Steps in MMPI-A and MMPI-A-RF Interpretation

1. Consideration of setting in which the test is administered
   a. Clinical/psychological/psychiatric
   b. School/academic evaluation
   c. Medical
   d. Neuropsychological
   e. Forensic
   f. Alcohol/drug treatment
2. Evaluation of history and background of patient
   a. Cooperativeness/motivation for treatment or evaluation
   b. Cognitive ability
   c. History of psychological adjustment
   d. History of stress factors
   e. History of academic performance
   f. History of interpersonal relationships
   g. Family history and characteristics
3. Validity Scale Interpretation

Validity Issue	MMPI-A Source	MMPI-A-RF Source
a. Omissions	CNS	CNS
b. Consistency	*VRIN, TRIN*	*VRIN-r, TRIN-r, CRIN*
c. Accuracy		
1. Overreporting	*F, Fb, F$_1$, F$_2$*	*F-r*
2. Underreporting	*L, K*	*L-r, K-r*

Chapter 4 of this text, based on the model proposed by Greene (2000, 2011). This process includes a review of the number of item omissions that occurred in the response process, and an evaluation of response consistency and response accuracy. As previously noted, response consistency is primarily evaluated using the MMPI-A Variable Response Inconsistency (*VRIN*) scale, and scores from the True Response Inconsistency (*TRIN*) scale may be used for assessing the presence of an acquiescence or "nay-saying" response style. Inferences concerning response consistency can also be derived by examining the T-score elevation difference between the MMPI-A F_1 and F_2 subscales, and the overall elevation of *F*. Conclusions regarding response consistency may be drawn for the MMPI-A-RF based on results for the *VRIN-r, TRIN-r,* and *CRIN* scales. As we have noted, consistency is a necessary, but not sufficient, condition for establishing protocol validity. The accuracy of an adolescent's MMPI-A response patterns may be evaluated using the traditional validity scales *F, L,* and *K* (or with the revised forms of these scales for the MMPI-A-RF), with particular attention to the overall configuration of these three validity measures. In addition to issues of technical validity, however, the MMPI-A and MMPI-A-RF Validity measures can provide valuable information concerning the adolescent's willingness to engage in the psychotherapeutic process. For example, the Validity scale configuration may indicate a technically valid profile, but also exhibit a level of *K* or *K-r* scale elevation indicative of a teenager who is likely to underreport psychiatric symptoms and to be guarded and defensive in the psychotherapy process. Thus, some MMPI-A and MMPI-A-RF Validity scales, (e.g., *L*, *F*, and *K* or *L-r*, *F-r* and *K-r*, respectively) provide information concerning technical validity *and* extra-test characteristics or correlates of the teenager that should be included in the overall interpretation of the adolescent's profile.

Steps in MMPI-A Interpretation

The steps in the interpretation of the MMPI-A are summarized in Table 8.2.

The interpretation of the MMPI-A profile involves an examination of the basic clinical scales, including an evaluation of the adolescent's codetype assignment based on their most elevated basic clinical scales. The process of evaluating the adolescent's MMPI-A codetype includes consideration of the degree of scale elevation manifested in the profile. The higher the adolescent's basic scale elevations, the more likely that adolescent is to display the symptoms or characteristics associated with a codetype classification. Additionally, the greater the degree to which the adolescent's specific MMPI-A profile corresponds to the prototypic profiles used in research investigations for that codetype, the more confidence we can place in the accuracy of the codetype correlates attributed to the obtained profile. The degree of correspondence between a particular MMPI-A codetype and the prototypic profile characteristics for a given codetype may be estimated, for example, by visual inspection of the Marks et al. (1974) modal MMPI profiles for adolescents. In contrast, the MMPI-A Interpretive System software (Version 5), distributed by Psychological Assessment Resources (Archer, 2013), illustrates a statistical approach to this issue. Specifically, this interpretive program provides a correlation coefficient that expresses the degree of association between an adolescent's MMPI-A profile and the mean MMPI-A profile characteristics for adolescents classified in that codetype grouping. Further, the program calculates the definition of the codetype, expressed in T-scores. The greater the degree to which the adolescent's codetype is clearly defined, that is, the two-point codetype demonstrates a substantial T-score elevation difference between the two most elevated scales and the third-highest elevation, the more likely that a particular codetype descriptor will be found to be accurate for that adolescent. In addition to high-point descriptors, it may also be useful to examine the low-point characteristics of the adolescent's MMPI-A profile for selected scales. Finally, a specific review of MMPI-A Basic scales *2* and *7* will provide information concerning the degree of affective distress currently experienced by the adolescent, permitting important inferences concerning the adolescent's motivation to engage in psychotherapy.

A review of MMPI-A Supplementary scales (Step 2 in Table 8.2) should provide substantial information to support and refine Basic scale interpretation.

TABLE 8.2 Steps in MMPI-A Interpretation

---

1. Basic Clinical Scale and/or codetype Interpretation
   a. Degree of match with prototype
      (1) Degree of elevation
      (2) Degree of definition
   b. Low-point scale interpretation
   c. Note elevation of scales 2 (*D*) and 7 (*Pt*)
2. Supplementary and PSY-5 scales (supplement and confirm interpretation)
   a. Supplementary scale dimensions
      (1) Welsh *A* and *R* scales and the *IMM* scale
   b. Substance abuse scales
      (1) *MAC-R*, *ACK* and *PRO*
   c. Personality Psychopathology Five (PSY-5) scales
      (1) Aggressiveness and Disconstraint
3. Content scales
   a. Supplement, refine, and confirm basic scale data
   b. Interpersonal functioning (*A-fam*, *A-cyn*, *A-aln*), treatment recommendations (*A-trt*), and academic difficulties (*A-sch* and *A-las*).
   c. Review scores on content component scales
   d. Consider effects of overreporting/underreporting
4. Review of Harris-Lingoes and *Si* subscales and critical item content
   a. Items endorsed can assist in understanding reasons for elevation of basic scales
   b. Review of Forbey and Ben-Porath MMPI-A critical items

Welsh's *A* and *R* scales indicate an overall level of maladjustment and the use of repression as a primary defense mechanism, respectively, and the adolescent's level of psychological maturity may be assessed through the use of the Immaturity (*IMM*) scale. Substance abuse screening information is available through the MMPI-A revision of the MacAndrew (1965) Alcoholism Scale (the *MAC-R*), as well as two additional Substance Abuse scales created for the MMPI-A (*ACK* and *PRO*) to evaluate alcohol and drug abuse problems (Weed, Butcher, & Williams, 1994). The Personality Psychopathology Five (PSY-5), extended to the MMPI-A by McNulty et al. (1997) also provides important data on personality dimensions (e.g., Aggressiveness and Disconstraint) of substantial usefulness in evaluating adolescents.

In addition to Supplemental scales, there are 15 MMPI-A Content scales that are also used to improve profile interpretation (see Step 3 in Table 8.2). Many of the MMPI-A Content scales may be used to refine the interpretation of Basic scales. For example, scale *A-anx* may be helpful in relation to scale *Pt*, scale *A-biz* may be useful in clarifying interpretations from scale *Sc*, and scales *A-con* and *A-fam* may be helpful in refining interpretations from MMPI scale *Pd*. Further, content scales such as *A-trt* may provide important information concerning the adolescent's probable initial response to therapy, and *A-sch* and *A-las* may signal the presence of academic problems. Content scales including *A-fam*, *A-cyn*, and *A-aln* are also relevant to descriptions of the adolescent's interpersonal functioning. The Content Component scales developed by Sherwood et al. (1997) for 13 of the 15 MMPI-A Content scales are quite valuable in refining the interpretation of the adolescent's protocol. For example, the *A-ang* component scales should provide important information discriminating the potential for explosive and aggressive behaviors from more benign irritability, and the *A-trt* components hold promise in providing a more detailed understanding of the reasons why initial obstacles to treatment may be present in the psychological functioning of the adolescent. In evaluating Content scale data, however, it is also important to consider the effects of overreporting or underreporting (i.e., response accuracy) on Content scale findings. Because Content scales are constructed based on obvious items, adolescents may easily suppress Content scale values when underreporting symptomatology, and grossly elevate Content scale values when consciously or unconsciously overreporting symptomatology.

In the next stage (Step 4) of MMPI-A profile analysis, the interpreter may wish to selectively examine the content of the adolescent's MMPI-A responses as manifested in the Harris–Lingoes (1955) subscales for the standard MMPI-A scales 2, 3, 4, 6, 8, and 9, and the *Si* subscales for 0, and as expressed in responses to the Forbey and Ben-Porath MMPI-A Critical Item list. A content review may refine interpretive hypotheses generated from examination of the MMPI-A Basic, Supplementary, and Content scales. This content-based information, however, should be used only as a means of refining or clarifying hypotheses generated based on results of the MMPI-A Basic Clinical scales. For example, it has been previously noted that Harris–Lingoes subscales should not be interpreted unless a clinical range elevation has occurred on the corresponding MMPI-A Basic scale and that findings for the Hy_1 (Denial of Social Anxiety) and Pd_3 (Social Imperturbability) subscales may not provide useful clinical information because clinical range elevations are not possible on these two subscales (Krishnamurthy et al., 1995). The MMPI-A critical item set by Forbey and Ben-Porath (1998) are useful as a means of identifying particular content themes, particularly as areas to clarify in post-test feedback with the adolescent.

Steps in MMPI-A-RF Interpretation

Table 8.3 illustrates the sequence of steps involved in the interpretation of the MMPI-A-RF substantive scales. This sequence has been modified slightly from the guidance in the MMPI-A-RF manual (Archer et al., 2016a) to clarify and emphasize the importance of interpreting the Higher-Order (*H-O*) scales prior to consideration of the Somatic-Cognitive scales.

As shown in Table 8.3, substantive scale interpretation following the evaluation of validity scale data begins with a review of scores for the Higher-Order

TABLE 8.3 Steps in MMPI-A-RF Substantive Scale Interpretation

Topic	MMPI-A-RF Sources
a. Emotional Dysfunction	1. EID
	2. RCd, HLP, SFD, NFC
	3. RC2, INTR-r
	4. RC7, STW, AXY, ANP, BRF, SPF, OCS, NEGE-r
b. Thought Dysfunction	1. THD
	2. RC6
	3. RCB
	4. PSYC-r
c. Behavioral Dysfunction	1. BXD
	2. RC4, NSA, ASA, CNP, SUB, NPI
	3. RC9, AGG
	4. AGGR-r, DISC-r
d. Somatic/Cognitive Dysfunction	RC1, MLS, GIC, HPC, NUC, COG
e. Interpersonal Functioning	1. FML
	2. RC3
	3. IPP
	4. SAV
	5. SHY
	6. DSF
f. Diagnostic Considerations	All Substantive Scales Results
g. Treatment Considerations	All Substantive Scale Results

Source: From the MMPI-A-RF Adminstration, Scoring, Interpretation, and Technical Manual by Archer et al. Copyright © 2016 by the Regents of the University of Minnesota. Reproduced with the permission of the University of Minnesota Press. All rights reserved. "Minnesota Multiphasic Personality Inventory" and "MMPI" are trademarks owned by the Regents of the University of Minnesota.

(*H-O*) scales. The specific manifestations of symptoms related to elevations in the Higher-Order scales are facilitated by a review of the elevated scores on the RC, SP, and PSY-5 scales that are associated with emotional dysfunction (*EID*), Thought Dysfunction (*THD*), or Behavioral Dysfunction (*BXD*). For example, manifestations of an elevation on the Thought Dysfunction (*THD*) Higher-Order scale are facilitated by the review of test findings for *RC6* and *RC8*, as well as the Psychoticism (*PSYC-r*) PSY-5 scale. After reviewing the H-O scales, the somatic-cognitive scores are considered next, with description of the adolescent along this latter dimension refined by consideration of scores in *RC1, MLS, GLC, HPC, NUC,* and *COG.* As shown in Section e of Table 8.3, interpersonal functioning is evaluated by consideration of the six scales related to interpersonal functioning, *FML, RC3, IPP, SAV, SHY,* and *DSF.* Elevations on Social Avoidance (*SAV*), for example, indicate the degree to which the adolescent may avoid social events and situations, and elevations on

Disaffiliativeness (*DSF*) provide valuable information concerning the degree to which the adolescent may be socially introverted, withdrawn, and manifest a poor self-esteem.

Following the interpretation of the Substantive scales, the interpretive process for the MMPI-A-RF proceeds to diagnostic and treatment issues. The interpretive process during these stages typically involves all of the test findings from the MMPI-A-RF Substantive scales, because all of these data are potentially relevant to diagnostic and treatment issues. Consideration of the Forbey and Ben-Porath MMPI-A-RF Critical Items during this stage also provides important information concerning the specific nature and characteristics of the psychopathology endorsed by the adolescent, as well as identifying important topics for test feedback for the adolescent.

Case Illustrations

Three cases were selected to illustrate recommended approaches for interpretation of the MMPI-A and MMPI-A-RF, using the test results from the same adolescents for both the MMPI-A and MMPI-A-RF to highlight both the similarities and the differences in the test interpretation. Specifically, these cases were selected from MMPI-A protocols obtained in three different settings, and the selected MMPI-A results were rescored in order to produce MMPI-A-RF scale test findings. For each clinical case example, the background information and Validity scale findings are presented initially for the adolescent. We will then present the results derived from the MMPI-A, followed by the MMPI-A-RF results for the case.

Clinical Case Example 1: Richard (Clinical Outpatient Setting)

Background and Validity Scale Findings:

Richard is a 16-year-old boy from a middle-class African-American family who was referred for outpatient evaluation with complaints of anxiety, depression, and increasing family conflict. Previously an excellent student, this adolescent has shown a pattern of decreasing academic performance over the past year. Additionally, Richard's parents expressed concern that he would break into angry and rebellious episodes with them without apparent reason, alternating with periods of apathy and lethargy. This adolescent showed a diminished interest in participating in school activities, and increasing conduct and behavioral problems in school. Richard reported problems sleeping, and complained of feelings of fatigue and loss of energy. Richard was placed in outpatient treatment, which included both individual and family therapy, with an initial diagnosis of Major Depressive Episode.

This adolescent's scores on the MMPI-A Validity scales appear in Figure 8.1 and for the MMPI-A-RF Validity scales in Figure 8.4. The first issue to be considered with either instrument relates to the number of omitted items on the Cannot Say (*CNS*) scale. In this case, the Cannot Say scale equals 0, a result which is consistent with valid interpretation on both tests. Richard's scores on measures of response consistency for both the MMPI-A (*VRIN* = 42 and *TRIN* = 51F) and the MMPI-A-RF (*VRIN-r* = 47, *TRIN-r* = 59F, and *CRIN* = 47) are within expected and normal ranges and demonstrate acceptable levels of response consistency across instruments. Finally, Richard's T-scores on MMPI-A measures of overreporting (F = 52, F_1 = 52, F_2 = 52) and his T-scores on the MMPI-A-RF scale related to overreporting (*F-r* = 48) are well within normal limits, and Richard's T-scores on MMPI-A measures of underreporting of symptomatology (*L* = 42 and *K* = 38) and MMPI-A-RF scales of underreporting (*L-r* = 44 and *K-r* = 39) are also well within normal limits.

In summary, the Validity scale findings from the MMPI-A and MMPI-A-RF indicate a reliable and accurate response pattern. Richard appears to neither be denying problems nor claiming an excessive number of unusual symptoms. His relatively low *K* scale scores on both instruments suggest that he is offering a frank self-appraisal, possibly presenting a more negative picture than may be warranted. His test results from both instruments appear to be subject to valid and meaningful interpretation.

Analysis of MMPI-A Findings

This adolescent's MMPI-A Basic Clinical Scale profile produced the two highest elevations on scales *D* (T = 79) and *Si* (T = 72). Approximately 3% of boys in clinical treatment programs produce clinical scale profiles with the *2-0* codetype. As noted in Chapter 5, adolescents who produce this MMPI-A clinical profile present with a high degree of psychological distress including feelings of depression, inferiority, anxiety, and social introversion and withdrawal. Many show strong evidence of social ineptitude or a general lack of age-appropriate social skills. An examination of Richard's Basic Clinical scale profile elevations indicates that his *2-0* profile was not well defined in that his second highest profile (*Si*) is only 2 T-score points higher than his T-score of 70 on the *Pd* scale (his third-highest elevation). This limited definition suggests that this two-point codetype profile may not be stable for Richard, and that some shifting among the most prominent scale elevations in this profile may occur if he were retested over a relatively short period. In particular, it is also important to consider the implications of Richard's elevation on the *Pd* scale (T = 70) and on the *Pt* scale (T = 69). The *Pd* scale elevation suggests that Richard may be considerably more rebellious, defiant, and impulsive than typically shown by adolescents with a *2-0* codetype, and his elevation on scale *Pt* indicates that Richard be described as not only depressed, but also anxious, tense, self-critical, and marked by strong feelings of inadequacy and inferiority. Finally, in terms of Richard's Basic Clinical scale profile, the relatively marked elevations on both *D* and *Pt* suggest that Richard

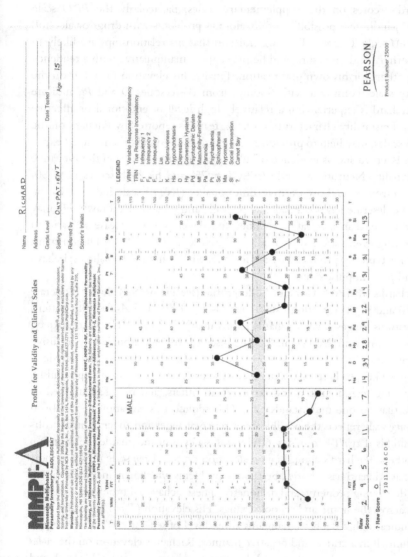

FIGURE 8.1 MMPI-A Profile for Scales for Clinical Case Example 1 (Richard).

Source: Reproduced with the permission of the University of Minnesota Press. All rights reserved. "Minnesota Multiphasic Personality Inventory®-Adolescent" and "MMPI®-A" are trademarks owned by the University of Minnesota.

experiences significant emotional distress which may serve as an important motivating factor for this adolescent in terms of increasing his willingness to participate actively in the psychotherapy process.

Figure 8.2 shows Richard's Supplementary and PSY-5 scale profile. Richard's scores on the Supplementary scales, particularly the *PRO* scale (T = 67) indicate a possibility of developing problems with drugs or alcohol. His *IMM* scale T-score (T = 70) indicates that his relationships are likely to be superficial and immature, and he may appear manipulative with a tendency to use others for his own gratification. Finally, his elevation (T = 69) on the Anxiety scale, consistent with findings from Basic scales *D* and *Pt*, indicate that Richard is experiencing a relatively high level of emotional or affective distress. Personality characteristics, that is, features reported by Richard on the PSY-5 scales, may help to provide a context to understand his emotional experience. Richard shows evidence of substantial negative affect on the Negative Emotionality/Neuroticism scale (*NEGE* = 75) and his high scores (T = 80) on the Introversion/Low Positive Emotionality (*INTR*) scale indicate that he might be described as pessimistic, anhedonic, and socially withdrawn. He may view the world in a negative manner and develop a worst case scenario in interpreting events around him. His elevated score (T = 71) on Disconstraint (*DISC*) is typically produced by adolescents who exhibit externalizing behaviors and poor impulse control.

Richard's MMPI-A Content Scale profile (see Figure 8.3) shows moderate (T ≥ 70 and < 80) elevations on *A-anx*, *A-obs*, *A-dep*, and *A-aln*. This pattern of elevations suggests that Richard reports many symptoms related to anxiety, tension, worry, and depression. He may also report being troubled by intrusive thoughts and disturbed by reoccurring worries or ruminations. His decision-making is likely to be problematic and he approaches decisions in a pessimistic manner. He feels alienated and distant from others, and may feel unliked or believe that no one understands him. This adolescent's elevation (T = 64) on the *A-ang* scale reflects the possible occurrence of anger and anger control problems and his *A-cyn* T-score (T = 60) indicates a cynical and guarded relationship with others. Richard's clinical range elevation on the *A-con* scale (T = 68) indicates that Richard has reported behavioral problems which may include stealing, lying, destroying property, and dishonesty. These behavioral problems are likely to cut across the home and school settings. His elevation (T = 79) on the *A-lse* scale indicates that Richard maintains a low level of self-esteem and is likely to view himself in a critical and negative manner. Richard's elevation on the *A-las* scale (T = 69) is similar to that of adolescents who have few, or no, life goals and his *A-sod* scale (T= 78) indicates that he might be described as an introverted individual who has difficulty meeting and interacting with others, and is shy, emotionally distant, and uncomfortable in social situations. Richard is unlikely to participate in social activities at school and might be described as socially isolated. His striking elevation on the *A-sch* scale (T = 91) strongly suggests that

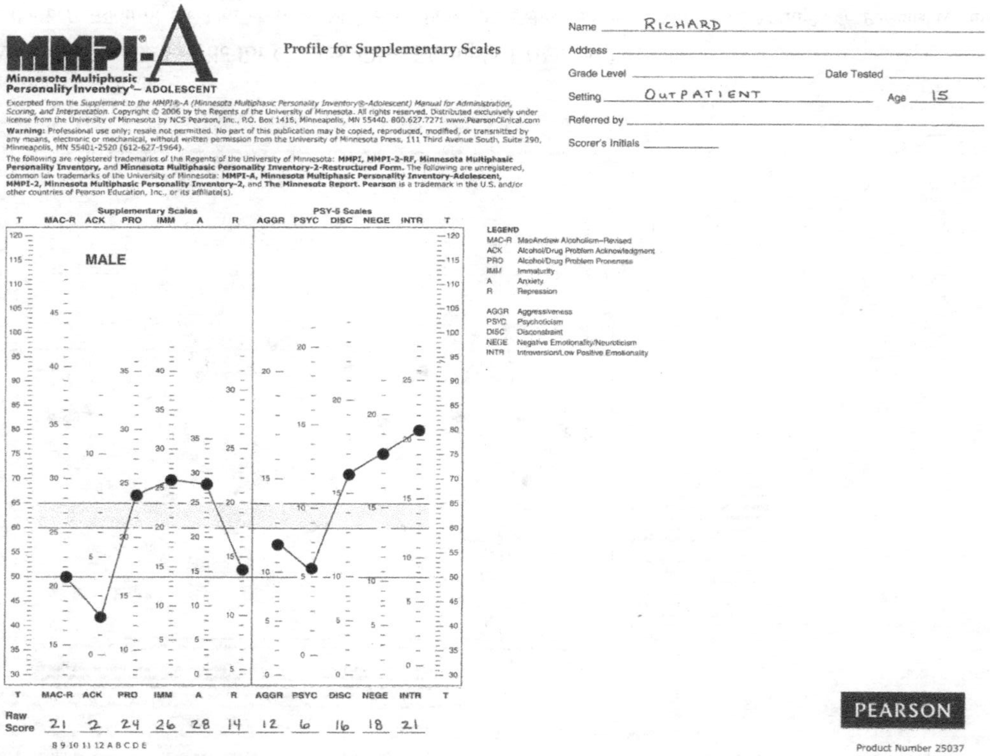

FIGURE 8.2 MMPI-A Supplementary Scale and PSY-5 Scale Profile for Clinical Case Example 1 (Richard).

Source: Reproduced with the permission of the University of Minnesota Press. All rights reserved. "Minnesota Multiphasic Personality Inventory®–Adolescent" and "MMPI®–A" are trademarks owned by the University of Minnesota.

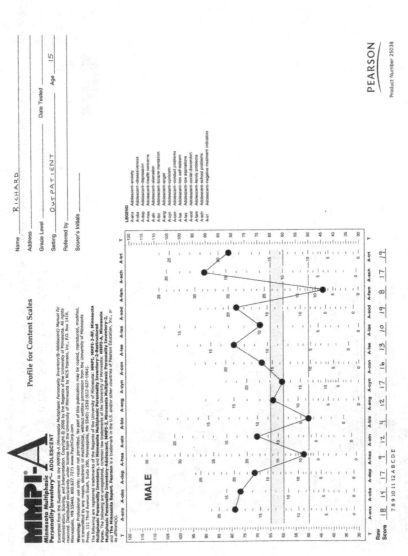

FIGURE 8.3 MMPI-A Content Scale Profile for Clinical Case Example 1 (Richard).

Source: Reproduced with the permission of the University of Minnesota Press. All rights reserved. "Minnesota Multiphasic Personality Inventory®–Adolescent" and "MMPI®-A" are trademarks owned by the University of Minnesota.

Richard has numerous difficulties in the school environment, probably including poor academic performance as well as behavioral problems in the classroom. He may have a history of truancy or school suspensions, and maintains very negative attitudes about school and has few goals or objectives related to his education. Finally, Richard's elevation on the A-trt scale (T = 81) is consistent with the view that Richard may be pessimistic concerning his ability to change, or cynical regarding the value of engaging in psychotherapy.

In summary, the MMPI-A profile produced by Richard is consistent with diagnoses related to depression combined with externalizing behaviors and/or conduct-disordered features. His likely history of academic underachievement and behavioral problems in the classroom indicates a need for assessment of possible academic skill deficits and/or learning disabilities. Further, his elevation on the *PRO* scales suggests the need for further evaluation for possible drug or alcohol problems.

Analysis of MMPI-A-RF Findings

Richard's MMPI-A-RF results appear in Figures 8.4 through 8.8. Substantive scale interpretation begins with a review of scores from the Higher-Order (H-O) scales (Figure 8.5). In Richard's case, scores show a clinical range elevation (T = 77) on the *EID* scale indicating that this adolescent is likely to experience emotional distress and dysfunction, including internalizing symptoms and problems. As discussed in Chapter 7, adolescents who produce T-score elevations equal to or greater than 75 on the *EID* scale typically endorse a broad range of symptoms associated with demoralization, low positive emotions, and negative emotional experiences. Their emotional distress frequently includes anxiety, unhappiness, depression, and hopelessness.

The specific manifestations of Richard's emotional/internalizing dysfunction scale elevations are indicated by a review of his elevated scale scores on related RC (Figure 8.5), SP (Figure 8.6 and 8.7), and PSY-5 (Figure 8.8) scales that are associated with this area of dysfunction (see Table 8.3). Among the RC scales, this adolescent produced a clinical range elevation (T = 70) on the *RCd* scale, indicative of considerable emotional distress. The nature of this distress may be further evaluated by considering his elevated scores on *HLP*, *SFD*, and *NFC* scales. A review of these scores in Figure 8.6 shows that all three of these SP scales are clinically elevated and indicate that this adolescent has feelings of hopelessness and helplessness (*HLP*, T = 67), reports self-doubts and poor self-esteem (*SFD*, T = 74), and indecisive and ineffective in coping with challenges or difficulties (*NFC*, T = 74).

In addition to the clinical range elevation in *RCd* noted above, Richard also produced elevated scores on *RC2* (T = 69) and *RC7* (T = 69). This adolescent's elevation on *RC2* is consistent with a lack of positive emotional

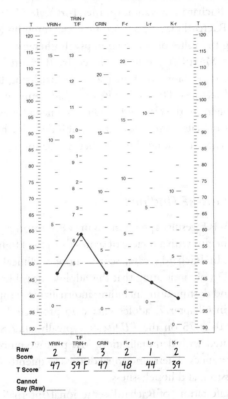

Excerpted from the *MMPI-A-RF™ (Minnesota Multiphasic Personality Inventory-Adolescent-Restructured Form™) Administration, Scoring, Interpretation, and Technical Manual.* Copyright © 2016 by the Regents of the University of Minnesota. All rights reserved. Distributed exclusively under license from the University of Minnesota by NCS Pearson, Inc., P.O. Box 1416, Minneapolis, MN 55440. 800.627.7271 www.PearsonClinical.com

Warning: Professional use only; resale not permitted. No part of this publication may be copied, reproduced, modified, or transmitted by any means, electronic or mechanical, without written permission from the University of Minnesota Press, 111 Third Avenue South, Suite 290, Minneapolis, MN 55401-2520 (612-627-1964).

The following are registered trademarks of the Regents of the University of Minnesota: **MMPI, MMPI-2-RF, Minnesota Multiphasic Personality Inventory,** and **Minnesota Multiphasic Personality Inventory-2-Restructured Form.** The following are unregistered, common law trademarks of the University of Minnesota: **MMPI-A, Minnesota Multiphasic Personality Inventory-Adolescent, MMPI-A-RF, Minnesota Multiphasic Personality Inventory-Adolescent-Restructured Form, MMPI-2, Minnesota Multiphasic Personality Inventory-2,** and **The Minnesota Report. Pearson** is a trademark, in the US and/or other countries, of Pearson Education, Inc., or its affiliate(s).

1 2 3 4 5 6 7 8 9 10 11 12 A B C D E   Product Number 25093

FIGURE 8.4   MMPI-A-RF Validity Scale Profile for Clinical Case Example 1 (Richard).

Source: Reproduced with the permission of the University of Minnesota Press. All rights reserved. "Minnesota Multiphasic Personality Inventory®-Adolescent-Restructured Form" and "MMPI®-A-RF" are trademarks owned by the University of Minnesota.

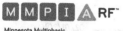

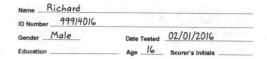

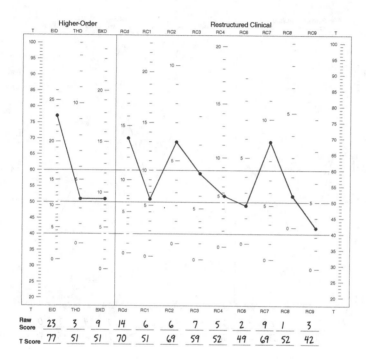

FIGURE 8.5   MMPI-A-RF Higher-Order (*H-O*) and Restructured Clinical (*RC*) Scale Profile for Clinical Case Example 1 (Richard).

Source: Adapted from the MMPI-A-RF Administration, Scoring, Interpretation and Technical Manual by Archer et al. Copyright © 2016 by the Regents of the University of Minnesota. Reproduced with the permission of the University of Minnesota Press. All rights reserved. "Minnesota Multiphasic Personality Inventory" and "MMPI" are trademarks owned by the Regents of the University of Minnesota.

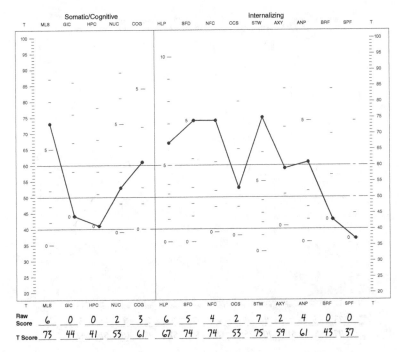

MMPI-A-RF T scores are nongendered.

Somatic/Cognitive Scales		Internalizing Scales			
MLS	Malaise	HLP	Helplessness/Hopelessness	AXY	Anxiety
GIC	Gastrointestinal Complaints	SFD	Self-Doubt	ANP	Anger Proneness
HPC	Head Pain Complaints	NFC	Inefficacy	BRF	Behavior-Restricting Fears
NUC	Neurological Complaints	OCS	Obsessions/Compulsions	SPF	Specific Fears
COG	Cognitive Complaints	STW	Stress/Worry		

FIGURE 8.6 MMPI-A-RF Somatic/Cognitive and Internalizing Scale Profile for Clinical Case Example 1 (Richard).

Source: Adapted from the MMPI-A-RF Administration, Scoring, Interpretation and Technical Manual by Archer et al. Copyright © 2016 by the Regents of the University of Minnesota. Reproduced with the permission of the University of Minnesota Press. All rights reserved. "Minnesota Multiphasic Personality Inventory" and "MMPI" are trademarks owned by the Regents of the University of Minnesota.

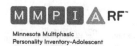

Name   _Richard_

ID Number _99914016_

Gender   _Male_   Date Tested   _02/01/2016_

Minnesota Multiphasic
Personality Inventory-Adolescent
Restructured Form™

Education _____   Age _16_   Scorer's Initials _____

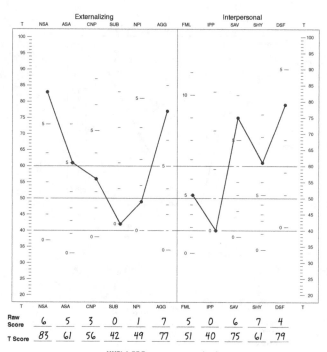

	NSA	ASA	CNP	SUB	NPI	AGG	FML	IPP	SAV	SHY	DSF
Raw Score	6	5	3	0	1	7	5	0	6	7	4
T Score	83	61	56	42	49	77	51	40	75	61	79

MMPI-A-RF T scores are nongendered.

Externalizing Scales		Interpersonal Scales	
NSA	Negative School Attitudes	FML	Family Problems
ASA	Antisocial Attitudes	IPP	Interpersonal Passivity
CNP	Conduct Problems	SAV	Social Avoidance
SUB	Substance Abuse	SHY	Shyness
NPI	Negative Peer Influence	DSF	Disaffiliativeness
AGG	Aggression		

FIGURE 8.7   MMPI-A-RF Externalizing and Interpersonal Scale Profile for Clinical Case Example 1 (Richard).

Source: Adapted from the MMPI-A-RF Administration, Scoring, Interpretation and Technical Manual by Archer et al. Copyright © 2016 by the Regents of the University of Minnesota. Reproduced with the permission of the University of Minnesota Press. All rights reserved. "Minnesota Multiphasic Personality Inventory" and "MMPI" are trademarks owned by the Regents of the University of Minnesota.

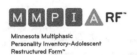

Name	Richard
ID Number	99914016
Gender	Male
Date Tested	02/01/2016
Education	
Age	16
Scorer's Initials	

Minnesota Multiphasic
Personality Inventory–Adolescent
Restructured Form™

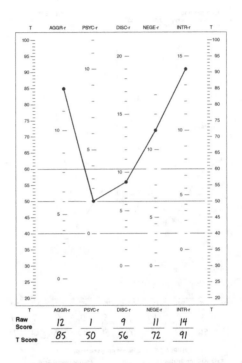

	AGGR-r	PSYC-r	DISC-r	NEGE-r	INTR-r
Raw Score	12	1	9	11	14
T Score	85	50	56	72	91

MMPI-A-RF T scores are nongendered.

AGGR-r Aggressiveness-Revised
PSYC-r Psychoticism-Revised
DISC-r Discontraint-Revised

NEGE-r Negative Emotionality/Neuroticism-Revised
INTR-r Introversion/Low Positive Emotionality-Revised

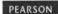

FIGURE 8.8 MMPI-A-RF Personality Psychopathology-Five (*PSY-5*) Profile for Clinical Case Example 1 (Richard).

Source: Adapted from the MMPI-A-RF Administration, Scoring, Interpretation and Technical Manual by Archer et al. Copyright © 2016 by the Regents of the University of Minnesota. Reproduced with the permission of the University of Minnesota Press. All rights reserved. "Minnesota Multiphasic Personality Inventory" and "MMPI" are trademarks owned by the Regents of the University of Minnesota.

experiences and a markedly elevated (T = 91) score on the PSY-5 *INTR-r* scale (see Figure 8.8), underscoring his report of a lack of positive emotional experiences and his avoidance of social situations. Empirical correlates associated with elevations on this latter scale include fatigue and low energy, depression, and anxiety. Richard's elevation (T = 69) on *RC7* can be refined by consideration of his scores on the SP scales *STW, ANX, ANP, BRF, SPF, OCS*, and the PSY-5 scale *NEGE-r*. Among the SP scales, Richard produced clinical range elevations on the Stress/Worry scale (T = 75) and on the *Anger Proneness* Scale (T = 61), indicating that Richard reports an above-average amount of stress and worry (including anxiety, sleeplessness, and a variety of internalizing symptoms) combined with a substantial degree of irritability and anger-proneness. His elevated scale on the *NEGE-r* PSY-5 scale (T = 72) is consistent with the report of strong negative emotional experiences including anxiety, stress, dread, and anger.

Richard's score on the Thought Dysfunction (*THD*) scale is well within normal limits, as are his scores on all related scales including *RC6* (T = 49), *RC8* (T = 52), and the PSY-5 *PSYC-r* scale (T = 50). Further, Richard's score on the Behavioral Dysfunction (*BXD*) scale is within normal limits (T = 51), as are Richard's scores on related RC scales (*RC4* and *RC9*), and among all of the related Externalizing scales with the exception of his clinical range elevations on the Negative School Attitude (*NSA*) scale (T = 83) and on the *AGG* scale (T = 77). Further, Richard also produced a clinical range elevation (T = 85) on the *AGGR-r* PSY-5 scale related to behavioral dysfunction. These elevations underscore Richard's substantial problems in the school environment as well as his problems with anger and use of aggression as a means of obtaining objectives and controlling others.

The *Somatic/Cognitive* scores are considered next in Table 8.3 (and shown in Figure 8.6) and display an elevated score (T = 73) on the *MLS* scale. This elevation indicates that Richard reports a generalized sense of poor physical health, including feelings of tiredness and fatigue. Richard also produced a clinical range elevation (T = 61) on the *COG* scale, a measure of cognitive complaints including memory problems, difficulties in concentration, and cognitive confusion. In contrast, Richard did not produce elevations on *Somatic/Cognitive* scales related to Gastrointestinal Complaints (*GIC*), Head Pain Complaints (*HPC*), or Neurological Complaints (*NUC*). On six MMPI-A-RF scales related to interpersonal functioning (*FML, RC3, IPP, SAV, SHY*, and *DSF*), Richard produced elevated scores on *DSF* (T = 79), *SAV* (T = 75), and *SHY* (T = 61). Richard's elevations on Disaffiliativeness (*DSF*) indicates that he reports disliking people and is likely to be socially introverted and socially withdrawn. Richard's elevation on the *SAV* scale (T = 75) is associated with adolescents who report the avoidance of social events and situations, including parties and crowds. Finally, Richard's elevation on the Shyness scale (*SHY*) underscores a view of Richard as socially anxious, and easily embarrassed.

Following the interpretation of the Substantive scales, the interpretive process outlined in Table 8.3 proceeds to diagnostic and treatment considerations. The MMPI-A-RF test results reviewed for Richard indicate a number of possible diagnoses for consideration. Richard should be further evaluated for the possibility of a significant Mood Disorder diagnosis, particularly those related to depression. Richard's overall high level of emotional distress may serve as an important motivation for him to actively engage in the treatment process. On the other hand, his relatively low level of positive emotions and his social disengagement and withdrawal may serve as barriers that diminish his ability or willingness to become actively involved in the treatment effort. Richard's degree of social disengagement may actively impede his ability to form a therapeutic relationship. Further, the current test findings would highlight the area of aggression and anger management as a potentially important treatment area for this adolescent. Finally, test results underscore the importance of evaluating Richard for possible learning disabilities or educational deficits which may contribute to his negative school attitudes as reflected in his elevation on the *NSA* scale.

Case Example Number 2: Joe (Forensic Setting)
Background and Validity Scale Information

Joe is a 16-year-old male adolescent from a lower socioeconomic status (SES) White family in a large urban area who was referred for an evaluation resulting from his forced entry, with two peers, into a public high school and associated vandalism and destruction of property. This adolescent was subsequently arrested, placed in detention, and released to the custody of his family pending his hearing. Following his conviction, this adolescent was referred by a Juvenile and Domestic Relations District Court for a psychological evaluation prior to sentencing. This teenager has a history of two prior school suspensions for fighting and an educational record which is marked by behavioral problems and academic underachievement.

The MMPI-A and MMPI-A-RF results for Joe indicate a consistent and interpretable test protocol. Joe did not omit any item responses. Joe's scores on MMPI-A measures of consistency (*VRIN* and *TRIN*), and MMPI-A-RF measures of consistency (*VRIN-r*, *TRIN-R* and *CRIN*) are consistently within normal limits or expectations. Joe's responses on measures of underreporting on the MMPI-A (*L* and *K*) and the MMPI-A-RF (*L-r* and *K-r*) are all consistently below 50, and Joe's scores on measures of overreporting (scale *F* and scale *F-r*, respectively) are well below critical levels. Interestingly, the 21 T-score difference between F_1 and F_2 suggests that Joe reported a higher frequency of unusual psychological symptoms in the first part of the MMPI-A test booklet, but these results do not raise a level of concern that would result in invalidating the test protocol. Both F_1 and F_2 T-scores are well below the T ≥ 90 cutoff recommended for identifying invalid profiles. Overall, this MMPI-A and MMPI-A-RF response pattern reflects a consistent and accurate self-report compatible with meaningful interpretation.

Analysis of MMPI-A Findings

Joe's MMPI-A Basic Scale profile (see Figure 8.9) may be classified as a 4-9 codetype. Scales *Pd* and *Ma* are elevated more frequently among adolescents than adults, and this 4-9 codetype is found in approximately 7% to 10% of adolescents in clinical settings. The marked elevations on scales *Pd* (T = 83) and *Ma* (T = 81) indicate this is a very well-defined two-point codetype with the third-highest clinical scale elevation found in a T-score of 63 on Scale *Pa*. Teenagers who obtain this 4-9 profile typically display a marked disregard for social standards and are likely to manifest problems related to acting out and impulsivity. They are described as egocentric, self-indulgent, and selfish and are often unwilling to accept responsibility for their behaviors. In social situations, these adolescents often appear extroverted, a hypothesis supported by Joe's T-score of 38 on the *Si* scale. While these adolescents typically make a good first impression, their egocentric and demanding interpersonal style usually results in chronic difficulties in establishing close and enduring friendships. They are usually referred for treatment because of defiance, disobedience, provocative behaviors, and school truancy. In youth correctional settings, their impulsive and disobedient behaviors are likely to evoke conflicts with staff and other residents. Further, their antisocial and self-indulgent characteristics are likely to decrease their motivation to engage in treatment or rehabilitation efforts, an impression further supported by Joe's relatively low scores on scales *D* (T = 51) and *Pt* (T = 60) reflecting relatively little emotional distress. Adolescents who produce the 4-9 codetype often receive diagnoses related to Conduct Disorder and their primary defense mechanisms typically consist of acting out. The prognosis for adolescents with this codetype is often seen as inversely related to their age at the time that therapy or rehabilitation efforts are undertaken.

Results from Joe's MMPI-A Supplementary and PSY-5 scales (see Figure 8.10) are involved in the second step of the MMPI-A interpretation as illustrated in Table 8.3. Joe's Supplementary scale findings emphasize likely problems in the areas of substance abuse as reflected in a T-score of 70 on the *MAC-R* scale and a T-score of 78 on the *PRO* scale. Further, Joe's T-score of 67 on the *IMM* scale suggests that Joe may be described as an easily frustrated adolescent who is impatience, defiant, and exploitive in interpersonal relationships. In contrast, Joe displays a relatively low level of emotional distress on the Anxiety (*A*) scale (T = 52). Joe's lack of internalizing defenses, such as repression, is reflected in his low T-score value (40) on the *R* scale. Joe's scores on the PSY-5 scales strongly emphasize his poor impulse control and use of externalizing behaviors (*DISC* = 83), and his use of aggression as a method of accomplishing goals or

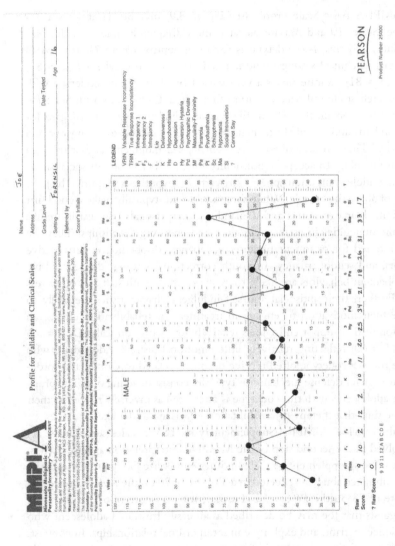

FIGURE 8.9 MMPI-A Profile for Basic Scales for Clinical Case Example 2 (Joe).

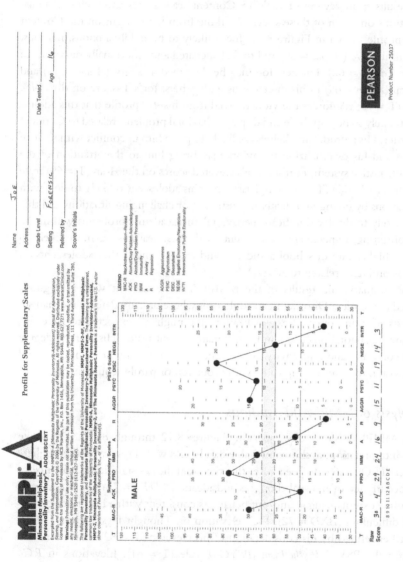

FIGURE 8.10 MMPI-A Supplementary Scale and PSY-5 Scale Profile for Clinical Case Example 2 (Joe).

objectives ($AGGR = 70$). The PSY-5 results also show, to a lesser extent, his tendency to exhibit behaviors perceived as odd or unusual by others ($PSYC = 67$) and to have mild clinical range experiences of some negative emotions such as worry or apprehension ($NEGE = 60$).

Results from review of Joe's 15 Content scale scores show clinical range elevations on seven of these scales. Working from left to right on the Content scale profile shown in Figure 8.11, Joe is likely to be mildly anxious, nervous, and ruminative (A-$anx = 69$) and to feel alienated and emotionally distant from others (A-$aln = 62$). Further, Joe may be described as angry (A-$ang = 74$) and cynical (A-$cyn = 69$) in his interactions with others. Joe's T-score on the A-con scale (T = 75) reinforces the view derived from his 4-9 profile that this adolescent is likely to be impulsive and display behavioral problems related to Conduct Disorder. His attitudes and beliefs are likely to place him in conflict with societal norms and his externalizing behaviors may bring him to the attention of the juvenile justice system. Further, Joe's elevated scores on the A-las (T = 69) scale and the A-sch scale (T = 65) emphasize that this adolescent is likely to deal with frustrations by giving up quickly in frustrating or challenging situations and that he is likely to display significant behavioral and academic problems within the school setting, respectively. Adolescents with these features are more likely to have a higher rate of school avoidance and truancy than other adolescents, as well as problems related to ADHD.

In summary, the results of the MMPI-A are consistent with a diagnosis related to Conduct Disorder in an adolescent whose primary defense mechanism consists of acting out and externalization. Joe might be expected to have significant behavioral problems and anger management issues. His marked degree of disconstraint and impulsivity indicate the need for consistent monitoring and supervision to ensure compliance with probation or parole requirements.

Analysis of MMPI-A-RF Findings

Joe's MMPI-A-RF results appear in Figures 8.12 through 8.16. Substantive scale interpretation, as shown in Table 8.3, begins with a review of the Higher-Order (H-O) scales. In Joe's case, this review indicates significant evidence of the occurrence of unusual thoughts and ideation ($THD = 76$) combined with extensive externalizing acting-out behaviors consistent with a history of behavioral difficulties ($BXD = 72$). Joe's elevation on Thought Dysfunction (THD) is further refined by his consideration of his elevated (T = 82) scores on $RC6$ and on the PSY-5 *Psychoticism* ($PSYC$-r) scale (T = 61). Elevations in $RC6$ has been found for adolescents who report significant persecutory ideas associated with external correlates including aggressiveness, assaultiveness, fighting, and a history of school suspension. These results underscore Joe's tendency to perceive the world around him in an idiosyncratic manner with particular emphasis on a sense of being treated unfairly and unkindly by others, potentially

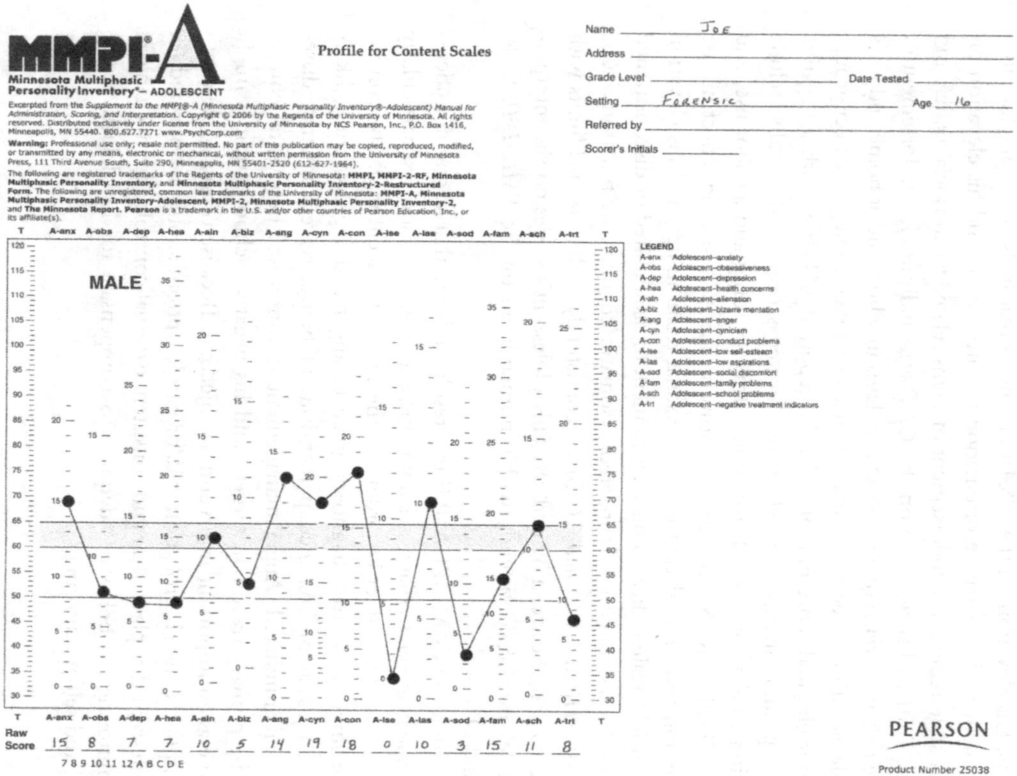

FIGURE 8.11 MMPI-A Content Scale Profile for Clinical Case Example 2 (Joe).

Source: Reproduced with the permission of the University of Minnesota Press. All rights reserved. "Minnesota Multiphasic Personality Inventory®-Adolescent" and "MMPI®-A" are trademarks owned by the University of Minnesota.

including persecutory and even delusional beliefs. Joe's clinical range elevation on the Behavioral/Externalizing (*BXD*) Higher-Order scale is also reflected in clinically significant elevations on *RC4* (T = 71), Externalizing scales *NSA* (T = 73), *ASA* (T = 73), *CNP* (T = 71), *NPI* (T = 62), *AGG* (T = 68), and PSY-5 scales *AGGR-r* (T = 78) and *DISC-r* (T = 73). This adolescent's *RC4* elevation indicates that Joe reported a significant history of conduct-disordered behaviors. His elevation on the *NSA* scale shows that Joe's beliefs and attitudes are consistent with a negative orientation toward school, and his elevation on the *ASA* scale reflects his endorsement of items related to antisocial beliefs and attitudes. Further, his elevation on the *CNP* scale indicates his endorsement of multiple behaviors reflecting conduct problems in school and at home and Joe's *NPI* scale elevation reflects his tendency to associate with a negative peer group. This latter elevated score indicates that he reported affiliation with a negative peer group, and empirical correlates of elevated scores on this scale include oppositional behavior, school suspension, truancy, drug and alcohol use, and fighting. Finally, his PSY-5 scale elevations on the *AGG-r* scale reflect his use of aggression and intimidation in interpersonal relationships, and his elevation on the *DISC-r* scale indicated his endorsement of disinhibited or disconstrained behaviors. Joe's scores on scales related to somatic/cognitive dysfunction (*RC1, MLS, GIC, HPC, NUC, and COG*) are consistently within normal limits with T-scores ranging between 39 and 58. This adolescent's scores on the interpersonal scales are also consistently within normal limits on the *FML, IPP, SAV, SHY,* and *DSF* scales.

This adolescent's MMPI-A-RF test results indicate that strong consideration should be given to diagnoses involving externalizing disorders, particularly various forms of Conduct Disorder. Further, this adolescent might be considered for impulse control diagnoses given to anger and aggressiveness, likely triggered by real or imagined perceptions of being treated unfairly, disrespected, or humiliated. Anger management and increased behavioral control would be primary treatment targets, and his negative school attitudes might also serve as an important intervention objective. Because of this adolescent's poor impulse control, probation and/or parole options should be pursued for this adolescent that place clear and consistent external controls and mechanisms for monitoring his behavior adequate to compensate for his defective self-control and self-monitoring.

Clinical Case Example 3: Emily (Inpatient Clinical Setting)

Background and Validity Scale Information:

Emily is a 15-year-old, White, female adolescent from a middle-class family who was evaluated shortly after admission to an adolescent psychiatric inpatient unit. Emily was hospitalized following rapidly increasing problems in concentration

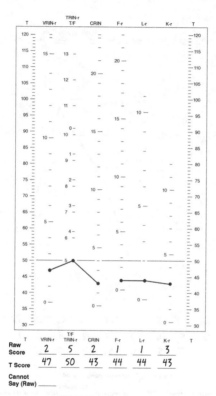

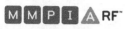

MMPI-A-RF T scores are nongendered.

VRIN-r   Variable Response Inconsistency   F-r   Infrequent Responses
TRIN-r   True Response Inconsistency   L-r   Uncommon Virtues
CRIN   Combined Response Inconsistency   K-r   Adjustment Validity

FIGURE 8.12   MMPI-A-RF Validity Scale Profile for Clinical Case Example 2 (Joe).

Source: Adapted from the MMPI-A-RF Administration, Scoring, Interpretation and Technical Manual by Archer et al. Copyright © 2016 by the Regents of the University of Minnesota. Reproduced with the permission of the University of Minnesota Press. All rights reserved. "Minnesota Multiphasic Personality Inventory" and "MMPI" are trademarks owned by the Regents of the University of Minnesota.

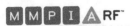

Minnesota Multiphasic
Personality Inventory-Adolescent
Restructured Form™

Name ___Joe___

ID Number ___99914394___

Gender ___Male___   Date Tested ___02/01/2016___

Education _____   Age ___16___   Scorer's Initials _____

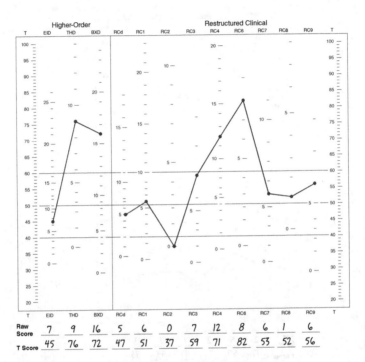

MMPI-A-RF T scores are nongendered.

	H-O Scales		RC Scales	
EID	Emotional/Internalizing Dysfunction	RCd	Demoralization	RC6	Ideas of Persecution
THD	Thought Dysfunction	RC1	Somatic Complaints	RC7	Dysfunctional Negative Emotions
BXD	Behavioral/Externalizing Dysfunction	RC2	Low Positive Emotions	RC8	Aberrant Experiences
		RC3	Cynicism	RC9	Hypomanic Activation
		RC4	Antisocial Behavior		

FIGURE 8.13   MMPI-A-RF Higher-Order (*H-O*) and Restructured Clinical (*RC*) Scale Profile for Clinical Case Example 2 (Joe).

Source: Adapted from the MMPI-A-RF Administration, Scoring, Interpretation and Technical Manual by Archer et al. Copyright © 2016 by the Regents of the University of Minnesota. Reproduced with the permission of the University of Minnesota Press. All rights reserved. "Minnesota Multiphasic Personality Inventory" and "MMPI" are trademarks owned by the Regents of the University of Minnesota.

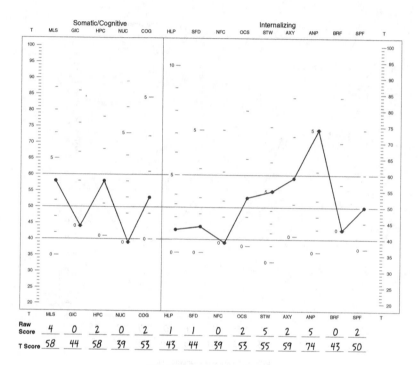

	MLS	GIC	HPC	NUC	COG	HLP	SFD	NFC	OCS	STW	AXY	ANP	BRF	SPF
Raw Score	4	0	2	0	2	1	1	0	2	5	2	5	0	2
T Score	58	44	58	39	53	43	44	39	53	55	59	74	43	50

MMPI-A-RF T scores are nongendered.

Somatic/Cognitive Scales
MLS Malaise
GIC Gastrointestinal Complaints
HPC Head Pain Complaints
NUC Neurological Complaints
COG Cognitive Complaints

Internalizing Scales
HLP Helplessness/Hopelessness
SFD Self-Doubt
NFC Inefficacy
OCS Obsessions/Compulsions
STW Stress/Worry

AXY Anxiety
ANP Anger Proneness
BRF Behavior-Restricting Fears
SPF Specific Fears

FIGURE 8.14 MMPI-A-RF Somatic/Cognitive and Internalizing Scale Profile for Clinical Case Example 2 (Joe).

Source: Adapted from the MMPI-A-RF Administration, Scoring, Interpretation and Technical Manual by Archer et al. Copyright © 2016 by the Regents of the University of Minnesota. Reproduced with the permission of the University of Minnesota Press. All rights reserved. "Minnesota Multiphasic Personality Inventory" and "MMPI" are trademarks owned by the Regents of the University of Minnesota.

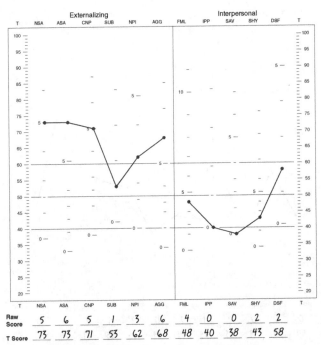

FIGURE 8.15   MMPI-A-RF Externalizing and Interpersonal Scale Profile for Clinical Case Example 2 (Joe).

Source: Adapted from the MMPI-A-RF Administration, Scoring, Interpretation and Technical Manual by Archer et al. Copyright © 2016 by the Regents of the University of Minnesota. Reproduced with the permission of the University of Minnesota Press. All rights reserved. "Minnesota Multiphasic Personality Inventory" and "MMPI" are trademarks owned by the Regents of the University of Minnesota.

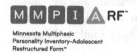

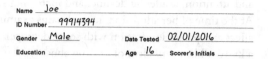

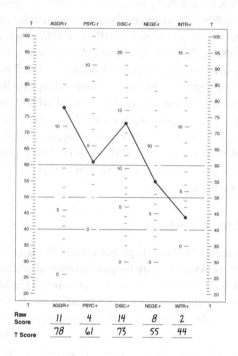

FIGURE 8.16 MMPI-A-RF Personality Psychopathology-Five (*PSY-5*) Profile for Clinical Case Example 2 (Joe).

Source: Adapted from the MMPI-A-RF Manual for Administration, Scoring, and Interpretation by Archer, et al. Copyright © 2016 by the Regents of the University of Minnesota. Reproduced with the permission of the University of Minnesota Press. All rights reserved. "Minnesota Multiphasic Personality Inventory" and "MMPI" are trademarks owned by the Regents of the University of Minnesota.

and attention, academic decline, and increasing social isolation and withdrawal. At the time of her admission, mental status examination revealed intensely angry affect and paranoid ideation with some delusional thinking. Emily did not have a known history of alcohol or drug abuse.

The results of Emily's MMPI-A and MMPI-A-RF Validity scale profiles (shown in Figures 8.17 and 8.20) indicate that Emily has produced valid and interpretable test findings. Emily omitted no test responses on either instrument. Her scores on measures of consistency (*VRIN* and *TRIN* on the MMPI-A, and *VRIN-r*, *TRIN-r* and *CRIN* on the MMPI-A-RF) were consistently within normal limits between T-score values of 40 and 60, and well below the recommended ranges associated with inconsistent responding on either test. Emily's scores on measures of defensiveness on both the MMPI-A and MMPI-A-RF are quite low (T ≤ 40), suggesting a relatively candid and open reporting style. Finally, on measures of overreporting of symptomatology (Scale *F* on the MMPI-A and Scale *F-r* on the MMPI-A-RF), Emily produced moderate clinical range elevations consistent with the view that Emily is experiencing significant psychopathology.

Analysis of MMPI-A Findings

Emily's MMPI-A Basic Clinical scale profile (shown in Figure 8.17) corresponds to a *4-6/6-4* codetype which is fairly frequent among adolescents, and occurs in roughly 5% of adolescent assessments in clinical settings. Emily displays a well-defined two-point codetype with an 11-point difference between her T-score elevations of 82 on scales *Pd* and *Pa*, and her next highest elevation (T = 71) on Scale *Sc*. Teenagers with the *4-6/6-4* codetype are often described as angry, resentful, and argumentative. They are generally suspicious and distrustful of the motives of others and characteristically avoid deep emotional attachments. They display little insight into their psychological problems, and their behaviors often result in rejection and anger by others. There are often large discrepancies between the way adolescents with a *4-6/6-4* codetype perceive themselves (frequently very positively) and the way they are described by others. These adolescents are often referred for psychotherapy as a result of repeated conflicts with parents, which may take the form of chronic and tense struggles. The *4-6/6-4* adolescents typically undercontrol their impulses and act without sufficient thought or deliberation. Problems with authority figures may also be present for these teenagers, and they are described as provocative by others. Histories involving drug abuse are relatively frequent among these adolescents. Diagnoses associated with this codetype often include Conduct Disorder or Oppositional-Defiant Disorder. Primary defense mechanisms typically involve denial, projection, rationalization, and acting out. These adolescents characteristically avoid responsibility for their behaviors and are difficult to motivate in psychotherapy and slow to develop a therapeutic relationship. Emily also produced secondary clinical range elevations on scales *Sc*

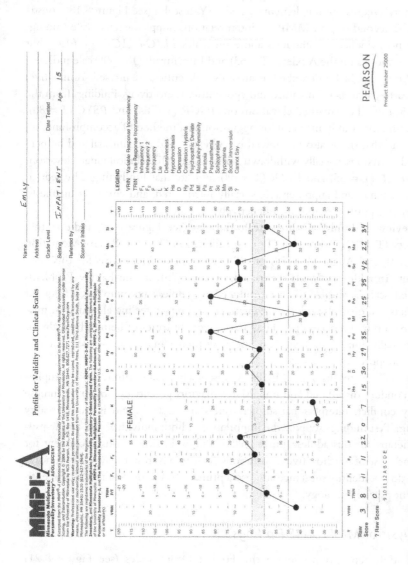

FIGURE 8.17 MMPI-A Profile for Basic Scales for Clinical Case Example 3 (Emily).

Source: Reproduced with the permission of the University of Minnesota Press. All rights reserved. "Minnesota Multiphasic Personality Inventory®-Adolescent" and "MMPI®-A" are trademarks owned by the University of Minnesota.

(T = 71), *Pt* (T = 70), and *D* (T = 67). These elevations indicate, respectively, that Emily may be typically described as disorganized, withdrawn, confused, and alienated (scale *Sc*, and seen by others as anxious, tense, self-critical, and indecisive (*Pt* scale). She also reported feeling depressed and hopeless (scale *D*).

Emily's scores on Supplementary and PSY-5 scales (see Figure 8.18) constitute the second step in MMPI-A interpretation. Supplementary scale findings show no evidence of substance abuse on scales *MAC-r*, *ACK*, or *PRO*, but mild elevations on the Anxiety (T = 63) and Immaturity (T = 60) scale indicates that Emily might be described as anxious, self-critical, depressed, ruminative, and fearful, as well as immature and egocentric, respectively. Findings from the PSY-5 scales show marked elevations on *AGGR* (T = 84) and *PSYC* (T = 86), indicating that Emily may employ aggression as a method of accomplishing her goals and that she is also be viewed by others as odd and unusual and be perceived as anxious, socially withdrawn, and strange. Mild clinical range elevations on *NEGE* (T = 65) and *INTR* (T = 64) indicate that Emily might be seen as anxious, tense, and apprehensive, socially introverted, and currently unable to experience positive emotions, respectively.

Review of Emily's Content scale findings (see Figure 8.19) indicate that Anxiety (T = 81), Depression (T = 76), Alienation (T = 73), Bizarre Mentation (T = 73), and Anger (T = 72) are all significant problem areas for this adolescent. In addition, Emily's elevated T-score (75) on the Family Problems (*A-fam*) scale is similar to that produced by adolescents who have frequent conflicts and quarrels with family members and report feeling alienated or misunderstood by their families. They may report histories of being physically or emotionally abused, and they do not view their families as a source of emotional support or nurturance.

Overall, the results of the MMPI-A present a portrait of Emily which emphasizes conduct-disordered and impulsive behaviors potentially driven by intense family conflict, interpersonal suspiciousness and distrust, and impaired reality testing. Test findings support the importance of both individual and family psychotherapy for this adolescent, as well as the evaluation of this adolescent for potential use of psychoactive medications. Test results from the MMPI-A, however, do not identify substance abuse as a primary component of this adolescent's current psychopathology.

Analysis of MMPI-A-RF Findings

This adolescent's responses to the Higher-Order scales (see Figure 8.21) produced a clinical range (T = 86) elevation on the Thought Dysfunction (*THD*) scale, as well as a clinical range elevation (T = 69) on the Emotional/Internalizing (*EID*) scale. This pattern indicates that Emily is reporting symptoms related to serious aspects of thought dysfunction which may include the presence of delusions and/or hallucinations (i.e., *THD*) *as* well as more

FIGURE 8.18 MMPI-A Supplementary Scale and PSY-5 Scale Profile for Clinical Case Example 3 (Emily).

Source: Reproduced with the permission of the University of Minnesota Press. All rights reserved. "Minnesota Multiphasic Personality Inventory®-Adolescent" and "MMPI®-A" are trademarks owned by the University of Minnesota.

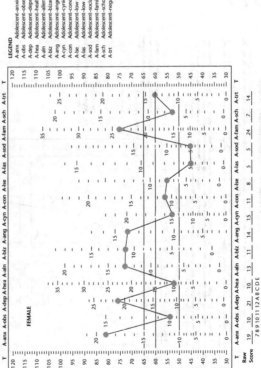

FIGURE 8.19 MMPI-A Content Scale Profile for Clinical Case Example 3 (Emily).

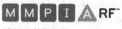

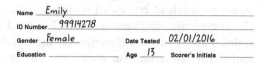

		Name	Emily				
		ID Number	99914278				
		Gender	Female		Date Tested	02/01/2016	
		Education			Age	13	Scorer's Initials

Minnesota Multiphasic
Personality Inventory-Adolescent
Restructured Form™

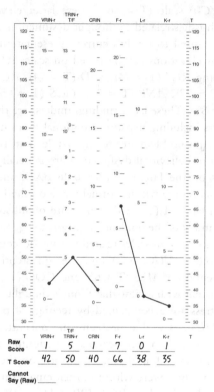

T	VRIN-r	TRIN-r T/F	CRIN	F-r	L-r	K-r
Raw Score	1	5	1	7	0	1
T Score	42	50	40	66	38	35

Cannot Say (Raw) _____

MMPI-A-RF T scores are nongendered.

VRIN-r	Variable Response Inconsistency	F-r	Infrequent Responses
TRIN-r	True Response Inconsistency	L-r	Uncommon Virtues
CRIN	Combined Response Inconsistency	K-r	Adjustment Validity

FIGURE 8.20   MMPI-A-RF Validity Scale Profile for Clinical Case Example 3 (Emily).

Source: Adapted from the MMPI-A-RF Administration, Scoring, Interpretation and Technical Manual by Archer et al. Copyright © 2016 by the Regents of the University of Minnesota. Reproduced with the permission of the University of Minnesota Press. All rights reserved. "Minnesota Multiphasic Personality Inventory" and "MMPI" are trademarks owned by the Regents of the University of Minnesota.

moderate levels of emotional distress and discomfort (i.e., *EID*). Following the interpretive structure shown in Table 8.3 for the MMPI-A Substantive scales, Emily's marked elevation on the *THD* scale is further evaluated by considering elevations on *RC6* (T = 76), *RC8* (T = 86), and the PSY-5 Psychoticism (*PSYC-r*) scale (T = 86). These latter elevations underscore the extent to which issues related to thought dysfunction and impaired reality testing may be central to Emily's current presentation of symptoms. In addition, significant elevations can be noted on scales related to emotional dysfunction including *RCd* (T = 74), *SFD* (T = 74), *RC7* (T = 76), *STW* (T = 75), *AXY* (T = 72), *ANP* (T = 74), *OCS* (T = 65), and the PSY-5 scale *NEGE-r* (T = 83). These latter findings underscore that emotional dysfunction and distress including negative emotional states such as anxiety and anger represent a major problem area for this adolescent. In contrast, Emily's scores on measures of behavioral dysfunction are generally within expected and normal ranges on the Higher-Order scale *BXD*, and RC scales *RC4* and *RC9*. Emily's scores are within normal range on the Externalizing scales with the exception of *ASA* (T = 61), a measure of antisocial attitudes, and *AGG* (T = 77), an index of the tendency to resort to aggression. As shown in Figure 8.22, Emily's scores on scales related to somatic/cognitive dysfunction (*RC1, MLS, GIC, HPC, NUC,* and *COG*) are consistently below a T-score of 60 with the exception of *MLS* (T = 65) and *COG* (T = 72). These latter elevations are consistent with a view that Emily's thought disorder symptoms and emotional distress are accompanied by feelings of poor health, weakness and fatigue (*MLS*), as well as problems in concentration and attention (*COG*). On scales related to interpersonal functioning (see Figure 8.23), Emily produced a notable clinical range elevation on the Family Problems scale (*FML*), but her scores were within normal ranges on all of the remaining interpersonal scales including *RC3, IPP, SAV, SHY* and *DSF*. Finally, her scores on the PSY-5 scales, shown in Figure 8.24, reflect clinical range elevations on measures of Psychoticism (*PSYC-r*), Negative Emotionality/Neuroticism (*NEGE-r*), and Aggressiveness (*AGG-r*).

The results of the MMPI-A indicate that diagnostic consideration should be primarily directed toward disorders associated with thought dysfunction, particularly if the effects of substance abuse may be ruled out as an important in this adolescent's report of unusual symptoms and experiences. Elevations on scales related to emotional dysfunction also indicate the consideration of mood disorders, particularly anxiety related disorders, as a primary treatment target. Finally, Emily's elevation on the *FML* scale emphasized the potential importance of family therapy as well as individual therapy in therapeutic interventions with this adolescent. The co-occurrence of thought disorder, including possible symptoms of delusions and hallucinations, with affective distress also raise the possibility of a first episode of Schizoaffective Disorder.

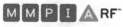

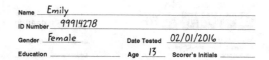

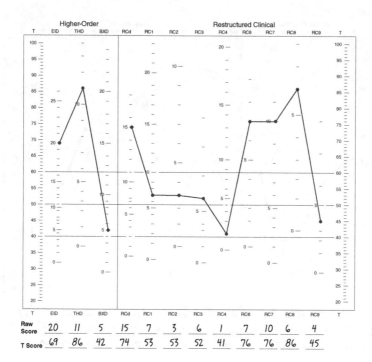

	EID	THD	BXD	RCd	RC1	RC2	RC3	RC4	RC6	RC7	RC8	RC9	
Raw Score	20	11	5	15	7	3	6	1	7	10	6	4	
T Score	69	86	42	74	53	53	52	41	76	76	86	45	

MMPI-A-RF T scores are nongendered.

H-O Scales

EID	Emotional/Internalizing Dysfunction	
THD	Thought Dysfunction	
BXD	Behavioral/Externalizing Dysfunction	

RC Scales

RCd	Demoralization		RC6	Ideas of Persecution
RC1	Somatic Complaints		RC7	Dysfunctional Negative Emotions
RC2	Low Positive Emotions		RC8	Aberrant Experiences
RC3	Cynicism		RC9	Hypomanic Activation
RC4	Antisocial Behavior			

FIGURE 8.21   MMPI-A-RF Higher-Order (*H-O*) and Restructured Clinical (*RC*) Scale Profile for Clinical Case Example 3 (Emily).

Source: Adapted from the MMPI-A-RF Administration, Scoring, Interpretation and Technical Manual by Archer et al. Copyright © 2016 by the Regents of the University of Minnesota. Reproduced with the permission of the University of Minnesota Press. All rights reserved. "Minnesota Multiphasic Personality Inventory" and "MMPI" are trademarks owned by the Regents of the University of Minnesota.

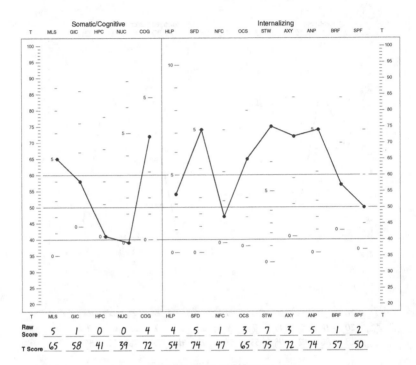

		Name	Emily			
		ID Number	99914278			
Minnesota Multiphasic Personality Inventory-Adolescent Restructured Form™		Gender	Female	Date Tested	02/01/2016	
		Education		Age	13	Scorer's Initials

	MLS	GIC	HPC	NUC	COG	HLP	SFD	NFC	OCS	STW	AXY	ANP	BRF	SPF
Raw Score	5	1	0	0	4	4	5	1	3	7	3	5	1	2
T Score	65	58	41	39	72	54	74	47	65	75	72	74	57	50

MMPI-A-RF T scores are nongendered.

Somatic/Cognitive Scales
MLS Malaise
GIC Gastrointestinal Complaints
HPC Head Pain Complaints
NUC Neurological Complaints
COG Cognitive Complaints

Internalizing Scales
HLP Helplessness/Hopelessness
SFD Self-Doubt
NFC Inefficacy
OCS Obsessions/Compulsions
STW Stress/Worry

AXY Anxiety
ANP Anger Proneness
BRF Behavior-Restricting Fears
SPF Specific Fears

FIGURE 8.22 MMPI-A-RF Somatic/Cognitive and Internalizing Scale Profile for Clinical Case Example 3 (Emily).

Source: Adapted from the MMPI-A-RF Administration, Scoring, Interpretation and Technical Manual by Archer et al. Copyright © 2016 by the Regents of the University of Minnesota. Reproduced with the permission of the University of Minnesota Press. All rights reserved. "Minnesota Multiphasic Personality Inventory" and "MMPI" are trademarks owned by the Regents of the University of Minnesota.

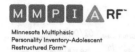

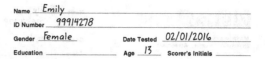

Minnesota Multiphasic
Personality Inventory-Adolescent
Restructured Form™

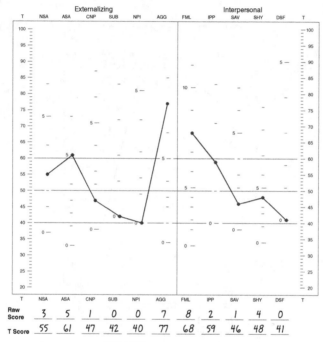

	NSA	ASA	CNP	SUB	NPI	AGG	FML	IPP	SAV	SHY	DSF
Raw Score	3	5	1	0	0	7	8	2	1	4	0
T Score	55	61	47	42	40	77	68	59	46	48	41

MMPI-A-RF T scores are nongendered.

Externalizing Scales		Interpersonal Scales	
NSA	Negative School Attitudes	FML	Family Problems
ASA	Antisocial Attitudes	IPP	Interpersonal Passivity
CNP	Conduct Problems	SAV	Social Avoidance
SUB	Substance Abuse	SHY	Shyness
NPI	Negative Peer Influence	DSF	Disaffiliativeness
AGG	Aggression		

FIGURE 8.23   MMPI-A-RF Externalizing and Interpersonal Scale Profile for Clinical Case Example 3 (Emily).

Source: Adapted from the MMPI-A-RF Administration, Scoring, Interpretation and Technical Manual by Archer et al. Copyright © 2016 by the Regents of the University of Minnesota. Reproduced with the permission of the University of Minnesota Press. All rights reserved. "Minnesota Multiphasic Personality Inventory" and "MMPI" are trademarks owned by the Regents of the University of Minnesota.

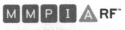

Name _Emily_

ID Number _99914278_

Gender _Female_   Date Tested _02/01/2016_

Education _____   Age _13_   Scorer's Initials _____

Minnesota Multiphasic
Personality Inventory-Adolescent
Restructured Form™

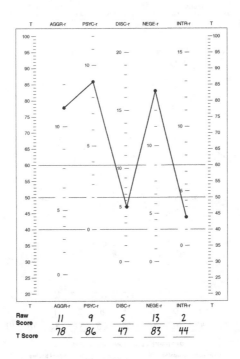

	AGGR-r	PSYC-r	DISC-r	NEGE-r	INTR-r
Raw Score	11	9	5	13	2
T Score	78	86	47	83	44

MMPI-A-RF T scores are nongendered.

AGGR-r Aggressiveness-Revised	NEGE-r Negative Emotionality/Neuroticism-Revised
PSYC-r Psychoticism-Revised	INTR-r Introversion/Low Positive Emotionality-Revised
DISC-r Disconstraint-Revised	

FIGURE 8.24   MMPI-A-RF Personality Psychopathology-Five (*PSY-5*) Profile for Clinical Case Example 3 (Emily).

Source: Adapted from the MMPI-A-RF Administration, Scoring, Interpretation and Technical Manual by Archer et al. Copyright © 2016 by the Regents of the University of Minnesota. Reproduced with the permission of the University of Minnesota Press. All rights reserved. "Minnesota Multiphasic Personality Inventory" and "MMPI" are trademarks owned by the Regents of the University of Minnesota.

Computer-Based Test Interpretation (CBTI) Systems

The use of computer technology to assist in the administration, scoring, or inter-pretation of psychological tests is a rapidly developing and evolving area. Butcher (1987b) edited a text overviewing the use of CBTI technology in relationship to a broad variety of assessment measures and tasks, and Moreland (1990) examined the use of computer-assisted technology for adolescent and child personality assessment. Reviews of CBTI products for the MMPI-2 and MMPI-2-RF are more recently available in Friedman et al. (2015) and in Graham (2012).

Butcher (1987a) noted that the MMPI served as the first subject of a com-puter scoring and interpretation system among psychological test instruments because of the extensive empirical literature available on the MMPI, and the strong conceptual basis for actuarial interpretation of MMPI test findings pro-vided by Meehl (1954, 1956, 1986) and others. Further, the MMPI was also the most widely used objective measure of personality in both adult (Lubin et al., 1984) and adolescent (Archer, Maruish, et al., 1991) settings. Thus, the MMPI provided sufficient commercial incentive to motivate individuals to develop CBTI packages for this instrument. The use of CBTI technology has spread far beyond the MMPI to include many diverse assessment instruments. Groth-Marnat and Schumaker (1989) reported that the Veterans Administration had computerized 62 psychological tests for general clinical use. These authors also noted that in a single 1987 edition of the American Psychological Association *Monitor*, there were 18 advertisements for psychological test software involving a total of 71 instruments. Krug (1993) provided a source book describing over 300 CBTI products involving various aspects of psychological assessment. As noted by Groth-Marnat (2003), however, the domain of CBTI products is subject to such rapid change that the best source for accurate product information is typi-cally the current catalogues of the major distributors for these products (e.g., Pearson Assessment and Psychological Assessment Resources).

The first application of CBTI to the MMPI was developed at the Mayo Clinic in Rochester, Minnesota (Rome et al., 1962; Swenson & Pearson, 1964). This computer-based system was designed to handle the large volume of patients seen at the Mayo Clinic. The first CBTI system to receive widespread professional use, however, was developed by Fowler (1964, 1985) and became operational in 1963. In 1965, the Roche Psychiatric Service Institute, a subdivision of Roche Laboratories, made the Fowler system commercially available on a national basis. Fowler (1985) reported that over the 17-year period that the report was nationally marketed, one-fourth of all clinical psychologists in the United States used this service and approximately 1.5 million MMPI computer-based reports were produced. Another widely used and popular MMPI interpretation sys-tem was developed by Alex Caldwell (1971), and revised for the MMPI-2, and is marketed as the *Caldwell Report*. In addition, James Butcher developed an interpretive system in the late 1970s, which was licensed by the University of Minnesota to (what is currently) Pearson Assessments as the *Minnesota Report* (Fowler, 1985). Both the *Caldwell Report* and the *Minnesota Report* are examples of narrative report services in CBTI software that are not sold directly to the consumer. In contrast, Roger Greene (1989b), in collaboration with Psychological Assessment Resources (PAR), Inc., developed an unlimited-use software system for the interpretation of the MMPI and repeatedly revised this product for the MMPI-2, currently marketed as the *MMPI-2 Adult Interpretive System, Version 4*. Examples of two of these reports (i.e., Caldwell's and Butcher's) may be found in Friedman et al.'s (2015) text. Each of these reports have been periodically revised and updated to include new MMPI-2 output following the release of major modifications to the instrument.

CBTI interpretive systems for adolescents' MMPI profiles were developed in the form of the *MMPI Adolescent Interpretive System*, developed by Archer (1987a) and marketed through PAR, and the *Marks Adolescent Clinical Report* developed by Philip Marks and Richard Lewak (1991) and distributed by Western Psychological Services. In addition, an MMPI-A interpretive report was originally released in 1992 that was developed by Archer in collaboration with PAR (the *MMPI-A Interpretive System*), and a fifth version of this report was released in 2013. An MMPI-A report was also developed by James Butcher and Carolyn Williams (1992), distributed through Pearson Assessments.

The PAR MMPI-A Adolescent Interpretive System, applied to the clinical case example presented at the end of this chapter, is given in Appendix 8.1. The output from this fifth version of the MMPI-A Interpretive System presents several unique features including the ability to graph both the clients' basic scale profile and an overlay of the modal or prototype *codetype* profile obtained by adolescents producing this two-point code, on the same profile form. The PAR MMPI-A program also presents specific interpretive output for adolescents in six assessment settings including outpatient psychiatric, inpatient psychiatric, medical/hospital, drug/alcohol treatment, school/academic, and correctional/juvenile justice. Most recently (2016), a CBTI report for the MMPI-A-RF has been developed by Archer, Handel, Ben-Porath, and Tellegen (2016b) and distributed by Pearson Assessments. At the current time, this is the only interpretive program available for the MMPI-A-RF. Appendix 8.2 provides an example of the output from the program.

The development of CBTI systems for the MMPI, as well as for other psychometric instruments, has been accompanied by considerable controversy and debate. Automated CBTI reports are based on varying combinations of clinical experience and research findings, resulting in what has been described as an actuarial-clinical approach to test interpretation (Graham, 2012). For certain instruments, particularly the MMPI-2, a wide variety of CBTI reports are available, which vary greatly in quality and accuracy. Several MMPI-2 CBTI systems have been written by individuals very knowledgeable in the use of this instrument who have augmented the available research literature with their expert judgment concerning test interpretation procedures. Unfortunately, other commercially available CBTI reports have been written by individuals less skilled in MMPI-2 interpretation procedures, and less knowledgeable concerning the existing MMPI-A and MMPI-2 research. In this latter regard, Graham (2012) has noted that the quality of interpretive programs has varied widely, making it imperative that clinicians carefully evaluate the adequacy of these services. Matarazzo (1983, 1986) and Lanyon (1987) expressed concerns regarding the absence of validation studies on automated interpretations of the MMPI. Matarazzo further noted that CBTI programs may give the appearance of accuracy and that inexperienced clinicians may be unaware of the limitations and potential for misuse of these services. The American Psychological Association (APA) published a set of guidelines for the development and use of CBTI products (APA, 1986). These guidelines include the provision that professionals limit their use of CBTI products to those instruments with which they are familiar and competent, and that such reports only be used in conjunction with professional judgment. Butcher (1987b) noted that the advantages of computer-based test interpretation (CBTI) reports include the following:

1. *Objectivity*. CBTI products are not subject to interpreter bias, and test rules are automatically and consistently applied to the interpretation of cases.
2. *Use as an Outside Opinion*. CBTI products may serve as a source of second opinion for clinical and forensic evaluations. The CBTI product is useful in this regard because test interpretation is not biased by any subjective preconceptions the interpreter may hold concerning a specific client.
3. *Rapid Turnaround*. CBTI reports can typically be generated within a few minutes after data is entered in the system.
4. *Cost Effectiveness*. The cost of CBTI products varies widely depending on the test distributor, test authors, and nature of the service (e.g., software vs. test report service). Nevertheless, almost all forms of CBTI reports compare favorably in terms of cost to clinician-generated reports.
5. *Reliability*. The reliability of a CBTI product should be invariant over repeated uses, in contrast to the errors and lapses in memory manifested by human beings.

In addition to these advantages, Butcher (1987a) also listed several disadvantages connected with CBTI products:

1. *The Question of Excessive Generality*. Computer-based reports are typically based on prototypic profiles, which may differ in many specifics from the individual patient who produced the MMPI profile being interpreted. As noted by Butcher (1987a), "The most valid computerized reports are those that most closely match the researched prototype" (p. 5). In the worst cases, CBTI reports may include numerous statements that are highly generalizable

and could apply to anyone. These types of reports, although appearing accurate to the novice test user, are of little use in attempting to identify the unique features of the individual.

2. *Potential for Misuse.* Because computerized reports are widely available and may be mass produced, the potential for abuse of this type of product may potentially be greater than that of clinically derived personality interpretation reports. This issue is also related to the need to establish that a computer-assisted test administration is equivalent to standard paper-and-pencil test administration procedures in terms of producing equivalent test results. Graham (2012) has noted that sufficient research attention has been directed to this latter issue to conclude that any differences observed in results produced by paper-and-pencil versus computer administrations are typically small and typically attributable to sampling error.

3. *Clinician Start-Up Time.* The use of computerized psychological testing requires a clinician to become familiar with various aspects of computer use. This task, depending on the degree of "user friendliness" of the CBTI product, may be accomplished quickly or be very time consuming and frustrating.

4. *Confusing Abundance of Packages.* Literally hundreds of CBTI products are currently available for clinician use, and it is often difficult for clinicians to determine the optimal CBTI products for their applications and setting. Not only must clinicians determine the quality of CBTI products, but there is also the question of "fit" between their particular utilization of tests and various CBTI products that are designed for particular settings, use volume, and methods of scoring or data transfer.

Added to these cautions might be the recommendation that the clinician becomes aware of the limitations of CBTI reports. Moreland (1985a, 1985b) noted that CBTI programs should be used as only one element in the assessment process, and should never be employed as a substitute for professional judgment. Even the best CBTI programs for the MMPI produce descriptive statements that show only modest relationships, in terms of statement accuracy, to clinician descriptions of the patient (Graham, 2012). Butcher, Perry and Atlis (2000), for example, concluded that only 60% of the interpretations in the narratives of CBTI reports typically were appropriate, with shorter narratives containing higher percentages of valid/accurate interpretations. In choosing a CBTI product, the following five guidelines are offered to clinicians:

1. All CBTI products represent a combination or blending of the author's clinical judgment with research findings that have been established for a particular instrument. The potential test user, therefore, should be aware of the identity and expertise of the individual or individuals who developed the CBTI package (Graham, 2012; Friedman et al. 2015). In a very

real sense, the clinician acquiring a CBTI product is purchasing/leasing the clinical and scientific judgment of the test developers.

2. Know how the CBTI report was written. Specifically, to what extent was the CBTI generated based on empirical findings, and how broad was the empirical base used for the development of the test instrument? The clinician should review the CBTI manual for this information prior to purchasing and using computerized reports.

3. To what degree does the company that markets the CBTI product support its use and application? Before purchasing a CBTI product it is reasonable for the consumer to request samples of interpretive output, and to check the history of the company in terms of customer satisfaction. Does the company have an 800 number available for product use support? Does the company provide a detailed and "user-friendly" manual or online support resource that contains sufficient detail to meaningfully assist the clinician in using the technical and clinical features of the product?

4. Is the CBTI product periodically revised or updated to reflect changes in interpretive practices based on new research findings? This point is particularly important for CBTI products related to the use of the MMPI-2-RF or the MMPI-A-RF, for which empirical support is rapidly evolving.

5. To what extent has this CBTI product been subject to empirical validation? Moreland (1985b) noted that CBTI products have generated two basic types of research studies. These include consumer satisfaction studies in which CBTI users rate the degree of accuracy and usefulness of the CBTI, and external criterion studies in which comparisons are made between CBTI-based descriptors and patient ratings/descriptions made on the basis of external sources including, for example, psychiatric diagnoses, medical records, and clinician judgments. Based on findings for the original form of the MMPI, it would be anticipated that the accuracy of MMPI-2 and MMPI-A interpretive statements will be found to vary considerably from product to product. In this regard, the Pearson Assessment MMPI-A-RF Interpretive Report (Archer et al. 2016b) has the innovative feature of identifying the source of each interpretive statement in the report output. Further, it is possible that the accuracy of interpretive statements within a particular CBTI product may be found to vary from scale to scale and/ or codetype to codetype. Also, Moreland (1984) noted that the accuracy of codetype descriptors for rare codetypes is likely to be less accurate than descriptors provided for commonly occurring codetypes that have received extensive research attention. The question is often raised concerning the "best" or most accurate CBTI for various forms of the MMPI. In this regard, Graham (2012) has the following thoughtful observation:

Each of the commercially available services has both strengths and weaknesses. It would be premature to recommend any particular service for general clinical use. What clearly is needed is more research concerning the external validity of computer-based MMPI-2 inferences.

In this latter regard, Graham reports a study by Williams and Weed (2004) that reviewed eight commercially available MMPI-2 CBTI services and found that while all exhibited both strengths and weaknesses, Pearson Assessments and PAR products were evaluated the most positively on a variety of dimensions such as ability to edit reports, ease of data entry, accuracy of documentation, and readability of reports.

Illustrations of MMPI-A and MMPI-A-RF Interpretive Reports

A practical method of illustrating the uses and limitations of computer-based test interpretation packages, as well as facilitating and understanding of the similarities and differences between the MMPI-A and MMPI-A-RF, can be provided by comparing the results of CBTI programs for these tests when applied to the same case (shown in Appendices 8.1 and 8.2).

Stephen is a 15-year-old boy whose mother died in an auto accident when he was 6 years old. Stephen was very close to his mother, and her death substantially affected his psychological functioning and subsequent adjustment. Stephen became anxious concerning the possibility of losing other family members, particularly his father, to accidents and he became tearful, anxious and upset when separated from his father. Stephen started receiving therapy services shortly after his mother's death, but these services lasted only three months. As Stephen grew older, he was seen as an anxious and fearful child who had few friends in school. Stephen became a target of school bullying, and as his social frustration increased he became increasingly withdrawn, anxious and depressed. After his father became concerned about Stephen's growing reluctance to participate in after-school activities, and his tendency to cry when discussing his frustration with his peers, Stephen was referred for outpatient evaluation and treatment. Stephen was evaluated, in part, with the MMPI-A (see Appendix 8.1), which was subsequently rescored to produce the MMPI-A-RF protocol interpreted in the Pearson Assessments output shown in Appendix 8.2.

APPENDIX 8.1 AND 8.2

Appendix 8.1

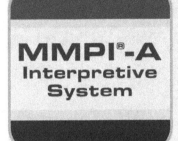

by Robert P. Archer, PhD and PAR Staff

Client Information

Name:	622932
Client ID:	622932
Gender:	Male
Date of birth:	07/01/2000
Age:	15
Grade level:	0
Setting:	Outpatient
Test date:	07/16/2015

This report is intended for use by qualified professionals only and is not to be shared with the examinee or any other unqualified persons.

Profile Matches and Scores

	Client profile	Highest scale codetype	Best-fit codetype
Codetype match:		2-0/0-2	2-0/0-2
Coefficient of fit:		0.888	0.888
Scores			
F (Infrequency)	55	53	53
L (Lie)	55	55	55
K (Correction)	32	48	48
Hs (Scale 1)	60	52	52
D (Scale 2)	79	75	75
Hy (Scale 3)	50	51	51
Pd (Scale 4)	62	56	56
Mf (Scale 5)	57	54	54
Pa (Scale 6)	52	52	52
Pt (Scale 7)	78	59	59
Sc (Scale 8)	54	55	55
Ma (Scale 9)	43	45	45
Si (Scale 0)	79	68	68
Codetype definition in *T*-score points	1	9	9
Mean clinical scale elevation	59.0	55.6	55.6
Mean excitatory scale elevation	53.0	52.2	52.2
Mean age - Females		15.8	15.8
Mean age - Males		16.1	16.1
Percent of cases		1.0	1.0

Configural clinical scale interpretation is provided in the report for the following codetype(s):
2-0/0-2

Unanswered (?) Items	3
Welsh code	027'+41-5863/9: FL/:K#

Validity and Clinical Scales

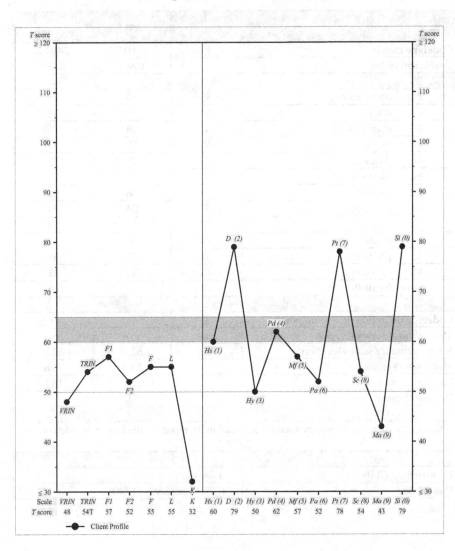

Scale	VRIN	TRIN	F1	F2	F	L	K	Hs (1)	D (2)	Hy (3)	Pd (4)	Mf (5)	Pa (6)	Pt (7)	Sc (8)	Ma (9)	Si (0)
T score	48	54T	57	52	55	55	32	60	79	50	62	57	52	78	54	43	79

● Client Profile

Content and Supplementary Scales

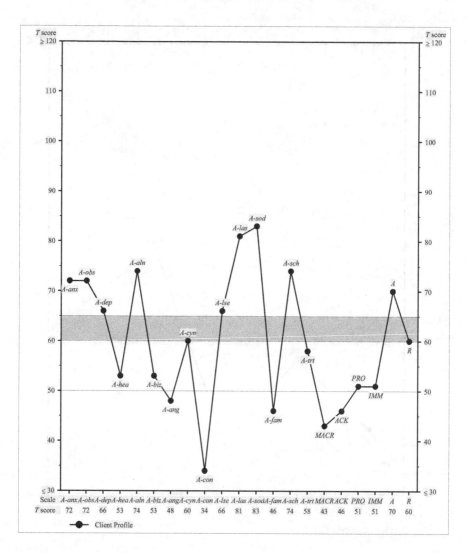

PSY-5 Scales

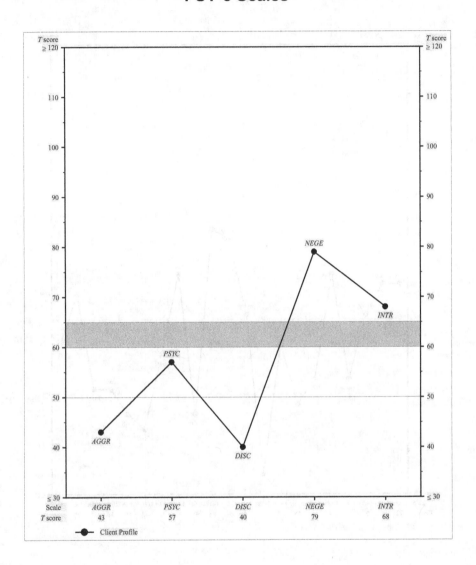

Scale	AGGR	PSYC	DISC	NEGE	INTR
T score	43	57	40	79	68

●— Client Profile

Harris-Lingoes and Si Subscales

Scale[a]	T score
Depression subscale	
Subjective Depression (D1)	79[a]
Psychomotor Retardation (D2)	61
Physical Malfunctioning (D3)	62
Mental Dullness (D4)	68[a]
Brooding (D5)	71[a]
Hysteria subscale	
Denial of Social Anxiety (Hy1)	38
Need for Affection (Hy2)	46
Lassitude-Malaise (Hy3)	74
Somatic Complaints (Hy4)	50
Inhibition of Aggression (Hy5)	36
Psychopathic Deviate subscale	
Familial Discord (Pd1)	48
Authority Problems (Pd2)	35
Social Imperturbability (Pd3)	30
Social Alienation (Pd4)	69[a]
Self-Alienation (Pd5)	69[a]
Paranoia subscales	
Persecutory Ideas (Pa1)	57
Poignancy (Pa2)	61
Naiveté (Pa3)	40
Schizophrenia subscale	
Social Alienation (Sc1)	62
Emotional Alienation (Sc2)	48
Lack of Ego Mastery, Cognitive (Sc3)	68
Lack of Ego Mastery, Conative (Sc4)	61
Lack of Ego Mastery, Defective Inhibition (Sc5)	48
Bizarre Sensory Experiences (Sc6)	47
Hypomania subscale	
Amorality (Ma1)	38
Psychomotor Acceleration (Ma2)	48
Imperturbability (Ma3)	30
Ego Inflation (Ma4)	48
Social Introversion subscale	
Shyness/Self-Consciousness (Si1)	69[a]

Social Avoidance (Si2)	77[a]
Alienation-Self and Others (Si3)	66[a]

[a] *T* scores for subscales printed in bold are *T* ≥ 65 and the corresponding Main Clinical scale is *T* ≥ 60.

Content Component Scales

Scale[a]	T score
Depression	
Dysphoria (A-dep1)	71[a]
Self-Depreciation (A-dep2)	66[a]
Lack of Drive (A-dep3)	60
Suicidal Ideation (A-dep4)	53
Health Concerns	
Gastrointestinal Symptoms (A-hea1)	59
Neurological Symptoms (A-hea2)	46
General Health Concerns (A-hea3)	64
Alienation	
Misunderstood (A-aln1)	64
Social Isolation (A-aln2)	70[a]
Interpersonal Skepticism (A-aln3)	64
Bizarre Mentation	
Psychotic Symptomatology (A-biz1)	57
Paranoid Ideation (A-biz2)	42
Anger	
Explosive Behavior (A-ang1)	44
Irritability (A-ang2)	59
Cynicism	
Misanthropic Beliefs (A-cyn1)	62
Interpersonal Suspiciousness (A-cyn2)	56
Conduct Problems	
Acting-Out Behaviors (A-con1)	35
Antisocial Attitudes (A-con2)	30
Negative Peer Group Influences (A-con3)	51
Low Self-Esteem	
Self-Doubt (A-lse1)	61
Interpersonal Submissiveness (A-lse2)	69[a]
Low Aspirations	
Low Achievement Orientation (A-las1)	69[a]
Lack of Initiative (A-las2)	61
Social Discomfort	
Introversion (A-sod1)	81[a]
Shyness (A-sod2)	66[a]

[a] T scores for subscales printed in bold are $T \geq 65$ and the corresponding Main Content scale is $T \geq 60$.

Content Component Scales (continued)

Scale[a]	T score
Family Problems	
Familial Discord (A-fam1)	50
Familial Alienation (A-fam2)	39
School Problems	
School Conduct Problems (A-sch1)	50
Negative Attitudes (A-sch2)	57
Negative Treatment Indicators	
Low Motivation (A-trt1)	58
Inability to Disclose (A-trt2)	53

[a] T scores for subscales printed in bold are $T \geq 65$ and the corresponding Main Content scale is $T \geq 60$.

Specified Setting

This adolescent was assessed in an outpatient setting.

Configural Validity Scale Interpretation

This adolescent has produced a consistent MMPI-A response pattern, reflected in acceptable values on validity scales VRIN and TRIN.

This F-L-K validity scale configuration is indicative of an adolescent who responded to the MMPI-A in a valid, accurate, and cooperative manner. The validity scale features produced by this teenager are characteristic of normal adolescents and are unusual for teenagers evaluated in psychiatric settings.

Both F1 and F2 T scores are below 90. T-score values of 90 or greater on either F1 or F2 are likely to indicate problems with profile validity.

Validity Scales

Raw (?) = 3

There were a few item responses omitted in completing this MMPI-A. These omissions may represent areas of limitation in the adolescent's life experience that rendered certain items unanswerable or limitations in the adolescent's reading ability. There is little probability of profile distortion as a result of these few item omissions.

Appendix 8.1

Variable Response Inconsistency (VRIN) = 48

VRIN scores in this range suggest that the adolescent responded to test items with an acceptable level of consistency.

True Response Inconsistency (TRIN) = 54T

TRIN scores in this range suggest that the adolescent responded to test items with an acceptable level of consistency.

Infrequency 1 (F1) = 57

Scores in this range suggest that the adolescent has responded in a valid manner to items that appear in the first part of the MMPI-A test booklet.

Infrequency 2 (F2) = 52

Scores in this range suggest that the adolescent has responded in a valid manner to items that appear in the latter part of the MMPI-A test booklet.

Infrequency (F) = 55

Scores in this range usually indicate that the respondent has answered the test items in a manner similar to most normal adolescents. Although some clinical scale scores may be elevated, this teenager has not reported many symptoms of highly deviant/unusual psychopathology.

Lie (L) = 55

Scores in this range suggest an appropriate balance between the admission and the denial of common social faults. These adolescents are often viewed as flexible and psychologically sophisticated.

Correction (K) = 32

Scores in this range are often produced by adolescents with poor self-concepts and limited resources for coping with stress. Adolescents in acute distress may produce similar scores, as well as teenagers who are attempting to "fake bad" or exaggerate their degree of psychopathology.

Configural Clinical Scale Interpretation

2-0/0-2 Codetype

This MMPI-A profile is classified as a 2-0/0-2 codetype, which occurs in roughly 3% of adolescents evaluated in psychiatric settings. These adolescents often present symptomatology that includes depression, feelings of inferiority, anxiety, social introversion, and withdrawal. They are described as being conforming, passive individuals who are unlikely to engage in antisocial or delinquent behaviors. Many show strong evidence of social ineptitude and a general lack of age-appropriate social skills. Findings for the A-sod content scale support the view that this adolescent is socially introverted and uncomfortable. Adolescents with the 2-0/0-2 profile are typically referred for psychiatric treatment with presenting problems that include anxiety and tension, apathy, shyness, lethargy, and interpersonal hypersensitivity. They describe themselves as being awkward, dull, gloomy, shy, cowardly, silent, and meek. They are isolated teenagers who are perceived as loners. The findings for this adolescent on the A-aln content scale further reflect substantial interpersonal isolation and alienation. Adolescents with the 2-0/0-2 codetype typically attempt to conform to parental demands.

These adolescents often present many symptoms related to the development of schizoid personality features. Psychiatric diagnoses associated with this codetype may include Schizoid Personality Disorder (301.20), Dysthymic Disorder (300.4), Major Depression (296.XX), and Generalized Anxiety Disorder (300.02). In therapy these adolescents often express concerns regarding feelings of inferiority, social rejection, and impaired body image. Findings from the A-lse content scale also indicate this adolescent lacks self-confidence and feels inadequate. Primary defense mechanisms appear to involve social withdrawal, denial, and obsessive-compulsive mechanisms. Findings from the A-obs content scale further support the view that this adolescent is obsessive and ruminative. The 2-0/0-2 adolescent may respond favorably to interventions involving skill training programs such as anxiety management and relaxation training. Adolescents who have sufficient ego strength to tolerate group intervention may respond well to group psychotherapies. These interventions may often be combined with more traditional supportive psychotherapies.

Clinical Scales

Scale 1 (Hs) = 60

The T-score value obtained for this basic MMPI-A scale is at a marginal or transitional level of elevation. Some of the following descriptors may not apply to this adolescent.

Scores in this range are frequently obtained by adolescents with a history of symptoms associated with hypochondriasis, including vague physical complaints and a preoccupation with body functioning, illness, and disease. Such elevated scores may also be obtained, however, by adolescents who are experiencing actual physical illness. The possibility of organic dysfunction should be carefully ruled out. High scores for adolescents on this scale often indicate the increased likelihood of neurotic diagnoses and the development of somatic responses to stress. These adolescents are typically seen by others as self-centered, dissatisfied, pessimistic, and demanding. The prognosis for psychological intervention is typically guarded, and these adolescents often display little insight in psychotherapy.

Scale 2 (D) = 79

Scores in this range are typically found for adolescents who are depressed, dissatisfied, hopeless, and self-depreciating. They often experience apathy, loss of interest in daily activities, loss of self-confidence, and feelings of inadequacy and pessimism. Additionally, these adolescents often experience substantial feelings of guilt, worthlessness, and self-criticism and may experience suicidal ideation. However, this degree of distress may serve as a positive motivator for psychotherapy efforts.

Scale 3 (Hy) = 50

The obtained score is within normal or expected ranges, and this adolescent probably has the capacity to acknowledge unpleasant issues or negative feelings.

Scale 4 (Pd) = 62

The T-score value obtained for this basic MMPI-A scale is at a marginal or transitional level of elevation. Some of the following descriptors may not apply to this adolescent.

Scale 4 high points are very common among adolescents, particularly among those in psychiatric or criminal justice settings. Scores in this range are typical for adolescents who are characterized as rebellious, hostile toward authority figures, and defiant. These adolescents often have histories of poor school adjustment and problems in school conduct. High scores on this scale present an increased probability of overtly delinquent behavior. These adolescents often show an inability to delay gratification and are described as being impulsive and having little tolerance for frustration and boredom.

Primary defense mechanisms typically involve acting-out, and such behaviors may be unaccompanied by feelings of guilt or remorse. Although these adolescents typically create a good first impression and maintain an extroverted and outgoing interpersonal style, their interpersonal relationships tend to be shallow and superficial. They are eventually viewed by others as selfish, self-centered, and egocentric.

Scale 5 (Mf) = 57

The obtained score is within normal or expected ranges and indicates standard interest patterns in the traditional masculine activities.

Scale 6 (Pa) = 52

The obtained score is within normal or expected ranges, and this adolescent appears to be capable of engaging in interpersonal exchanges without excessive suspiciousness or distrust.

Scale 7 (Pt) = 78

Scores in this range are typically obtained by adolescents who are described as anxious, tense, indecisive, self-critical, and perfectionistic. They often have marked feelings of insecurity, inadequacy, and inferiority and maintain unrealistically high standards for their performance. At extreme elevations, the score may indicate clear patterns of intense ruminations and obsessions.

Scale 8 (Sc) = 54

The obtained score is within normal or expected ranges and suggests intact reality testing and coherent thought processes.

Scale 9 (Ma) = 43

The obtained score is within normal or expected ranges and reflects a typical energy or activity level for normal adolescents.

Scale 0 (Si) = 79

Adolescents who produce scores in this range are socially introverted, insecure, and uncomfortable in social situations. They tend to be shy, timid, submissive, and lacking in self-confidence. They are unlikely to engage in impulsive behaviors and are at low risk for acting-out or delinquency.

Additional Scales

Content and Content Component Scales

The MMPI-A content component scales should not be viewed as "stand alone" scales, but rather should be interpreted in relation to elevated scores on the corresponding content scales. Specifically, the content component scales should be interpreted only in the presence of a T score of 60 or greater on the content scale. Further, content component scales should not be interpreted even under these circumstances unless the specific content component scale T score is 65 or greater. Examination of the content component scales under appropriate circumstances can identify the most important and salient components associated with an elevated score for a given content scale. If most or all of the content component scale scores are elevated in the presence of an elevated score on the parent content scale, it is possible to assume with greater certainty that the adolescent endorsed items associated with the entire range of content for that content scale. Therefore, in the following sections, interpretations for content component scales will be provided only if the content component scale score is greater than or equal to 65 and the corresponding content scale score is greater than or equal to 60.

Anxiety (A-anx) = 72

Scores in this range are often produced by adolescents who are tense, anxious, nervous, and ruminative. Concentration and low endurance or rapid fatigue may also be problem areas.

Obsessiveness (A-obs) = 72

Scores in this range are produced by adolescents experiencing obsessiveness. These adolescents are ambivalent and have difficulty making decisions. They may ruminate and worry excessively. These teenagers may also have problems in concentration and report intrusive thoughts.

Depression (A-dep) = 66

Scores in this range are often produced by adolescents who are depressed and despondent. These teenagers may be apathetic and easily fatigued. Their depression may include the occurrence of suicidal ideation and a sense of hopelessness or despair.

An elevated score on the Dysphoria content component scale indicates that this adolescent has reported a number of symptoms related to depressed mood and may meet the criteria for a diagnosis of depressed mood associated with a major depressive episode (296.XX).

An elevated score on the Self-Depreciation content component scale suggests that this adolescent experiences a negative self-concept and is likely to feel helpless and ineffectual. These adolescents typically have little self-confidence and may experience feelings of worthlessness and poor self-esteem.

Health Concerns (A-hea) = 53

The obtained score on this content scale is within normal or expected ranges.

Alienation (A-aln) = 74

Scores in this range are often produced by adolescents who are interpersonally isolated and alienated. They do not believe others understand them, and they perceive their lives to be harsh or unfair. They may be socially withdrawn and feel they cannot turn to, or depend on, anyone.

This adolescent's elevated score on the Social Isolation content component scale reflects feelings of social discomfort and isolation that may be related to social skills deficits.

Bizarre Mentation (A-biz) = 53

The obtained score on this content scale is within normal or expected ranges.

Anger (A-ang) = 48

The obtained score on this content scale is within normal or expected ranges.

Cynicism (A-cyn) = 60

Scores in this range represent a marginal elevation on the Cynicism scale, which may reflect a tendency to be guarded in relationships and suspicious of the motives of others.

Conduct Problems (A-con) = 34

The obtained score on this content scale is within normal or expected ranges.

Low Self-Esteem (A-lse) = 66

Scores in this range may be produced by adolescents who feel inadequate, incompetent, or useless. They lack self-confidence and believe they have many faults and flaws. These teenagers may be interpersonally passive and socially uncomfortable.

This adolescent produced a significantly elevated score on the Interpersonal Submissiveness content component scale, typically found among adolescents who are easily influenced by others and show little interpersonal assertiveness or initiative. Such adolescents are likely to be viewed by others as passive and dependent.

Low Aspirations (A-las) = 81

Scores in this range are produced by adolescents who have few, or no, educational or life goals or objectives. These adolescents often have patterns of poor academic achievement. They tend to become frustrated quickly and give up, and they do not apply themselves in challenging situations.

This adolescent produced a significantly elevated score on the Low Achievement Orientation content component scale, indicating he or she does not endorse attitudes or behaviors associated with strong academic performance. These adolescents often have difficulty performing in school and may have a higher rate of school avoidance and truancy than other adolescents.

Social Discomfort (A-sod) = 83

Scores in this range are produced by adolescents who are uncomfortable in social situations and may be described as introverted and shy. They avoid social events and find it difficult to interact with others.

This adolescent produced an elevated score on the Introversion content component scale, indicating discomfort or dislike of interpersonal contact and a tendency to be distant and withdrawn from others.

This adolescent produced an elevated score on the Shyness content component scale, indicating a general discomfort in social situations. He may find it difficult to interact with others and may wish that he were more outgoing and comfortable around people.

Family Problems (A-fam) = 46

> The obtained score on this content scale is within normal or expected ranges.

School Problems (A-sch) = 74

> Scores in this range are produced by adolescents who are encountering significant behavioral and/or academic problems within the school setting. These adolescents often have developed a negative attitude toward academic achievement and activities. The possibility of learning disabilities or developmental delays should be evaluated.

Negative Treatment Indicators (A-trt) = 58

> The obtained score on this content scale is within normal or expected ranges.

Supplementary Scales

MacAndrew Alcoholism (MAC-R) = 43

> Adolescents who score in this range are not likely to abuse alcohol or drugs. The most notable exception are adolescents who are primarily neurotic in terms of their personality configuration and who employ alcohol and drugs as a means of "self-medication."

Alcohol-Drug Problem Acknowledgement (ACK) = 46

> This score is in within acceptable or normal ranges on the ACK scale. Because an adolescent may underreport drug or alcohol use, related attitudes, or related symptoms, MAC-R and PRO scale scores should also be carefully reviewed to optimally screen for alcohol- and drug-related problems.

Alcohol-Drug Problem Proneness (PRO) = 51

> This scores is within acceptable or normal ranges on the PRO scale.

Immaturity (IMM) = 51

> The obtained score on the IMM scale is within normal or expected ranges.

Anxiety (A) = 70

> Adolescents who score in this range may be described as maladjusted, anxious, self-critical, depressed, pessimistic, ruminative, overwhelmed, and uncomfortable. Because of their degree of emotional discomfort, however, such adolescents often demonstrate positive motivation to engage in psychological treatment.

Repression (R) = 60

> Adolescents who score in this range are often unexcitable, inhibited, submissive, and conventional and tend to show little feeling. Scores in this range are infrequently obtained by adolescents evaluated in psychiatric settings.

The Personality Psychopathology-Five (PSY-5) Scales

The interpretation of the PSY-5 scales is provided in this report in order to complement interpretive data derived from the MMPI-A basic and content scales. The correlates of these research scales have received limited investigation in adolescent populations, and the interpreter is urged to apply caution in using these scales with adolescents.

Aggression (AGGR) = 43

> The obtained score is within normal or expected ranges.

Psychoticism (PSYC) = 57

> The obtained score is within normal or expected ranges.

Disconstraint (DISC) = 40

> The obtained score is within normal or expected ranges.

Negative Emotionality/Neuroticism (NEGE) = 79

> Adolescents who produce elevated scores on the Negative Emotionality/Neuroticism scale are likely to be described by others as anxious, tense, worried, and apprehensive. These adolescents may have a history of internalizing behaviors and may be seen as dependent or excessively reliant on others for direction and reassurance. In addition to anxiety and withdrawal, substantial guilt and remorse are likely to be experienced by these adolescents.

Introversion/Low Positive Emotionality (INTR) = 68

> Adolescents who produce elevated scores on the Introversion/Low Positive Emotionality scale are often described as socially withdrawn, isolated, and uncommunicative. In addition, they are often described by others as depressed, with few or no friends, and they are less likely than other adolescents to have histories of externalizing behaviors or Conduct Disorder problems. These adolescents typically show little capacity to experience positive emotions including joy or happiness.

Harris-Lingoes and Si Subscales

The interpretation of Harris-Lingoes and Si subscales is provided in this program because of the potential relevance of these data to adolescent profiles. The correlates of these research scales have not been examined in adolescent populations, however, and the user is cautioned that the following interpretive statements are based on findings in adult populations.

Subjective Depression (D1) = 79

> High D1 scorers feel depressed, unhappy, and nervous. They lack energy and interest and are not coping well with their problems. They show deficits in concentration and attention, lack self-confidence, and feel shy and uneasy in social situations.

Psychomotor Retardation (D2) = 61

> The obtained score is within normal or expected ranges.

Physical Malfunctioning (D3) = 62

> The obtained score is within normal or expected ranges.

Mental Dullness (D4) = 68

> High D4 scorers lack energy to cope with the problems of everyday life. They report difficulties with concentration and they complain of poor memory and judgment. They lack self-confidence, feel inferior to others, get little enjoyment out of life, and may feel that life is no longer worthwhile.

Brooding (D5) = 71

> High D5 scorers lack energy and brood and ruminate excessively about life not being worthwhile. They feel inferior and are easily hurt by

criticism. At times, they report feeling like they are losing control of their thought processes.

Denial of Social Anxiety (Hy1) = 38

Low Hy1 scorers tend to be socially introverted and bashful and are greatly influenced by social standards and customs.

Need for Affection (Hy2) = 46

The obtained score is within normal or expected ranges.

Lassitude-Malaise (Hy3) = 74

High Hy3 scorers generally feel unhappy and uncomfortable and believe they are not in good health. They present vague somatic complaints, including weakness and fatigue, and complain about functioning below par both physically and mentally. They may have a poor appetite and report problems with sleeping.

Somatic Complaints (Hy4) = 50

The obtained score is within normal or expected ranges.

Inhibition of Aggression (Hy5) = 36

Low Hy5 scorers openly admit to experiencing hostile and aggressive impulses.

Familial Discord (Pd1) = 48

The obtained score is within normal or expected ranges.

Authority Problems (Pd2) = 35

Low Pd2 scorers are socially conforming and accepting of authority. They are reluctant to express their personal beliefs and opinions, and they are easily influenced by others. They deny academic or legal difficulties.

Social Imperturbability (Pd3) = 30

Low Pd3 scorers are uncomfortable and anxious in social situations. They are socially conforming, and they do not express their opinions and beliefs openly.

Social Alienation (Pd4) = 69

> High Pd4 scorers feel misunderstood, alienated, isolated, and estranged from others. They are lonely, unhappy, and uninvolved people who blame others for their own problems and shortcomings. They are often insensitive and inconsiderate in relationships and will later verbalize regret and remorse for their actions.

Self-Alienation (Pd5) = 69

> High Pd5 scorers describe themselves as feeling uncomfortable and unhappy. They have problems with concentration and attention, and they do not find their life to be especially interesting or rewarding. They verbalize guilt and regret and display negative emotions in an exhibitionistic manner. Excessive alcohol abuse may be a problem.

Persecutory Ideas (Pa1) = 57

> The obtained score is within normal or expected ranges.

Poignancy (Pa2) = 61

> The obtained score is within normal or expected ranges.

Naiveté (Pa3) = 40

> The obtained score is within normal or expected ranges.

Social Alienation (Sc1) = 62

> The obtained score is within normal or expected ranges.

Emotional Alienation (Sc2) = 48

> The obtained score is within normal or expected ranges.

Lack of Ego Mastery-Cognitive (Sc3) = 68

> High Sc3 scorers admit to strange thought processes, feelings of unreality, and problems with concentration and attention. At times, they may feel that they are "losing their minds."

Lack of Ego Mastery-Conative (Sc4) = 61

> The obtained score is within normal or expected ranges.

Lack of Ego Mastery-Defective Inhibition (Sc5) = 48

The obtained score is within normal or expected ranges.

Bizarre Sensory Experiences (Sc6) = 47

The obtained score is within normal or expected ranges.

Amorality (Ma1) = 38

Low Ma1 scorers see other people and themselves as honest and concerned.

Psychomotor Acceleration (Ma2) = 48

The obtained score is within normal or expected ranges.

Imperturbability (Ma3) = 30

Low Ma3 scorers report being uncomfortable around others. They are easily influenced by others. They deny anger and resentment toward other people.

Ego Inflation (Ma4) = 48

The obtained score is within normal or expected ranges.

Shyness/Self-Consciousness (Si1) = 69

Scores in this range are produced by adolescents who may be described as shy around others and easily embarrassed. These adolescents are ill at ease in social situations.

Social Avoidance (Si2) = 77

Adolescents who produce scores in this range dislike or avoid group activities, and they may often seek to minimize social contacts or involvements.

Alienation-Self and Others (Si3) = 66

Adolescents who produce elevated scores on the Si3 subscale may have symptomatology that interferes in their relationships with others. They may be anxious and indecisive or fearful and suspicious, or they may maintain low self-concepts or self-esteem.

End of Report

Appendix 8.2

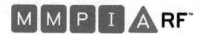

Minnesota Multiphasic
Personality Inventory-Adolescent
Restructured Form™

Interpretive Report

MMPI-A-RF™

Minnesota Multiphasic Personality Inventory-Adolescent-Restructured Form™

Robert P. Archer, PhD, Richard W. Handel, PhD, Yossef S. Ben-Porath, PhD, & Auke Tellegen, PhD

Name:	Stephen
ID Number:	622932
Age:	15
Gender:	Male
Years of Education:	Not reported
Date Assessed:	10/01/2015

MMPI-A-RF Validity Scales

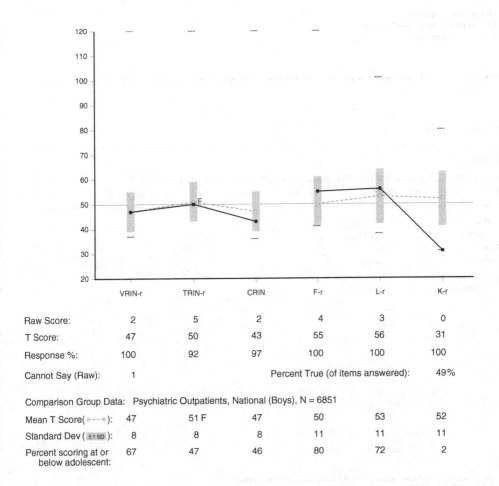

	VRIN-r	TRIN-r	CRIN	F-r	L-r	K-r
Raw Score:	2	5	2	4	3	0
T Score:	47	50	43	55	56	31
Response %:	100	92	97	100	100	100

Cannot Say (Raw): 1   Percent True (of items answered): 49%

Comparison Group Data: Psychiatric Outpatients, National (Boys), N = 6851

	VRIN-r	TRIN-r	CRIN	F-r	L-r	K-r
Mean T Score(◇- - -◇):	47	51 F	47	50	53	52
Standard Dev (±1 SD):	8	8	8	11	11	11
Percent scoring at or below adolescent:	67	47	46	80	72	2

The highest and lowest T scores possible on each scale are indicated by a "---"; MMPI-A-RF T scores are non-gendered.

VRIN-r	Variable Response Inconsistency	F-r	Infrequent Responses
TRIN-r	True Response Inconsistency	L-r	Uncommon Virtues
CRIN	Combined Response Inconsistency	K-r	Adjustment Validity

MMPI-A-RF Higher-Order (H-O) and Restructured Clinical (RC) Scales

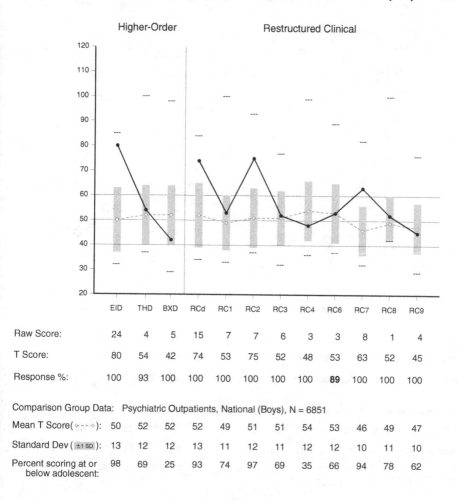

	EID	THD	BXD	RCd	RC1	RC2	RC3	RC4	RC6	RC7	RC8	RC9
Raw Score:	24	4	5	15	7	7	6	3	3	8	1	4
T Score:	80	54	42	74	53	75	52	48	53	63	52	45
Response %:	100	93	100	100	100	100	100	100	89	100	100	100

Comparison Group Data: Psychiatric Outpatients, National (Boys), N = 6851

Mean T Score(◇--◇):	50	52	52	52	49	51	51	54	53	46	49	47
Standard Dev (±1 SD):	13	12	12	13	11	12	11	12	12	10	11	10
Percent scoring at or below adolescent:	98	69	25	93	74	97	69	35	66	94	78	62

The highest and lowest T scores possible on each scale are indicated by a "---"; MMPI-A-RF T scores are non-gendered.

EID   Emotional/Internalizing Dysfunction
THD   Thought Dysfunction
BXD   Behavioral/Externalizing Dysfunction

RCd   Demoralization
RC1   Somatic Complaints
RC2   Low Positive Emotions
RC3   Cynicism
RC4   Antisocial Behavior

RC6   Ideas of Persecution
RC7   Dysfunctional Negative Emotions
RC8   Aberrant Experiences
RC9   Hypomanic Activation

MMPI-A-RF Somatic/Cognitive and Internalizing Scales

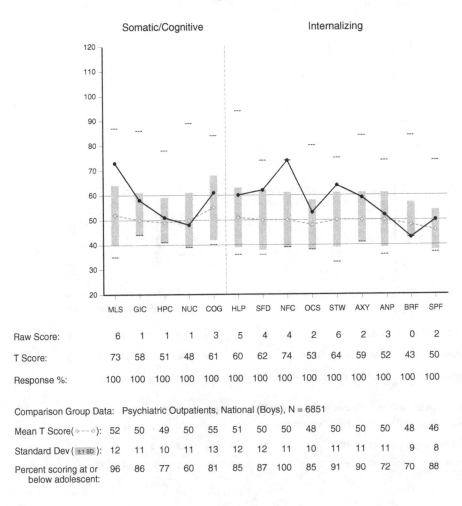

	MLS	GIC	HPC	NUC	COG	HLP	SFD	NFC	OCS	STW	AXY	ANP	BRF	SPF
Raw Score:	6	1	1	1	3	5	4	4	2	6	2	3	0	2
T Score:	73	58	51	48	61	60	62	74	53	64	59	52	43	50
Response %:	100	100	100	100	100	100	100	100	100	100	100	100	100	100

Comparison Group Data: Psychiatric Outpatients, National (Boys), N = 6851

	MLS	GIC	HPC	NUC	COG	HLP	SFD	NFC	OCS	STW	AXY	ANP	BRF	SPF
Mean T Score(◇‑‑‑◇):	52	50	49	50	55	51	50	50	48	50	50	50	48	46
Standard Dev (±1 SD):	12	11	10	11	13	12	12	11	10	11	11	11	9	8
Percent scoring at or below adolescent:	96	86	77	60	81	85	87	100	85	91	90	72	70	88

The highest and lowest T scores possible on each scale are indicated by a "---"; MMPI-A-RF T scores are non-gendered.

MLS	Malaise	HLP	Helplessness/Hopelessness
GIC	Gastrointestinal Complaints	SFD	Self-Doubt
HPC	Head Pain Complaints	NFC	Inefficacy
NUC	Neurological Complaints	OCS	Obsessions/Compulsions
COG	Cognitive Complaints	STW	Stress/Worry

AXY	Anxiety
ANP	Anger Proneness
BRF	Behavior-Restricting Fears
SPF	Specific Fears

MMPI-A-RF Externalizing and Interpersonal Scales

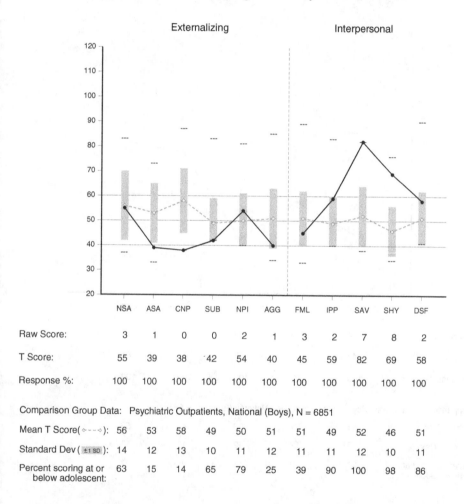

Externalizing   Interpersonal

	NSA	ASA	CNP	SUB	NPI	AGG	FML	IPP	SAV	SHY	DSF
Raw Score:	3	1	0	0	2	1	3	2	7	8	2
T Score:	55	39	38	42	54	40	45	59	82	69	58
Response %:	100	100	100	100	100	100	100	100	100	100	100

Comparison Group Data: Psychiatric Outpatients, National (Boys), N = 6851

	NSA	ASA	CNP	SUB	NPI	AGG	FML	IPP	SAV	SHY	DSF
Mean T Score(◇---◇):	56	53	58	49	50	51	51	49	52	46	51
Standard Dev (±1 SD):	14	12	13	10	11	12	11	11	12	10	11
Percent scoring at or below adolescent:	63	15	14	65	79	25	39	90	100	98	86

The highest and lowest T scores possible on each scale are indicated by a "---"; MMPI-A-RF T scores are non-gendered.

NSA	Negative School Attitudes		FML	Family Problems
ASA	Antisocial Attitudes		IPP	Interpersonal Passivity
CNP	Conduct Problems		SAV	Social Avoidance
SUB	Substance Abuse		SHY	Shyness
NPI	Negative Peer Influence		DSF	Disaffiliativeness
AGG	Aggression			

MMPI-A-RF Personality Psychopathology Five (PSY-5) Scales

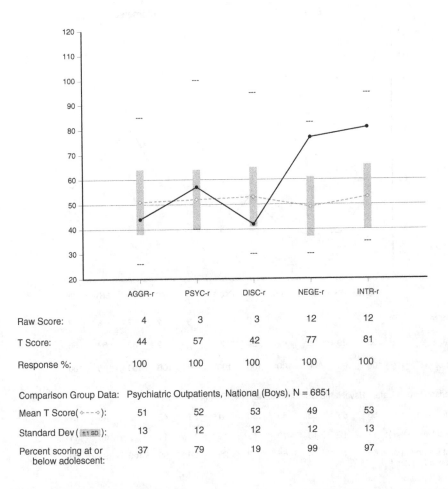

	AGGR-r	PSYC-r	DISC-r	NEGE-r	INTR-r
Raw Score:	4	3	3	12	12
T Score:	44	57	42	77	81
Response %:	100	100	100	100	100

Comparison Group Data: Psychiatric Outpatients, National (Boys), N = 6851

Mean T Score(◇---◇):	51	52	53	49	53
Standard Dev (±1 SD):	13	12	12	12	13
Percent scoring at or below adolescent:	37	79	19	99	97

The highest and lowest T scores possible on each scale are indicated by a "---"; MMPI-A-RF T scores are non-gendered.

AGGR-r   Aggressiveness-Revised
PSYC-r   Psychoticism-Revised
DISC-r   Disconstraint-Revised
NEGE-r   Negative Emotionality/Neuroticism-Revised
INTR-r   Introversion/Low Positive Emotionality-Revised

MMPI-A-RF T SCORES (BY DOMAIN)

PROTOCOL VALIDITY

Content Non-Responsiveness

1	47	50	43
CNS	VRIN-r	TRIN-r	CRIN

Over-Reporting

55
F-r

Under-Reporting

56	31
L-r	K-r

SUBSTANTIVE SCALES

Somatic/Cognitive Dysfunction

53	**73**	58	51	48	**61**
RC1	**MLS**	GIC	HPC	NUC	**COG**

Emotional Dysfunction

80
EID

74	60	62	74
RCd	HLP	SFD	NFC

75	81
RC2	INTR-r

63	53	64	59	52	43	50	77
RC7	OCS	STW	AXY	ANP	BRF	SPF	NEGE-r

Thought Dysfunction

54
THD

53*
RC6

52
RC8

57
PSYC-r

Behavioral Dysfunction

42
BXD

48	55	39	**38**	42	54
RC4	NSA	ASA	**CNP**	SUB	NPI

45	40	44	42
RC9	AGG	AGGR-r	DISC-r

Interpersonal Functioning

45	52	59	**82**	**69**	58
FML	RC3	IPP	**SAV**	**SHY**	DSF

---

*The adolescent provided scorable responses to less than 90% of the items scored on this scale. See the relevant profile page for the specific percentage.
Scale scores shown in bold font are interpreted in the report.

Note. This information is provided to facilitate interpretation following the recommended structure for MMPI-A-RF interpretation in Chapter 7 of the *MMPI-A-RF Administration, Scoring, Interpretation, and Technical Manual*, which provides details in the text and an outline in Table 7-1.

*This interpretive report is intended for use by a professional qualified to interpret the MMPI-A-RF.
The information it contains should be considered in the context of the adolescent's background, the
circumstances of the assessment, and other available information.*

SYNOPSIS

This is a valid MMPI-A-RF protocol. Scores on the substantive scales indicate somatic and cognitive
complaints, and emotional and interpersonal dysfunction. Somatic complaints relate to malaise.
Cognitive complaints include difficulties in memory and concentration. Emotional-internalizing findings
include **suicidal ideation**, demoralization, depression, generalized negative emotions, helplessness and
hopelessness, self-doubt, feelings of inefficacy, and stress and worry. Interpersonal difficulties include
social avoidance and social anxiety.

PROTOCOL VALIDITY

Content Non-Responsiveness

Unscorable Responses
The adolescent answered less than 90% of the items on the following scale. The resulting score may
therefore be artificially lowered. In particular, the absence of elevation on this scale is not interpretable.
A list of all items for which the adolescent provided unscorable responses appears under the heading
"Item-Level Information."

    Ideas of Persecution (RC6): 89%

Inconsistent Responding
The adolescent responded to the items in a consistent manner, indicating that he responded relevantly.

Over-Reporting

There are no indications of over-reporting in this protocol.

Under-Reporting

There are no indications of under-reporting in this protocol.

SUBSTANTIVE SCALE INTERPRETATION

Clinical symptoms, personality characteristics, and behavioral tendencies of the adolescent are described in this section and organized according to an empirically guided framework. Statements containing the word "reports" are based on the item content of MMPI-A-RF scales, whereas statements that include the word "likely" are based on empirical correlates of scale scores, as reported in Appendix G of the MMPI-A-RF manual. Specific sources for each statement can be accessed with the annotation features of this report.

Somatic/Cognitive Dysfunction

The adolescent reports experiencing poor health, weakness, and/or fatigue[1]. He likely presents with multiple somatic complaints[2] and complains of sleeplessness[3] and low energy and fatigue[4].

He reports a diffuse pattern of cognitive complaints[5] and indeed likely experiences attention problems[6], difficulties with concentration[7], and slow speech[6].

Emotional Dysfunction

The adolescent has responded in the keyed direction to one or more of the MMPI-A-RF items related to suicidal ideation or preoccupation with death. Please refer to the Critical Items section of the report. In addition, he received elevated scores on one or more scales that are correlated with suicidal ideation[8] and with suicide attempts or gestures[9].

His responses indicate considerable and pervasive emotional distress that is likely to be perceived as a crisis[10]. More specifically, he reports a lack of positive emotional experiences and being socially disengaged[11]. He likely experiences anhedonia[12] and psychomotor retardation[12]. He is likely difficult to motivate[13] and self-punishing[13].

The adolescent reports feeling sad and being dissatisfied with his current life circumstances[14]. He indeed likely feels sad and/or depressed[15] and that life is a strain[16] and has low self-esteem[17]. He also reports being indecisive and ineffective in coping with difficulties[18] and likely procrastinates[19]. In addition, he reports self-doubt, feelings of uselessness, and poor self-esteem[20]. He likely feels inferior[21] and is self-defeating[9], self-degrading[22], and passive[23]. He also reports feeling hopeless and helpless[24] and indeed likely feels hopeless[25] and like a failure[26] and believes he gets a raw deal from life[26] and cannot be helped[27]. He likely gives up easily[26]. He may engage in self-mutilation[26].

He reports an above-average level of negative emotional experiences including remorse and apprehensiveness[28]. He likely experiences anxiety[29], nightmares[30], and insecurity[30]. He also reports an above-average level of stress and worry[31].

Thought Dysfunction

There are no indications of disordered thinking in this protocol.

Behavioral Dysfunction

There are no indications of maladaptive externalizing behavior in this protocol. The adolescent reports a below-average number of conduct problems[32].

Interpersonal Functioning Scales

The adolescent reports substantial social avoidance and withdrawal[33] and very likely has few or no friends[34]. He very likely is introverted[35] and socially withdrawn and isolated[36]. He also very likely is socially awkward[37], may be bullied by peers[37], and may be uncomfortable with the opposite sex[37]. He also reports being shy, easily embarrassed, and uncomfortable around others[38]. He indeed likely is shy[39].

DIAGNOSTIC CONSIDERATIONS

This section provides recommendations for psychodiagnostic assessment based on the adolescent's MMPI-A-RF results. It is recommended that he be evaluated for the following:

Emotional-Internalizing Disorders

- Somatic Symptom Disorder and related disorders, if physical origins for malaise have been ruled out[40]
- Internalizing disorders[41]
- Depression-related disorders[42] and other conditions characterized by anhedonia[43]
- Anxiety-related disorders[44]
- Stress-related disorders[45]

Behavioral-Externalizing Disorders

- Attention Deficit/Hyperactivity Disorder (ADHD) and related neurodevelopmental disorders[46]

Interpersonal Disorders

- Disorders associated with social avoidance[47]
- Social Anxiety Disorder[48]

TREATMENT CONSIDERATIONS

This section provides inferential treatment-related recommendations based on the adolescent's MMPI-A-RF scores.

Areas for Further Evaluation

- **Evaluate risk for self-harm[49].**
- May require inpatient treatment due to significant depression[43].
- Evaluate need for antidepressant medication[43].
- Explore origin of cognitive complaints[46]. This may require a neuropsychological evaluation.

Psychotherapy Process Issues

- Malaise may impede his willingness or ability to engage in treatment[40].
- Emotional difficulties may motivate him for treatment[50].
- Significant lack of positive emotions and social isolation may interfere with engagement in therapy[43].

Possible Targets for Treatment

- Pronounced anhedonia[43]
- Psychological distress as an initial target[51]
- Passivity and indecisiveness[52]
- Low self-esteem and lack of confidence[53]
- Feelings of hopelessness and helplessness[54]
- Dysfunctional negative emotions[55]
- Stress management[45]
- Social avoidance[47]
- Social anxiety[48]

Special Note:
The content of the test items
is included in the actual reports.
To protect the integrity of the test,
the item content does not appear
in this sample report.

ITEM-LEVEL INFORMATION

Unscorable Responses

Following is a list of items to which the adolescent did not provide scorable responses. Unanswered or double answered (both True and False) items are unscorable. The scales on which the items appear are in parentheses following the item content.

26. Item Content Omitted. (TRIN-r, CRIN, THD, RC6)

Critical Responses

Six MMPI-A-RF scales--Helplessness/Hopelessness (HLP), Anxiety (AXY), Ideas of Persecution (RC6), Aberrant Experiences (RC8), Substance Abuse (SUB), and Aggression (AGG)--have been designated by the test authors as having critical item content that may require immediate attention and follow-up. Items answered by the adolescent in the keyed direction (True or False) on a critical scale are listed below if his T score on that scale is 60 or higher. The percentage of the MMPI-A-RF normative sample (NS) and of the Psychiatric Outpatients, National (Boys) comparison group (CG) that answered each item in the keyed direction are provided in parentheses following the item content.

Helplessness/Hopelessness (HLP, T Score = 60)
56. Item Content Omitted. (False; NS 31.6%, CG 28.1%)
60. Item Content Omitted. (True; NS 39.9%, CG 30.2%)
169. Item Content Omitted. (False; NS 17.1%, CG 19.0%)
228. Item Content Omitted. (True; NS 35.6%, CG 33.3%)
239. Item Content Omitted. (True; NS 40.9%, CG 49.1%)

Critical Items (Forbey & Ben-Porath)

The MMPI-A-RF contains a number of items whose content may indicate the presence of psychological problems when endorsed in the deviant direction. These "critical items" are adopted from the ones designated by Forbey and Ben-Porath for the MMPI-A (for details, see Forbey, J.D., & Ben-Porath, Y.S. [1998] A critical item set for the MMPI-A. Minneapolis, MN: University of Minnesota Press). Responses to critical items may provide an additional source of hypotheses about the adolescent; however, they should be used with caution because single item responses are unreliable. The percentage of the MMPI-A-RF normative sample (NS) and of the Psychiatric Outpatients, National (Boys) comparison group (CG) that answered each item in the keyed direction are provided in parentheses following the item content.

Anxiety
    170. Item Content Omitted.   (True; NS 12.4%, CG 23.3%)

Cognitive Problems
    126. Item Content Omitted.   (True; NS 17.0%, CG 20.2%)

Conduct Problems
    111. Item Content Omitted.   (True; NS 24.6%, CG 25.5%)

Depression/Suicidal Ideation
    46. Item Content Omitted. (True; NS 30.3%, CG 23.9%)
    69. Item Content Omitted.   (True; NS 20.1%, CG 26.0%)

Hallucinatory Experiences
    108. Item Content Omitted.   (True; NS 12.0%, CG 12.9%)

School Problems
    40. Item Content Omitted.   (True; NS 22.3%, CG 36.7%)

ENDNOTES

This section lists for each statement in the report the MMPI-A-RF score(s) that triggered it. In addition, each statement is identified as a Test Response (if based on item content), a Correlate (if based on empirical correlates), or an Inference (if based on the report authors' judgment). This information can also be accessed on-screen by placing the cursor on a given statement. Validity data supporting the correlate-based statements may be found in the MMPI-A-RF Administration, Scoring, Interpretation, and Technical Manual.

[1] Test Response: MLS=73
[2] Correlate: MLS=73; COG=61
[3] Correlate: MLS=73; STW=64
[4] Correlate: RC2=75; MLS=73; INTR-r=81
[5] Test Response: COG=61
[6] Correlate: COG=61
[7] Correlate: RCd=74; RC7=63; MLS=73; COG=61; STW=64; NEGE-r=77
[8] Correlate: RC7=63; HLP=60; SFD=62; NEGE-r=77
[9] Correlate: SFD=62
[10] Correlate: EID=80
[11] Test Response: RC2=75; INTR-r=81
[12] Correlate: RC2=75; INTR-r=81
[13] Correlate: RC2=75
[14] Test Response: RCd=74
[15] Correlate: RCd=74; RC2=75; HLP=60; SFD=62; NEGE-r=77; INTR-r=81
[16] Correlate: RCd=74
[17] Correlate: RCd=74; RC2=75; RC7=63; HLP=60; NEGE-r=77; INTR-r=81
[18] Test Response: NFC=74
[19] Correlate: NFC=74
[20] Test Response: SFD=62
[21] Correlate: SFD=62; SHY=69
[22] Correlate: RC2=75; SFD=62
[23] Correlate: SFD=62; NFC=74
[24] Test Response: HLP=60
[25] Correlate: RC2=75; HLP=60
[26] Correlate: HLP=60
[27] Correlate: HLP=60; INTR-r=81
[28] Test Response: RC7=63; NEGE-r=77
[29] Correlate: RCd=74; RC7=63; HLP=60; NFC=74; STW=64; NEGE-r=77
[30] Correlate: RC7=63
[31] Test Response: STW=64
[32] Test Response: CNP=38
[33] Test Response: SAV=82
[34] Correlate: SAV=82; SHY=69
[35] Correlate: RC2=75; SFD=62; SAV=82; SHY=69; INTR-r=81
[36] Correlate: RC2=75; SAV=82; SHY=69; INTR-r=81

[37] Correlate: SAV=82
[38] Test Response: SHY=69
[39] Correlate: SHY=69
[40] Inference: MLS=73
[41] Inference: EID=80
[42] Inference: RCd=74; RC2=75; HLP=60; SFD=62; NEGEr-r=77; INTR-r=81
[43] Inference: RC2=75
[44] Inference: RC7=63; NEGE-r=77; INTR-r=81
[45] Inference: STW=64
[46] Inference: COG=61
[47] Inference: SAV=82
[48] Inference: SHY=69
[49] Inference: RC7=63; HLP=60; SFD=62
[50] Inference: EID=80; RCd=74; RC7=63; NEGE-r=77
[51] Inference: RCd=74
[52] Inference: NFC=74
[53] Inference: SFD=62
[54] Inference: HLP=60
[55] Inference: RC7=63; NEGE-r=77

End of Report

REFERENCES

Achenbach, T. M. (1978). Psychopathology of childhood: Research problems and issues. *Journal of Consulting and Clinical Psychology, 46,* 759–776.

Achenbach, T. M., & Edelbrock, C. S. (1983). *Manual for the Child Behavior Checklist and revised child behavior profile.* Burlington: University of Vermont.

Albert, D., Chein, J., & Steinberg, L. (2013). The teenage brain: Peer influences on adolescent decision making. *Current Directions in Psychological Science, 22,* 114–120.

Alperin, J. J., Archer, R. P., & Coates, G. D. (1996). Development and effects of an MMPI-A K-correction procedure. *Journal of Personality Assessment, 67,* 155–168.

American Psychiatric Association. (1994). *Diagnostic and statistical manual of mental disorders* (4th ed.). Washington, DC: Author.

American Psychological Association. (1986). Committee on psychological tests and assessment (CPTA). *Guidelines for computer-based tests and interpretations.* Washington, DC: Author.

American Psychological Association (2002). *Developing adolescents: A reference for professionals.* Washington: DC: American Psychological Association.

Anastasi, A. (1982). *Psychological testing* (5th ed.). New York: MacMillan.

Andrucci, G. L., Archer, R. P., Pancoast, D. L., & Gordon, R. A. (1989). The relationship of MMPI and sensation seeking scales to adolescent drug use. *Journal of Personality Assessment, 53,* 253–266.

Anthony, N. (1976). Malingering as role taking. *Journal of Clinical Psychology, 32,* 32–41.

Archer, R. P. (1984). Use of the MMPI with adolescents: A review of salient issues. *Clinical Psychology Review, 4,* 241–251.

Archer, R. P. (1987a). MMPI adolescent interpretive system [Computer program]. Odessa, FL: Psychological Assessment Resources, Inc.

Archer, R. P. (1987b). *Using the MMPI with adolescents.* Hillsdale, NJ: Lawrence Erlbaum Associates.

Archer, R. P. (1989). *MMPI assessment of adolescent clients* (Clinical notes on the MMPI, Monograph No. 12). Minneapolis, MN: National Computer Systems.

Archer, R. P. (1990). Responses of adolescents on the MMPI-2: Comparisons with MMPI findings. In R. C. Colligan (Chair), *The MMPI and adolescents: Historical perspective, current research, and future developments.* Symposium conducted at the annual convention of the American Psychological Association, Boston, MA.

Archer, R. P. (1992). Review of the Minnesota Multiphasic Personality Inventory-2 (MMPI-2). In *The Eleventh Mental Measurements Yearbook* (pp. 558–562). Lincoln: Buros Institute of Mental Measurements, University of Nebraska.

Archer, R. P. (1995). *MMPI-A interpretive system* (Version 2) [Computer program]. Odessa, FL: Psychological Assessment Resources, Inc.

Archer, R. P. (1997a). Future directions for the MMPI-A: Research and Clinical Issues. *Journal of Personality Assessment, 68,* 95–109.

Archer, R. P. (1997b). *MMPI-A: Assessing adolescent psychopathology (2nd edition).* Mahwah, NJ: Lawrence Erlbaum Associates.

Archer, R. P. (2003). *MMPI-A interpretive system (Version 3).* [computer program]. Odessa: FL. Psychological Assessment Resources, Inc.

Archer, R.P. (2005). Implications of MMPI/MMPI-A findings for understanding adolescent development and psychopathology. *Journal of Personality Assessment, 8,* 257–270.

Archer, R. P. (2006). A perspective on the Restructured Clinical (RC) scale project. *Journal of Personality Assessment, 87(2),* 179–185.

Archer, R.P. (2013). *MMPI-A interpretive system (Version 5).* [Computer program]. Lutz, FL: Psychological Assessment Resources, Inc.

Archer, R. P., Aiduk, R., Griffin, R., & Elkins, D. E. (1996). Incremental validity of the MMPI-2 content scales in a psychiatric sample. *Assessment, 3,* 79–90.

Archer, R. P., Ball, J. D., & Hunter, J. A. (1985). MMPI characteristics of borderline psychopathology in adolescent inpatients. *Journal of Personality Assessment, 49,* 47–55.

Archer, R.P., Buffington-Vollum, J.K., Stredny, R.V., & Handel, R.W. (2006). A survey of psychological test use patterns among forensic psychologists. *Journal of Personality Assessment, 87,* 84–94.

Archer, R. P., & Elkins, D. E. (1999). Identification of random responding on the MMPI-A. *Journal of Personality Assessment, 73,* 407–421.

Archer, R. P., Fontaine, J., & McCrae, R. R. (1998). Effects of two MMPI-2 validity scales on basic scale relations to external criteria. *Journal of Personality Assessment, 70,* 87–102.

Archer, R. P., & Gordon, R. A. (1988). MMPI and Rorschach indices of schizophrenic and depressive diagnoses among adolescent inpatients. *Journal of Personality Assessment, 52,* 276–287.

Archer, R. P., & Gordon, R. A. (1991a). [Correlational analysis of the MMPI-A normative dataset]. Unpublished raw data.

Archer, R. P., & Gordon, R. A. (1991b, August). Use of content scales with adolescents: Past and future practices. In R. C. Colligan (Chair), *MMPI and MMPI-2 supplementary scales and profile interpretation – content scales revisited.* Symposium conducted at the annual convention of the American Psychological Association, San Francisco, CA.

Archer, R. P., & Gordon, R. A. (1994). Psychometric stability of MMPI-A item modifications. *Journal of Personality Assessment, 62,* 416–426.

Archer, R. P., Gordon, R. A., Anderson, G. L., & Giannetti, R. A. (1989). MMPI special scale clinical correlates for adolescent inpatients. *Journal of Personality Assessment, 53,* 654–664.

Archer, R. P., Gordon, R. A., Giannetti, R. A., & Singles, J. M. (1988). MMPI scale clinical correlates for adolescent inpatients. *Journal of Personality Assessment, 52,* 707–721.

Archer, R. P., Gordon, R. A., & Kirchner, F. H. (1987). MMPI response-set characteristics among adolescents. *Journal of Personality Assessment, 51,* 506–516.

Archer, R. P., Gordon, R. A., & Klinefelter, D. (1991). [Analyses of the frequency of MMPI and MMPI-A profile assignments for 1762 adolescent patients]. Unpublished raw data.

Archer, R. P., Griffin, R., & Aiduk, R. (1995). MMPI-2 clinical correlates for ten common codes. *Journal of Personality Assessment, 65,* 391–407.

Archer, R. P., Handel, R. W., Ben-Porath, Y. S., & Tellegen, A. (2016a). *Minnesota Multiphasic Personality Inventory – Adolescent – Restructured Form (MMPI-A-RF): Administration, Scoring, Interpretation, and Technical Manual.* Minneapolis: University of Minnesota Press.

Archer, R. P., Handel, R. W., Ben-Porath, Y. S., & Tellegen, A. (2016b). *Minnesota Multiphasic Personality Inventory – Adolescent – Restructured Form (MMPI-A-RF): User's Guide for Reports.* Minneapolis: University of Minnesota Press.

Archer, R. P., Handel, R. W., & Lynch, K. D. (2001). The effectiveness of MMPI-A items in discriminating between normative and clinical samples. *Journal of Personality Assessment, 77,* 420–435.

Archer, R. P., Handel, R. W., Lynch, K. D., & Elkins, D. E. (2002). MMPI-A validity scale uses and limitations in detecting varying levels of random responding. *Journal of Personality Assessment, 78,* 417–431.

Archer, R. P., & Jacobson, J. M. (1993). Are critical items "critical" for the MMPI-A? *Journal of Personality Assessment, 61,* 547–556.

Archer, R. P., & Klinefelter, D. (1991). MMPI factor analytic findings for adolescents: Item- and scale-level factor structures. *Journal of Personality Assessment, 57,* 356–367.

Archer, R. P., & Klinefelter, D. (1992). Relationships between MMPI codetypes and *MAC* scale elevations in adolescent psychiatric samples. *Journal of Personality Assessment, 58,* 149–159.

Archer, R. P., & Krishnamurthy, R. (2002). *Essentials of MMPI-A Assessment.* New York: John Wiley & Sons.

Archer, R. P., Maruish, M., Imhof, E. A., & Piotrowski, C. (1991). Psychological test usage with adolescent clients: 1990 survey findings. *Professional Psychology: Research and Practice, 22,* 247–252.

Archer, R. P., & Newsom, C. R. (2000). Psychological test usage with adolescent clients: Survey update. *Assessment, 7,* 227–235.

Archer, R. P., Pancoast, D. L., & Gordon, R. A. (1994). The development of the MMPI-A Immaturity (IMM) scale: Findings for normal and clinical samples. *Journal of Personality Assessment, 62,* 145–156.

Archer, R. P., Pancoast, D. L., & Klinefelter, D. (1989). A comparison of MMPI code types produced by traditional and recent adolescent norms. *Psychological Assessment: A Journal of Consulting and Clinical Psychology, 1,* 23–29.

Archer, R. P., & Slesinger, D. (1999). MMPI-A patterns related to the endorsement of suicidal ideation. *Assessment, 6,* 51–59.

Archer, R. P., Stolberg, A. L., Gordon, R. A., & Goldman, W. R. (1986). Parent and child MMPI responses: Characteristics among families with adolescents in inpatient and outpatient settings. *Journal of Abnormal Child Psychology, 14,* 181–190.

Archer, R. P., Tirrell, C. A., & Elkins, D. E. (2001). Evaluation of an MMPI-A short form: Implications for adaptive testing. *Journal of Personality Assessment, 76,* 76–89.

Archer, R. P., White, J. L., & Orvin, G. H. (1979). MMPI characteristics and correlates among adolescent psychiatric inpatients. *Journal of Clinical Psychology, 35,* 498–504.

Arita, A. A., & Baer, R. (1998). Validity of selected MMPI-A content scales. *Psychological Assessment, 10,* 59–63.

Baer, R. A., Ballenger, J., Berry, D. T. R., & Wetter, M. W. (1997). Detection of random responding on the MMPI-A. *Journal of Personality Assessment, 68,* 139–151.

Baer, R. A., Wetter, M. W., & Berry, D. T. R. (1995). Effects of information about validity scales on underreporting of symptoms on the MMPI-2: An analogue investigation. *Assessment, 2,* 189–200.

Bagby, R. M., Buis, T., & Nicholson, R. A. (1995). Relative effectiveness of the standard validity scales in detecting fake-bad and fake-good responding: Replication and extension. *Psychological Assessment, 7,* 84–92.

Bagby, R. M., Rogers, R., & Buis, T. (1994). Detecting malingering and defensive responding on the MMPI-2 on a forensic inpatient sample. *Journal of Personality Assessment, 62,* 191–203.

Bagby, R. M., Rogers, R., Buis, T., Nicholson, R. A., Cameron, S. L., Rector, N. A., Schuller, D. R., & Seeman, M. V. (1997). Detecting feigned depression and schizophrenia on the MMPI-2. *Journal of Personality Assessment, 68,* 650–664.

Bagdade, P. S. (2004). *Malingering on the MMPI-A: An investigation of the standard validity scales and the infrequency-psychopathology scale – adolescent version (fp-A)* (Doctoral dissertation). Available from ProQuest Dissertations & Theses Global. (UMI No. 3098566).

Ball, J. C. (1960). Comparison of MMPI profile differences among Negro-white adolescents. *Journal of Clinical Psychology, 16,* 304–307.

Ball, J. C. (1962). *Social deviancy and adolescent personality: An analytical study with the MMPI.* Lexington: University of Kentucky Press.

Ball, J. C., & Carroll, D. (1960). Analysis of MMPI Cannot Say scores in an adolescent population. *Journal of Clinical Psychology, 16,* 30–31.

Ball, J. D., Archer, R. P., & Imhof, E. A. (1994). Time requirements of psychological testing: A survey of practitioners. *Journal of Personality Assessment, 63,* 239–249.

Ball, J. D., Archer, R. P., Struve, F. A., Hunter, J. A., & Gordon, R. A. (1987). MMPI correlates of a controversial EEG pattern among adolescent psychiatric patients. *Journal of Clinical Psychology, 43,* 708–714.

Bandura, A. (1964). The stormy decade: Fact or fiction? *Psychology in the School, 1,* 224–231.

Barron, F. (1953). An ego-strength scale which predicts response to psychotherapy. *Journal of Consulting Psychology, 17,* 327–333.

Basham, R. B. (1992). Clinical utility of the MMPI research scales in the assessment of adolescent acting out behaviors. *Psychological Assessment, 4,* 483–492.

Baum, L.J., Archer, R.P., Forbey, J.D., & Handel, R.W. (2009). A review of the Minnesota Multiphasic Personality Inventory-Adolescent (MMPI-A) and the Millon Adolescent Clinical Inventory (MACI) with an emphasis on juvenile justice samples. *Assessment, 16,* 384–400.

Bell, H. M. (1934). *Adjustment Inventory.* Stanford, CA: Stanford University Press.

Bence, V. M., Sabourin, C., Luty, D. T., & Thackrey, M. (1995). Differential sensitivity of the MMPI-2 depression scales and subscales. *Journal of Clinical Psychology, 51,* 375–377.

Ben-Porath, Y. S. (1990). MMPI-2 items. In J. N. Butcher (Ed.), *MMPI-2 news and profiles: A newsletter of the MMPI-2 workshops and symposia* (Vol. 1, No 1, (pp. 8–9). Minneapolis: University of Minnesota Press.

Ben-Porath, Y. S. (1994). The ethical dilemma of coached malingering research. *Psychological Assessment, 6,* 14–15.

Ben-Porath, Y.S. (2012). *Interpreting the MMPI-2-RF*. Minneapolis: University of Minnesota Press.

Ben-Porath, Y. S., Butcher, J. N., & Graham, J. R. (1991). Contribution of the MMPI-2 content scales to the differential diagnosis of schizophrenia and major depression. *Psychological Assessment, 3*, 634–640.

Ben-Porath, Y. S., & Forbey, J. D. (2003). *Non-gendered norms for the MMPI-2*. Minneapolis: University of Minnesota Press.

Ben-Porath, Y.S., Graham, J.R., Archer, R.P., Tellegen, A., & Kaemmer, B. (2006). *Supplement to the MMPI-A manual for administration, scoring, and interpretation.* Minneapolis: University of Minnesota Press.

Ben-Porath, Y. S., Hostetler, K., Butcher, J. N., & Graham, J. R. (1989). New subscales for the MMPI-2 Social Introversion (Si) scale. *Psychological Assessment: A Journal of Consulting and Clinical Psychology, 1*, 169–174.

Ben-Porath, Y. S., McCully, E., & Almagor, M. (1993). Incremental validity of the MMPI-2 content scales in the assessment of personality and psychopathology by self-report. *Journal of Personality Assessment, 61*, 557–575.

Ben-Porath, Y. S., & Sherwood, N. E. (1993). *The MMPI-2 content component scales* (MMPI-2/MMPI-A Test Reports, No. 1) Minneapolis: University of Minnesota Press.

Ben-Porath, Y. S., Slutske, W. S., & Butcher, J. N. (1989). A real-data simulation of computerized adaptive administration of the MMPI. *Psychological Assessment: A Journal of Consulting and Clinical Psychology, 1*, 18–22.

Ben-Porath, Y. S., & Tellegen, A. (1995). How (not) to evaluate the comparability of MMPI and MMPI-2 profile configurations: A reply to Humphrey and Dahlstrom. *Journal of Personality Assessment, 65*, 52–58.

Ben-Porath, Y. S., & Tellegen, A. (2008/2011). *MMPI-2-RF (Minnesota Multiphasic Personality Inventory-2 Restructured Form): Manual for administration, scoring, and interpretation*. Minneapolis, MN: University of Minnesota Press.

Bernreuter, R. G. (1933). The theory and construction of the Personality Inventory. *Journal of Social Psychology, 4*, 387–405.

Berry, D. T. R., Wetter, M. W., Baer, R. A., Larsen, L., Clark, C., & Monroe, K. (1992). MMPI-2 random responding indices: Validation using a self-report methodology. *Psychological Assessment, 4*, 340–345.

Berry, D. T. R., Wetter, M. W., Baer, R. A., Widiger, T. A., Sumpter, J. C., Reynolds, S. K., & Hallam, R. A. (1991). Detection of random responding on the MMPI-2: Utility of F, back F and VRIN scales. *Psychological Assessment: A Journal of Consulting and Clinical Psychology, 3*, 418–423.

Bertelson, A. D., Marks, P. A., & May, G. D. (1982). MMPI and race: A controlled study. *Journal of Consulting and Clinical Psychology, 50*, 316–318.

Black, K. (1994). A critical review of the MMPI-A. *Child Assessment News, 4*, 9–12.

Blais, M. A. (1995). MCMI-II personality traits associated with the MMPI-2 masculinity-femininity scale. *Assessment, 2*, 131–136.

Blos, P. (1962). *On adolescence: A psychoanalytic interpretation*. New York: The Free Press.

Blos, P. (1967). The second individuation process of adolescence. *Psychoanalytic Study of the Child, 22*, 162–186.

Bolinskey, P. K., Arnau, R. C., Archer, R. P., & Handel, R. W. (2004) A replication of the MMPI-A PSY-5 scales and development of facet subscales. *Assessment, 11(1)*, 40–48.

Bonfilio, S. A., & Lyman, R. D. (1981). Ability to simulate normalcy as a function of differential psychopathology. *Psychological Reports, 49*, 15–21.

Bonnie, R.J., & Scott, E.S. (2013). The teenage brain: Adolescent brain research and the law. *Current Directions in Psychological Science, 22,* 158–161.

Boone, D. (1994). Reliability of the MMPI-2 subtle and obvious scales with psychiatric inpatients. *Journal of Personality Assessment, 62,* 346–351.

Boone, D. (1995). Differential validity of the MMPI-2 subtle and obvious scales with psychiatric inpatients: Scale 2. *Journal of Clinical Psychology, 51,* 526–531.

Brandenburg, N. A., Friedman, R. M., & Silver, S. E. (1989). The epidemiology of childhood psychiatric disorders: Prevalence findings from recent studies. *Journal of the American Academy of Child and Adolescent Psychiatry, 29,* 76–83.

Brauer, B. A. (1992). The signer effect on MMPI performance of deaf respondents. *Journal of Personality Assessment, 58,* 380–388.

Brems, C., & Johnson, M. E. (1991). Subtle-Obvious scales of the MMPI: Indicators of profile validity in a psychiatric population. *Journal of Personality Assessment, 56,* 536–544.

Breton, J. J., Bergeron, L., Valla, J. P., Berthiaume, C., Gaudet, N., Lambert, J., Saint-Georges, M., Houde, L., & Lepine, S. (1999). Quebec child mental health survey: Prevalence of DSM-III-R mental health disorders. *Journal of Child Psychology and Psychiatry and Allied Disciplines, 40,* 375–384.

Briggs, P. F., Wirt, R. D., & Johnson, R. (1961). An application of prediction tables to the study of delinquency. *Journal of Consulting Psychology, 25,* 46–50.

Brophy, A.L. (2005). Note on Meunier and Bodkins's (2005) "Interpretation of MMPI-A Scale 5 with female patients." *Psychological Reports, 97,* 673–674.

Burke, K. C., Burke, J. D., Regier, D. A., & Rae, D. S. (1990). Age at onset of selected mental disorders in five community populations. *Archives of General Psychiatry, 47,* 511–518.

Butcher, J. N. (1985). Why MMPI short forms should not be used for clinical predictions. In J. N. Butcher & J. R. Graham (Eds.), *Clinical applications of the MMPI* (pp. 10–11). Minneapolis: University of Minnesota Department of Conferences.

Butcher, J. N. (1987a). Computerized clinical and personality assessment using the MMPI. In J. N. Butcher (Ed.), *Computerized psychological assessment: A practitioner's guide* (pp. 161–197). New York: Basic Books.

Butcher, J. N. (Ed.) (1987b). *Computerized psychological assessment: A practitioner's guide.* New York: Basic Books.

Butcher, J. N. (1990). *MMPI-2 in psychological treatment.* New York: Oxford University Press.

Butcher, J. N. (2005). Exploring universal personality characteristics: An objective approach. *International journal of clinical and health psychology, 5,* 554–566.

Butcher, J.N., Cabiya, J., Lucio, E., & Garrido, M. (2007). Assessing Hispanic clients with the MMPI-A. In *Assessing Hispanic clients using the MMPI-2 and MMPI-A* (pp. 163–198). Washington, DC: American Psychological Association.

Butcher, J. N., Dahlstrom, W. G., Graham, J. R., Tellegen, A., & Kaemmer, B. (1989). *Minnesota Multiphasic Personality Inventory-2 (MMPI-2): Manual for administration and scoring.* Minneapolis: University of Minnesota Press.

Butcher, J. N., Graham, J. R., & Ben-Porath, Y. S. (1995). Methodological problems and issues in MMPI, MMPI-2, and MMPI-A research. *Psychological Assessment, 7,* 320–329.

Butcher, J. N., Graham, J. R., Ben-Porath, Y. S., Tellegen, A., Dahlstrom, W. G., & Kaemmer, B. (2001). *Minnesota Multiphasic Personality Inventory–2 (MMPI-2). Manual for administration, scoring, and interpretation (rev. ed.).* Minneapolis: University of Minnesota Press.

Butcher, J. N., Graham, J. R., Williams, C. L., & Ben-Porath, Y. S. (1990). *Development and use of the MMPI-2 content scales.* Minneapolis: University of Minnesota Press.

Butcher, J. N., & Hostetler, K. (1990). Abbreviating MMPI item administration: What can be learned from the MMPI for the MMPI-2? *Psychological Assessment: A Journal of Consulting and Clinical Psychology, 2,* 12–21.

Butcher, J. N., & Owen, P. L. (1978). Objective personality inventories: Recent research and some contemporary issues. In B. B. Wolman (Ed.), *Clinical diagnosis of mental disorders: A handbook* (pp. 475–545). New York: Plenum.

Butcher, J. N., Perry, J. N., & Atlis, M. M. (2000). Validity and utility of computer-based test interpretation. *Psychological Assessment, 12,* 6–18.

Butcher, J. N., & Tellegen, A. (1978). Common methodological problems in MMPI research. *Journal of Consulting and Clinical Psychology, 46,* 620–628.

Butcher, J. N., & Williams, C. L. (1992). *The Minnesota report: Adolescent interpretive system* [Computer program]. Minneapolis, MN: National Computer Systems.

Butcher, J. N., & Williams, C. L. (2000). *Essentials of MMPI-2 and MMPI-A interpretation (2nd ed.).* Minneapolis: University of Minnesota Press.

Butcher, J. N., Williams, C. L., Graham, J. R., Archer, R. P., Tellegen, A., Ben-Porath, Y. S., & Kaemmer, B. (1992). *MMPI-A (Minnesota Multiphasic Personality Inventory–Adolescent): Manual for administration, scoring, and interpretation.* Minneapolis: University of Minnesota Press.

Caldwell, A. B. (1969). *MMPI critical items.* Unpublished mimeograph. (Available from Caldwell Report, 1545 Sawtelle Boulevard, Ste. 14, Los Angeles, CA 90025.)

Caldwell, A. B. (1971, April). *Recent advances in automated interpretation of the MMPI.* Paper presented at the sixth annual MMPI Symposium, Minneapolis, MN.

Caldwell, A. B. (1977a). *Questions people ask when taking the MMPI.* (Special Bulletin No. 3, available from Caldwell Report, 1545 Sawtelle Blvd., Ste. 14, Los Angeles, CA 90025.)

Caldwell, A. B. (1988). *MMPI supplemental scale manual.* Los Angeles: Caldwell Report.

Calvin, J. (1975). *A replicated study of the concurrent validity of the Harris subscales for the MMPI.* Unpublished doctoral dissertation, Kent State University, Kent, OH.

Cantwell, D. P., Lewinsohn, P. M., Rohde, P., & Seeley, J. R. (1997). Correspondence between adolescent report and parent report of psychiatric diagnostic data. *Journal of the American Academy of Child and Adolescent Psychiatry, 36,* 610–619.

Capwell, D. F. (1945a). Personality patterns of adolescent girls. I. Girls who show improvement in IQ. *Journal of Applied Psychology, 29,* 212–228.

Capwell, D. F. (1945b). Personality patterns of adolescent girls. II. Delinquents and non-delinquents. *Journal of Applied Psychology, 29,* 284–297.

Carlson, D. A. (2001). *Computerized vs. written administration of the MMPI-A in clinical and non-clinical settings* (Doctoral dissertation). Available from ProQuest Dissertations & Theses Global (UMI No. 3006665).

Casey, B.J., & Caudle, K. (2013). The teenage brain: Self-control. *Current Directions in Psychological Science, 22,* 82–87.

Cashel, M. L., Rogers, R., Sewell, K. W., & Holliman, N. G. (1998). Preliminary validation of the MMPI-A for a male delinquent sample. An investigation of clinical correlates and discriminant validity. *Journal of Personality Assessment, 71,* 46–69.

Center for Disease Control and Prevention (2007). *Suicide trends among youths and young adults aged 10–24 years—United States, 1990–2004* [Online]. Available: http://www.cdc.gov/mmwr/preview/mmwrhtml/mm5635a2.htm.

Center for Disease Control and Prevention (2009). *Suicide rates among persons ages 10 years and older, by race/ethnicity, United States, 2005–2009 [Online]. Available:* http://www.cdc.gov/violenceprevention/suicide/statistics/rates01.html.

Center for Disease Control and Prevention (2009). *Trends in suicide rates among persons ages 10 years and older, by sex, United States, 1991–2009* [Online]. Available: http://www.cdc.gov/violenceprevention/suicide/statistics/trends01.html.

Center for Disease Control and Prevention (2012). *Suicide facts at a glance* [Online]. Available: http://www.cdc.gov/violenceprevention/pdf/Suicide-DataSheet-a.pdf

Cheung, F. M., Song, W., & Butcher, J. N. (1991). An infrequency scale for the Chinese MMPI. *Psychological Assessment: A Journal of Consulting and Clinical Psychology, 3,* 648–653.

Choi, H., Kurtz, E.G., & Proctor, T.B. (2012). Concurrent evidence for validity of the MMPI-A substance abuse scales in a school setting. *The International Journal of Educational and Psychological Assessment, 11,* 108–119.

Clark, M. E. (1994). Interpretive limitations of the MMPI-2 anger and cynicism content scales. *Journal of Personality Assessment, 63,* 89–96.

Clavelle, P. R. (1992). Clinicians' perceptions of the comparability of the MMPI and MMPI-2. *Psychological Assessment, 4,* 466–472.

Clopton, J. R. (1978). MMPI scale development methodology. *Journal of Personality Assessment, 42,* 148–151.

Clopton, J. R. (1979). Development of special MMPI scales. In C. S. Newmark (Ed.), *MMPI: Clinical and research trends* (pp. 354–372). New York: Praeger.

Clopton, J. R. (1982). MMPI scale development methodology reconsidered. *Journal of Personality Assessment, 46,* 143–146.

Clopton, J. R., & Neuringer, C. (1977). MMPI Cannot Say scores: Normative data and degree of profile distortion. *Journal of Personality Assessment, 41,* 511–513.

Cohn, L. D. (1991). Sex differences in the course of personality development: A meta-analysis. *Psychological Bulletin, 109,* 252–266.

Colligan, R. C. (Chair). (1988, August). *MMPI subscales and profile interpretation: Harris and Lingoes revisited.* Symposium conducted at the annual convention of the American Psychological Association, Atlanta, GA.

Colligan, R. C., & Offord, K. P. (1985). Revitalizing the MMPI: The development of contemporary norms. *Psychiatric Annals, 15,* 558–568.

Colligan, R. C., & Offord, K. P. (1989). The aging MMPI: Contemporary norms for contemporary teenagers. *Mayo Clinic Proceedings, 64,* 3–27.

Colligan, R. C., & Offord, K. P. (1991). Adolescents, the MMPI, and the issue of K-correction: A contemporary normative study. *Journal of Clinical Psychology, 47,* 607–631.

Colligan, R. C., & Offord, K. P. (1992). Age, stage, and the MMPI: Changes in response patterns over an 85-year age span. *Journal of Clinical Psychology, 48,* 476–493.

Colligan, R. C., & Osborne, D. (1977). MMPI profiles from adolescent medical patients. *Journal of Clinical Psychology, 33,* 186–189.

Colligan, R. C., Osborne, D., & Offord, K. P. (1980). Linear transformation and the interpretation of MMPI T-scores. *Journal of Clinical Psychology, 36,* 162–165.

Colligan, R. C., Osborne, D., & Offord, K. P. (1984). Normalized transformations and the interpretation of MMPI T-scores: A reply to Hsu. *Journal of Consulting and Clinical Psychology, 52,* 824–826.

Colligan, R. C., Osborne, D., Swenson, W. M., & Offord, K. P. (1983). *The MMPI: A contemporary normative study.* New York: Praeger.

Conkey, V. A. (2000). *Determining the sensitivity of the MMPI-A to random responding and malingering in adolescents* (Doctoral dissertation). Available from ProQuest Dissertations & Theses Global. (UMI No. 9935389).

Corrales, M. L., Cabiya, J. J., Gomes, F., Ayala, G. X., Mendoza, S., & Velasquez, R. J. (1998). MMPI-2 and MMPI-A research with U.S. Latinos: A bibliography. *Psychological Reports, 83,* 1027–1033.

Costello, E. J., Angold, A., Borns, B. J., Stangl, D. K., Tweed, D. L., Erkanli, A., & Worthman, C. M. (1996). The great smoky mountain study of youth: Goals, design, methods, and the prevalence of DSM-III-R disorders. *Archives of General Psychiatry, 53,* 1129–1137.

Costello, E.J., Copeland, W., & Angold, A.A. (2012). Trends in psychopathology across the adolescent years: What changes when children become adolescents, and when adolescents become adults? *Journal of Child Psychology and Psychiatry, 52,* 1015–1025.

Cross, T.L., Adams, C., Dixon, F., & Holland, J. (2004). Psychological characteristics of academically gifted adolescents attending a residential academy: A longitudinal study. *Journal for the Education of the Gifted, 28,* 159–181.

Cross, T.L., Cassady, J.C., Dixon, F.A., & Adams, C.M. (2008). The psychology of gifted adolescents as measured by the MMPI-A. *Gifted Child Quarterly, 52,* 326–339.

Cumella, E. J., Wall, A. D., & Kerr-Almeida, N. (1999). MMPI-A in the inpatient assessment of adolescents with eating disorders. *Journal of Personality Assessment, 73,* 31–44.

Dahlstrom, W. G. (1992). Comparability of two-point high-point code patterns from original MMPI norms to MMPI-2 norms for the restandardization sample. *Journal of Personality Assessment, 59,* 153–164.

Dahlstrom, W. G., Archer, R. P., Hopkins, D. G., Jackson, E., & Dahlstrom, L. E. (1994). *Assessing the readability of the Minnesota Multiphasic Personality Inventory instruments: The MMPI, MMPI-2, MMPI-A* (MMPI-2/MMPI-A Test Reports No. 2). Minneapolis: University of Minnesota Press.

Dahlstrom, W. G., & Dahlstrom, L. E. (Eds.) (1980). Basic *readings on the MMPI: A new selection on personality measurement.* Minneapolis: University of Minnesota Press.

Dahlstrom, W. G., Lachar, D., & Dahlstrom, L. E. (1986). *MMPI patterns of American minorities.* Minneapolis: University of Minnesota Press.

Dahlstrom, W. G., & Welsh, G. S. (1960). *An MMPI handbook: A guide to use in clinical practice and research.* Minneapolis: University of Minnesota Press.

Dahlstrom, W. G., Welsh, G. S., & Dahlstrom, L. E. (1972). *An MMPI handbook: Vol. I. Clinical interpretation* (rev. ed.). Minneapolis: University of Minnesota Press.

Dahlstrom, W. G., Welsh, G. S., & Dahlstrom, L. E. (1975). *An MMPI handbook: Vol. II. Research applications* (rev. ed.). Minneapolis: University of Minnesota Press.

Dannenbaum, S. E., & Lanyon, R. I. (1993). The use of subtle items in detecting deception. *Journal of Personality Assessment, 61,* 501–510.

Dodrill, C. B., & Clemmons, D. (1984). Use of neuropsychological tests to identify high school students with epilepsy who later demonstrate inadequate performances in life. *Journal of Consulting and Clinical Psychology, 52,* 520–527.

Drake, L. E. (1946). A social I-E Scale for the MMPI. *Journal of Applied Psychology, 30,* 51–54.

Edwards, D. W., Morrison, T. L., & Weissman, H. N. (1993a). The MMPI and MMPI-2 in an outpatient sample: Comparisons of code types, validity scales, and clinical scales. *Journal of Personality Assessment, 61,* 1–18.

Edwards, D. W., Morrison, T. L., & Weissman, H. N. (1993b). Uniform versus linear T-scores on the MMPI-2/MMPI in an outpatient psychiatric sample: Differential contributions. *Psychological Assessment, 5,* 499–500.

Ehrenworth, N. V. (1984). *A comparison of the utility of interpretive approaches with adolescent MMPI profiles.* Unpublished doctoral dissertation, Virginia Consortium for Professional Psychology, Norfolk, VA.

Ehrenworth, N. V., & Archer, R. P. (1985). A comparison of clinical accuracy ratings of interpretive approaches for adolescent MMPI responses. *Journal of Personality Assessment, 49,* 413–421.

Elkind, D. (1978). Understanding the young adolescent. *Adolescence, 13,* 127–134.

Elkind, D. (1980). Egocentrism in adolescence. In R. E. Muuss (Ed.), *Adolescent behavior and society: A book of readings* (3rd ed., pp. 79–88). New York: Random House.

Elkind, D., & Bowen, R. (1979). Imaginary audience behavior in children and adolescents. *Developmental Psychology, 15,* 38–44.

Endicott, J., & Spitzer, R. L. (1978). A diagnostic interview: the schedule for affective disorders and schizophrenia. *Archives of general psychiatry, 35,* 837–844.

Erikson, E. H. (1956). The concept of ego identity. *The Journal of the American Psychoanalytic Association, 4,* 56–121.

Exner, J. E., Jr., McDowell, E., Pabst, J., Stackman, W., & Kirk, L. (1963). On the detection of willful falsifications in the MMPI. *Journal of Consulting Psychology, 27,* 91–94.

Finlay, S. W., & Kapes, J. T. (2000). Scale 5 of the MMPI and MMPI-2: Evidence of disparity. *Assessment, 7,* 97–101.

Finn, S. E. (1996). *Manual for using the MMPI-2 as a therapeutic intervention.* Minneapolis: University of Minnesota Press.

Finn, S. E., & Tonsager, M. E. (1992). Therapeutic effects of providing MMPI-2 test feedback to college students awaiting therapy. *Psychological Assessment, 4,* 278–287.

Flesch, R. (1948). A new readability yardstick. *Journal of Applied Psychology, 32,* 221–233.

Foerstner, S. B. (1986). *The factor structure and factor stability of selected Minnesota Multiphasic Personality Inventory (MMPI) subscales: Harris and Lingoes subscales, Wiggins content scales, Wiener subscales, and Serkownek subscales.* Unpublished doctoral dissertation, University of Akron, Akron, OH.

Fontaine, J. L., Archer, R. P., Elkins, D. E., & Johansen, J. (2001). The effects of MMPI-A T-score elevation on classification accuracy for normal and clinical adolescent samples. *Journal of Personality Assessment, 76,* 264–281.

Forbey, J. D., & Ben-Porath, Y. S. (1998). *A critical item set for the MMPI-A (MMPI-2/MMPI-A test reports #4).* Minneapolis: University of Minnesota Press.

Forbey, J. D., & Ben-Porath, Y. S. (2003). Incremental validity of the MMPI-A content scales in a residential treatment facility. *Assessment, 10(2),* 191–202.

Forbey, J.D., Ben-Porath, Y.S., & Graham, J.R. (2005, April). *MMPI-A critical item endorsement frequencies across settings.* Poster session presented at the 40th Annual Symposium on Recent Research with the MMPI-2/MMPI-A. Fort Lauderdale, FL.

Forbey, J. D., Handel, R. W., & Ben-Porath, Y. S. (2000). Real data simulation of computerized adaptive administration of the MMPI-A. *Computers in Human Behavior, 16,* 83–96.

Fowler, R. D. (1964, September). *Computer processing and reporting of personality test data.* Paper presented at the annual meeting of the American Psychological Association, Los Angeles, CA.

Fowler, R. D. (1985). Landmarks in computer-assisted psychological assessment. *Journal of Consulting and Clinical Psychology, 53,* 748–759.

Freud, A. (1958). Adolescence. *Psychoanalytic Study of the Child, 13,* 255–278.

Friedman, A.F., Archer, R.P., & Handel, R.W. (2005). Minnesota Multiphasic Personality Inventories (MMPI/MMPI-2, MMPI-A) and suicide. In R.I. Yufit & D. Lester (Eds.), *Assessment, treatment, and prevention of suicidal behavior* (pp. 63–91). Hoboken: John Wiley & Sons.

Friedman, A.F., Bolinskey, P.K., Levak, R.W., & Nichols, D.S. (2015). *Psychological assessment with the MMPI-2/MMPI-2-RF.* New York: Routledge.

Friedman, A. F., Lewak, R., Nichols, D. S. & Webb, J. T. (2001). *Psychological assessment with the MMPI-2.* Mahwah, NJ: Lawrence Erlbaum Associates.

Friedman, A.F., Webb, J.T., & Lewak, R. (1989). *Psychological assessment with the MMPI.* Hillsdale, NJ: Lawrence Erlbaum Associates.

Friedman, J. M. H., Asnis, G. M., Boeck, M., & DiFiore, J. (1987). Prevalence of specific suicidal behaviors in a high school sample. *American Journal of Psychiatry, 144,* 1203–1206.

Gallucci, N. T. (1994). Criteria associated with clinical scales and Harris–Lingoes subscales of the Minnesota Multiphasic Personality Inventory with adolescent inpatients. *Psychological Assessment, 6,* 179–187.

Gallucci, N. T. (1997a). Correlates of MMPI-A substance abuse scales. *Assessment, 4,* 87–94.

Gallucci, N. T. (1997b). On the identification of patterns of substance abuse with the MMPI-A. *Psychological Assessment, 3,* 224–232.

Gantner, A., Graham, J., & Archer, R. P. (1992). Usefulness of the *MAC* scale in differentiating adolescents in normal, psychiatric, and substance abuse settings. *Psychological Assessment, 4,* 133–137.

Gilberstadt, H., & Duker, J. (1965). *A handbook for clinical and actuarial MMPI interpretation.* Philadelphia: Saunders.

Gocka, E. F., & Holloway, H. (1963). *Normative and predictive data on the Harris and Lingoes subscales for a neuropsychiatric population* (Rep. No. 7). American Lake, WA: Veterans Administration Hospital.

Goldberg, L. R. (1965). Diagnosticians vs. diagnostic signs: The diagnosis of psychosis vs. neurosis from the MMPI. *Psychological Monographs, 79* (9, Whole No. 602).

Goldberg, L. R. (1972). Man vs. mean: The exploitation of group profiles for the construction of diagnostic classification systems. *Journal of Abnormal Psychology, 79,* 121–131.

Goldman, V. J., Cooke, A., & Dahlstrom, W. G. (1995). Black-white differences among college students: A comparison of MMPI and MMPI-2 norms. *Assessment, 2,* 293–299.

Gottesman, I. I., Hanson, D. R., Kroeker, T. A., & Briggs, P. F. (1987). New MMPI normative data and power-transformed T-score tables for the Hathaway-Monachesi Minnesota cohort of 14,019 fifteen-year-olds and 3,674 eighteen-year-olds. In R. P. Archer, *Using the MMPI with adolescents* (pp. 241–297). Hillsdale, NJ: Lawrence Erlbaum Associates.

Gottesman, I. I., & Prescott, C. A. (1989). Abuses of the MacAndrew Alcoholism scale: A critical review. *Clinical Psychology Review, 9,* 223–242.

Gough, H. G. (1947). Simulated patterns on the MMPI. *Journal of Abnormal and Social Psychology, 42,* 215–225.

Gough, H. G. (1954). Some common misconceptions about neuroticism. *Journal of Consulting Psychology, 18,* 287–292.

Gould, M. S., Wunsch-Hitzig, R., & Dohrenwend, B. (1981). Estimating the prevalence of child psychopathology: A critical review. *Journal of the American Academy of Child Psychiatry, 20,* 462–476.

Graham, J. R. (2000). *MMPI-2: Assessing personality and psychopathology* (3rd ed.). New York: Oxford University Press.

Graham, J.R. (2012). *MMPI-2: Assessing personality and psychopathology* (5th ed.). New York: University of Oxford Press, Inc.

Graham, J. R., Ben-Porath, Y. S., & McNulty, J. L. (1999). *MMPI-2 Correlates for Outpatient Community Mental Health Settings.* Minneapolis: University of Minnesota Press.

Graham, J. R., Schroeder, H. E., & Lilly, R. S. (1971). Factor analysis of items on the Social Introversion and Masculinity-Femininity scales of the MMPI. *Journal of Clinical Psychology, 27,* 367–370.

Graham, J. R., Timbrook, R. E., Ben-Porath, Y. S., & Butcher, J. N. (1991). Code-type congruence between MMPI and MMPI-2: Separating fact from artifact. *Journal of Personality Assessment, 57,* 205–215.

Graham, J. R., Watts, D., & Timbrook, R. E. (1991). Detecting fake-good and fake-bad MMPI-2 profiles. *Journal of Personality Assessment, 57,* 264–277.

Graham, P., & Rutter, M. (1985). Adolescent disorders. In M. Rutter & L. Hovsov (Eds.), *Child and adolescent psychiatry: Modern approaches* (pp. 351–367). Oxford, England: Blackwell. *

Graham v. Florida, 130 S. Ct. 2011, 560 U.S. 48, 176 L. Ed. 2d 825 (2010).

Grayson, H. M. (1951). *A psychological admissions testing program and manual.* Los Angeles: Veterans Administration Center, Neuropsychiatric Hospital.

Grayson, H. M., & Olinger, L. B. (1957). Simulation of "normalcy" by psychiatric patients on the MMPI. *Journal of Consulting Psychology, 21,* 73–77.

Green, S. B., & Kelley, C. K. (1988). Racial bias in prediction with the MMPI for a juvenile delinquent population. *Journal of Personality Assessment, 52,* 263–275.

Greene, R.L. (1980). *The MMPI: An interpretive manual.* New York: Grune & Stratton.

Greene, R. L. (1982). Some reflections on "MMPI short forms: A literature review." *Journal of Personality Assessment, 46,* 486–487.

Greene, R. L. (1987). Ethnicity and MMPI performance: A review. *Journal of Consulting and Clinical Psychology, 55,* 497–512.

Greene, R. L. (1988). Introduction. In R. L. Greene (Ed.), *The MMPI: Use with specific populations* (pp. 1–21). San Antonio, TX: Grune & Stratton.

Greene, R. L. (1989a). *Assessing the validity of MMPI profiles in clinical settings* (Clinical notes on the MMPI, Monograph No. 11). Minneapolis, MN: National Computer Systems.

Greene, R. L. (1989b). *MMPI adult interpretive system* [Computer program]. Odessa, FL: Psychological Assessment Resources, Inc.

Greene, R. L. (1991). *The MMPI-2/MMPI: An interpretive manual.* Boston: Allyn & Bacon.

Greene, R. L. (1994). Relationships among MMPI codetype, gender, and setting in the MacAndrew Alcoholism Scale. *Assessment, 1,* 39–46.

Greene, R. L. (2000). *MMPI-2: An interpretive manual* (2nd ed.). Boston: Allyn & Bacon.

Greene, R.L. (2011). *The MMPI-2/MMPI-2-RF: An interpretive manual* (3rd ed.). Boston: Allyn & Bacon.

Greene, R. L., Arredondo, R., & Davis, H. G. (1990, August). *The comparability between the MacAndrew Alcoholism Scale-Revised (MMPI-2) and the MacAndrew Alcoholism Scale*

(MMPI). Paper presented at the annual meeting of the American Psychological Association, Boston, MA.

Greene, R. L., & Garvin, R. D. (1988). Substance abuse/dependence. In R. L. Greene (Ed.), *The MMPI: Use in specific populations* (pp. 157–197). San Antonio, TX: Grune & Stratton.

Grossman, H. Y., Mostofsky, D. I., & Harrison, R. H. (1986). Psychological aspects of Gilles de la Tourette Syndrome. *Journal of Clinical Psychology, 42*, 228–235.

Groth-Marnat, G. (2003). *Handbook of psychological assessment* (4th ed.). New York: John Wiley and Sons.

Groth-Marnat, G., & Schumaker, J. (1989). Computer-based psychological testing: Issues and guidelines. *American Journal of Orthopsychiatry, 59*, 257–263.

Gumbiner, J. (1997). Comparison of scores on the MMPI-A and the MMPI-2 for young adults. *Psychological Reports, 81*, 787–794.

Gumbiner, J. (1998). MMPI-A profiles of Hispanic adolescents. *Psychological Reports, 82*, 659–672.

Gumbiner, J. (2000). Limitations in ethnic research on the MMPI-A. *Psychological Reports, 87*, 1229–1230.

Gynther, M. D. (1972). White norms and black MMPIs: A prescription for discrimination? *Psychological Bulletin, 78*, 386–402.

Gynther, M. D. (1989). MMPI comparisons of blacks and whites: A review and commentary. *Journal of Clinical Psychology, 45*, 878–883.

Hall, G. S. (1904). *Adolescence: Its psychology and its relationship to physiology, anthropology, sociology, sex, crime, religion, and education.* New York: Appleton.

Hand, C.G., Archer, R.P., Handel, R.W., & Forbey, J.D. (2007). The classification accuracy of the Minnesota Multiphasic Personality Inventory-Adolescent: Effects of modifying the normative sample. *Assessment, 14*, 80–85.

Handel, R.W., Archer, R.P., Elkins, D.E., Mason, J.A., & Simonds-Bisbee, E.C. (2011). Psychometric properties of the Minnesota Multiphasic Personality Inventory-Adolescent (MMPI-A) clinical, content, and supplementary scales in a forensic sample. *Journal of Personality Assessment, 93*, 566–581.

Handel, R.W., Arnau, R.C., Archer, R.P., & Dandy, K.L. (2006). An evaluation of the MMPI-2 and MMPI-A True Response Inconsistency (TRIN) Scales. *Assessment, 13*, 98–106.

Hanson, D. R., Gottesman, I. I., & Heston, L. L. (1990). Long-range schizophrenia forecasting: Many a slip twixt cup and lip. In J. E. Rolf, A. Masten, D. Cicchetti, K. Neuchterlein, & S. Weintraub (Eds.), *Risk and protective factors in the development of psychopathology* (pp. 424–444). New York: Cambridge University Press.

Harkness, A.R., Finn, J.A., McNulty, J.L., & Shields, S.M. (2012). The Personality Psychopathy-Five (PSY-5): Recent constructive replication and assessment literature review. *Psychological Assessment, 24*, 432–443.

Harkness, A. R., & McNulty, J. L. (1994). The Personality Psychopathology Five (PSY-5): Issues from the pages of a diagnostic manual instead of a dictionary. In S. Strack and M. Lorr, *Differentiating normal and abnormal personality.* New York, NY: Springer Publishing Co.

Harkness, A. R., McNulty., J. L., & Ben-Porath, Y. S. (1995). The Personality Psychopathology Five (PSY-5): Constructs and MMPI-2 Scales. *Psychological Assessment, 7(1)*, 104–114.

Harkness, A. R., McNulty, J. L., Ben-Porath, Y. S., & Graham, J. R. (2002). *MMPI-2 Personality Psychopathology Five (PSY-5) Scales: Graining an overview for case conceptualization and treatment planning* (MMPI-2/MMPI-A Test Reports). Minneapolis: The University of Minnesota Press.

Harper, D. C. (1983). Personality correlates and degree of impairment in male adolescents with progressive and nonprogressive physical disorders. *Journal of Clinical Psychology, 39,* 859–867.

Harper, D. C., & Richman, L. C. (1978). Personality profiles of physically impaired adolescents. *Journal of Clinical Psychology, 34,* 636–642.

Harrell, T. H., Honaker, L. M., & Parnell, T. (1992). Equivalence of the MMPI-2 with the MMPI in psychiatric patients. *Psychological Assessment, 4,* 460–465.

Harris, R. E., & Christiansen, C. (1946). Prediction of response to brief psychotherapy. *Journal of Psychology, 21,* 269–284.

Harris, R. E., & Lingoes, J. C. (1955). *Subscales for the MMPI: An aid to profile interpretation.* Department of Psychiatry, University of California School of Medicine and the Langley Porter Clinic, mimeographed materials.

Hathaway, S. R. (1939). The personality inventory as an aid in the diagnosis of psychopathic inferiors. *Journal of Consulting Psychology, 3,* 112–117.

Hathaway, S. R. (1947). A coding system for MMPI profiles. *Journal of Consulting Psychology, 11,* 334–337.

Hathaway, S. R. (1956). Scales 5 (Masculinity-Femininity), 6 (Paranoia), and 8 (Schizophrenia). In G. S. Welsh & W. G. Dahlstrom (Eds.), *Basic readings on the MMPI in psychology and medicine* (pp. 104–111). Minneapolis: University of Minnesota Press.

Hathaway, S. R. (1964). MMPI: Professional use by professional people. *American Psychologist, 19,* 204–210.

Hathaway, S. R. (1965). Personality inventories. In B. B. Wolman (Ed.), *Handbook of clinical psychology* (pp. 451–476). New York: McGraw-Hill.

Hathaway, S. R., & Briggs, P. F. (1957). Some normative data on new MMPI scales. *Journal of Clinical Psychology, 13,* 364–368.

Hathaway, S. R., & McKinley, J. C. (1940). A multiphasic personality schedule (Minnesota): 1. Construction of the schedule. *Journal of Psychology, 10,* 249–254.

Hathaway, S. R., & McKinley, J. C. (1942). A multiphasic personality schedule (Minnesota): 3. The measurement of symptomatic depression. *Journal of Psychology, 14,* 73–84.

Hathaway, S. R., & McKinley, J. C. (1943). *The Minnesota Multiphasic Personality Inventory* (rev. ed.). Minneapolis: University of Minnesota Press.

Hathaway, S. R., & McKinley, J. C. (1967). *Minnesota Multiphasic Personality Inventory manual* (rev. ed.). New York: Psychological Corporation.

Hathaway, S. R., & Monachesi, E. D. (1951). The prediction of juvenile delinquency using the Minnesota Multiphasic Personality Inventory. *American Journal of Psychiatry, 108,* 469–473.

Hathaway, S. R., & Monachesi, E. D. (1952). The Minnesota Multiphasic Personality Inventory in the study of juvenile delinquents. *American Sociological Review, 17,* 704–710.

Hathaway, S. R., & Monachesi, E. D. (Eds.). (1953). *Analyzing and predicting juvenile delinquency with the MMPI.* Minneapolis: University of Minnesota Press.

Hathaway, S. R., & Monachesi, E. D. (1961). *An atlas of juvenile MMPI profiles.* Minneapolis: University of Minnesota Press.

Hathaway, S. R., & Monachesi, E. D. (1963). *Adolescent personality and behavior: MMPI patterns of normal, delinquent, dropout, and other outcomes.* Minneapolis: University of Minnesota Press.

Hathaway, S. R., Monachesi, E. D., & Salasin, S. (1970). A follow-up study of MMPI high 8, schizoid children. In M. Roff & D. F. Ricks (Eds.), *Life history research in psychopathology* (pp. 171–188). Minneapolis: University of Minnesota Press.

Hathaway, S. R., Reynolds, P. C., & Monachesi, E. D. (1969). Follow-up of the later careers and lives of 1,000 boys who dropped out of high school. *Journal of Consulting and Clinical Psychology, 33,* 370–380.

Hays, S. K. (2003). *A computer-administered version versus paper-and-pencil administered version of the MMPI-A* (Doctoral dissertation). Available from ProQuest Dissertations & Theses Global (UMI No. 3075545).

Hays, S., & McCallum, R.S. (2005). A comparison of the pencil-and-paper and computer-administrated Minnesota Multiphasic Personality Inventory-Adolescent. *Psychology in the Schools,* 605–613.

Hedlund, J. L., & Won Cho, D. (1979). [MMPI data research tape for Missouri Department of Mental Health patients]. Unpublished raw data.

Henry, L.M. (1999). *Comparison of MMPI and MMPI-A response patterns of African American adolescents* (Doctoral dissertation). Available from ProQuest Dissertations & Theses Global (UMI No. 9933767).

Herkov, M. J., Archer, R. P., & Gordon, R. A. (1991). MMPI response sets among adolescents: An evaluation of the limitations of the Subtle-Obvious subscales. *Psychological Assessment: A Journal of Consulting and Clinical Psychology, 3,* 424–426.

Herkov, M.J., Gordon, R.A., Gynther, M.D., & Greer, R.A. (1994). Perceptions of MMPI item subtlety: Influences of age and ethnicity. *Journal of Personality Assessment, 62,* 9–16.

Herman-Giddens, M. E., Slora, E. J., Wasserman, R. C., Bourdony, C. J., Bhapkar, M. B., Koch, G. G., & Hasemeier, C. M. (1997). Secondary sexual characteristics and menses in young girls seen in office practice: A study from the pediatric research in office settings network. *Pediatrics, 99,* 505–512.

Hillard, J. R., Slomowitz, M., & Levi, L. S. (1987). A retrospective study of adolescents' visits to a general hospital psychiatric emergency service. *American Journal of Psychiatry, 144,* 432–436.

Hilts, D., & Moore, J. M. (2003). Normal range MMPI profiles among psychiatric inpatients. *Assessment, 10,* 266–272.

Hoffmann, A. D., & Greydanus, D. E. (1997). *Adolescent Medicine.* Stamford, CT: Appleton & Lange.

Hoffmann, N. G., & Butcher, J. N. (1975). Clinical limitations of three MMPI short forms. *Journal of Consulting and Clinical Psychology, 43,* 32–39.

Hofstra, M. B., van der Ende, J., & Verhulst, F. C. (2002). Child and adolescent problems predict DSM-IV disorders in adulthood: A 14-year follow-up of a Dutch epidemiological sample. *Journal of the American Academy of Child & Adolescent Psychiatry, 41,* 182–189.

Hollrah, J. L., Schlottmann, R. S., Scott, A. B., & Brunetti, D. G. (1995). Validity of the MMPI subtle scales. *Journal of Personality Assessment, 65,* 278–299.

Holmbeck, G. N., & Updegrove, A. L. (1995). Clinical-development interface: Implications of developmental research for adolescent psychotherapy. *Psychotherapy, 32,* 16–33.

Holt, R. R. (1980). Loevinger's measure of ego development: Reliability and national norms for male and female short forms. *Journal of Personality and Social Psychology, 39,* 909–920.

Honaker, L. M. (1990). MMPI and MMPI-2: Alternate forms or different tests? In M. E. Maruish (Chair), *The MMPI and MMPI-2: Comparability examined from different perspectives.* Symposium conducted at the annual convention of the American Psychological Association, Boston, MA.

Huesmann, L. R., Lefkowitz, M. M., & Eron, L. D. (1978). Sum of MMPI Scales *F*, *4*, and *9* as a measure of aggression. *Journal of Consulting and Clinical Psychology, 46*, 1071–1078.

Humm, D. G., & Wadsworth, G. W. (1935). The Humm-Wadsworth Temperament Scale. *American Journal of Psychiatry, 92*, 163–200.

Humphrey, D. H., & Dahlstrom, W. G. (1995). The impact of changing from the MMPI to the MMPI-2 on profile configurations. *Journal of Personality Assessment, 64*, 428–439.

Husband, S. D., & Iguchi, M. Y. (1995). Comparison of MMPI-2 and MMPI clinical scales and high-point scores among methadone maintenance patients. *Journal of Personality Assessment, 64*, 371–375.

Imhof, E. A., & Archer, R. P. (1997). Correlates of the MMPI-A immaturity (IMM) scale in an adolescent psychiatric sample. *Assessment, 5*, 169–179.

Janus, M. D., de Grott, C., & Toepfer, S. M. (1998). The MMPI-A and 13-year-old inpatients: How young is too young? *Assessment, 5*, 321–332.

Janus, M. D., Toepfer, S., Calestro, K., & Tolbert, H. (1996). *Within normal limits profiles and the MMPI-A.* Unpublished manuscript.

Janus, M. D., Tolbert, H., Calestro, K., & Toepfer, S. (1996). Clinical accuracy ratings of MMPI approaches for adolescents: Adding ten years and the MMPI-A. *Journal of Personality Assessment, 67*, 364–383.

Johnson, R. H., & Bond, G. L. (1950). Reading ease of commonly used tests. *Journal of Applied Psychology, 34*, 319–324.

Kaplowitz, P. B., & Oberfield, S. E. (1999). Reexamination of the age limit for defining when puberty is precocious in girls in the United States: Implications for evaluation and treatment. *Pediatrics, 104*, 936–941.

Kashani, J. H., Beck, N., Hoeper, E. W., Fallahi, C., Corcoran, C. M., McAllister, J. A., Rosenberg, T. K., & Reid, J. C. (1987). Psychiatric disorders in a community sample of adolescents. *American Journal of Psychiatry, 144*, 584–589.

Kashani, J. H., & Orvaschel, H. (1988). Anxiety disorders in mid-adolescence: A community sample. *American Journal of Psychiatry, 145*, 960–964.

Kaufman, J., Birmaher, B., Brent, D., Rao, U. M. A., Flynn, C., Moreci, P., & Ryan, N. (1997). Schedule for affective disorders and schizophrenia for school-age children-present and lifetime version (K-SADS-PL): Initial reliability and validity data. *Journal of the American Academy of Child & Adolescent Psychiatry, 36*, 980–988.

Kazdin, A. E. (2000). Adolescent development, mental disorders, and decision making of delinquent youths in P. Grisso and R. G. Schwartz (Eds.), *Youth on trial: A developmental perspective on juvenile justice* (pp. 33–65). Chicago: University of Chicago Press.

Kelley, C. K., & King, G. D. (1979). Cross-validation of the 2-8/8-2 MMPI codetype for young adult psychiatric outpatients. *Journal of Personality Assessment, 43*, 143–149.

Kimmel, D. C., & Weiner, I. B. (1985). *Adolescence: A developmental transition.* Hillsdale, NJ: Lawrence Erlbaum Associates.

Kincannon, J. C. (1968). Prediction of the standard MMPI scale scores from 71 items: The Mini-Mult. *Journal of Consulting and Clinical Psychology, 32*, 319–325.

King, G. D., & Kelley, C. K. (1977). MMPI behavioral correlates of spike-5 and two-point codetypes with Scale 5 as one elevation. *Journal of Clinical Psychology, 33*, 180–185.

Klinge, V., Lachar, D., Grissell, J., & Berman, W. (1978). Effects of scoring norms on adolescent psychiatric drug users' and nonusers' MMPI profiles. *Adolescence, 13,* 1–11.

Klinge, V., & Strauss, M. E. (1976). Effects of scoring norms on adolescent psychiatric patients' MMPI profiles. *Journal of Personality Assessment, 40,* 13–17.

Kohutek, K. J. (1992a). The location of items of the Wiggins content scales on the MMPI-2. *Journal of Clinical Psychology, 48,* 617–620.

Kohutek, K. J. (1992b). Wiggins content scales and the MMPI-2. *Journal of Clinical Psychology, 48,* 215–218.

Kopper, B. A., Osman, A., Osman, J. R., & Hoffman, J. (1998). Clinical utility of the MMPI-A content scales and Harris–Lingoes subscales in the assessment of suicidal risk factors in psychiatric adolescents. *Journal of Clinical Psychology, 54,* 191–200.

Koss, M. P., & Butcher, J. N. (1973). A comparison of psychiatric patients' self-report with other sources of clinical information. *Journal of Research in Personality, 7,* 225–236.

Krakauer, S. (1991). *Assessing reading-deficit patterns among adolescents' MMPI profiles.* Unpublished doctoral dissertation, Virginia Consortium for Professional Psychology, Norfolk.

Krishnamurthy, R., Archer, R. P., & Huddleston, E. N. (1995). Clinical research note on psychometric limitations of two Harris–Lingoes subscales for the MMPI-2. *Assessment, 2,* 301–304.

Krug, S. E. (1993). *Psychware Sourcebook (4th ed.).* Kansas City, MO: Test Corporation of America.

Lachar, D. (1974). *The MMPI: Clinical assessment and automated interpretation.* Los Angeles: Western Psychological Services.

Lachar, D., Klinge, V., & Grissell, J. L. (1976). Relative accuracy of automated MMPI narratives generated from adult norm and adolescent norm profiles. *Journal of Consulting and Clinical Psychology, 44,* 20–24.

Lachar, D., & Wrobel, T. A. (1979). Validating clinicians' hunches: Construction of a new MMPI critical item set. *Journal of Consulting and Clinical Psychology, 47,* 277–284.

Lachar, D., & Wrobel, N. H. (1990, August). Predicting adolescent MMPI correlates: Comparative efficacy of self-report and other-informant assessment. In R. C. Colligan (Chair) *The MMPI and adolescents: Historical perspectives, current research, and future developments.* A symposium presented to the annual convention of the American Psychological Association, Boston, MA.

Lamb, D. G., Berry, D. T. R., Wetter, M. W., & Baer, R. A. (1994). Effects of two types of information on malingering of closed head injury on the MMPI-2: Analogue investigation. *Psychological Assessment, 6,* 8–13.

Landis, C., & Katz, S. E. (1934). The validity of certain questions which purport to measure neurotic tendencies. *Journal of Applied Psychology, 18,* 343–356.

Lanyon, R. I. (1967). Simulation of normal and psychopathic MMPI personality patterns. *Journal of Consulting Psychology, 31,* 94–97.

Lanyon, R. I. (1987). The validity of computer-based personality assessment products: Recommendations for the future. *Computers in Human Behavior, 3,* 225–238.

Lees-Haley, P. R., Smith, H. H., Williams, C. W., & Dunn, J. T. (1996). Forensic neuropsychological test usage: An empirical survey. *Archives of Clinical Neuropsychology, 11,* 41–51.

Levitt, E. E. (1989). *The clinical application of MMPI special scales.* Hillsdale, NJ: Lawrence Erlbaum Associates.

Levitt, E. E., Browning, J. M., & Freeland, L. J. (1992). The effect of MMPI-2 on the scoring of special scales derived from MMPI-1. *Journal of Personality Assessment, 59,* 22–31.

Levitt, E. E., & Gotts, E. E. (1995). *The clinical applications of MMPI special scales* (2nd ed.). Hillsdale, NJ: Lawrence Erlbaum Associates.

Lewak, R. W., Marks, P. A., & Nelson, G. E. (1990). *Therapist guide to the MMPI & MMPI-2: Providing feedback and treatment.* Muncie, IN: Accelerated Development, Inc.

Lewandowski, D., & Graham, J. R. (1972). Empirical correlates of frequently occurring two-point code types: A replicated study. *Journal of Consulting and Clinical Psychology, 39,* 467–472.

Lewinsohn, P. M., Hops, H., Roberts, R. E., Seeley, J. R., & Andrews, J. A. (1993). Adolescent psychopathology: I. Prevalence and incidence of depression in other DSM-III-R disorders in high school students. *Journal of Abnormal Psychology, 102,* 133–144.

Lewinsohn, P. M., Klein, D. N., & Seeley, J. R. (1995). *Journal of the American Academy of Child and Adolescent Psychiatry, 34,* 454–463.

Lindsay, K. A., & Widiger, T. A. (1995). Sex and gender bias in self-report personality disorder inventories: Item analyses of the MCMI-II, MMPI, and PDQ-R. *Journal of Personality Assessment, 65,* 1–20.

Loevinger, J. (1976). *Ego development: Conceptions and theories.* San Francisco: Jossey-Bass.

Loevinger, J., & Wessler, R. (1970). *Measuring ego development: Vol. I. Construction and use of a Sentence Completion Test.* San Francisco: Jossey-Bass.

Long, K. A., & Graham, J. R. (1991). The masculinity-femininity scale of MMPI-2: Is it useful with normal men in an investigation conducted with the MMPI-2? *Journal of Personality Assessment, 57,* 46–51.

Losada-Paisey, G. (1998). Use of the MMPI-A to assess personality of juvenile male delinquents who are sex offenders and non-sex offenders. *Psychological Reports, 83,* 115–122.

Lowman, J., Galinsky, M. D., & Gray-Little, B. (1980). *Predicting achievement: A ten-year follow-up of black and white adolescents.* Chapel Hill: The University of North Carolina at Chapel Hill, Institute for Research in Social Science (IRSS Research Reports).

Lubin, B., Larsen, R. M., & Matarazzo, J. D. (1984). Patterns of psychological test usage in the United States: 1935–1982. *American Psychologist, 39,* 451–454.

Lubin, B., Larsen, R. M., Matarazzo, J. D., & Seever, M. F. (1985). Psychological test usage patterns in five professional settings. *American Psychologist, 40,* 857–861.

Lubin, B., Wallis, R. R., & Paine, C. (1971). Patterns of psychological test usage in the United States: 1935–1969. *Professional Psychology, 2,* 70–74.

Lueger, R. J. (1983). The use of the MMPI-168 with delinquent adolescents. *Journal of Clinical Psychology, 39,* 139–141.

Lumry, A. E., Gottesman, I. I., & Tuason, V. B. (1982). MMPI state dependency during the course of bipolar psychosis. *Psychiatric Research, 7,* 59–67.

Luty, D., & Thackrey, M. (1993). Graphomotor interpretation of the MMPI-2? *Journal of Personality Assessment, 60,* 604.

Lynch, K. D., Archer, R. P., & Handel, R. W. (2004). The relationship of MMPI-A item effectiveness to item content, diagnostic category, and classification accuracy. Manuscript in review.

MacAndrew, C. (1965). The differentiation of male alcoholic out-patients from non-alcoholic psychiatric patients by means of the MMPI. *Quarterly Journal of Studies on Alcohol, 26,* 238–246.

MacAndrew, C. (1979). On the possibility of psychometric detection of persons prone to the abuse of alcohol and other substances. *Addictive Behaviors, 4,* 11–20.

MacAndrew, C. (1981). What the MAC scale tells us about men alcoholics: An interpretive review. *Journal of Studies on Alcohol, 42,* 604–625.

MacBeth, L., & Cadow, B. (1984). Utility of the MMPI-168 with adolescents. *Journal of Clinical Psychology, 40,* 142–148.

Marcia, J. E. (1966). Development and validation of ego identity status. *Journal of Personality and Social Psychology, 3,* 551–558.

Marks, P. A., & Briggs, P. F. (1972). Adolescent norm tables for the MMPI. In W. G. Dahlstrom, G. S. Welsh, & L. E. Dahlstrom, *An MMPI handbook: Vol. 1. Clinical interpretation* (rev. ed., pp. 388–399). Minneapolis: University of Minnesota Press.

Marks, P. A., & Haller, D. L. (1977). Now I lay me down for keeps: A study of adolescent suicide attempts. *Journal of Clinical Psychology, 33,* 390–400.

Marks, P. A., & Lewak, R. W. (1991). *The Marks MMPI adolescent feedback and treatment report* [Computer program]. Los Angeles: Western Psychological Services.

Marks, P. A., & Seeman, W. (1963). *The actuarial description of personality: An atlas for use with the MMPI.* Baltimore: Williams & Wilkins.

Marks, P. A., Seeman, W., & Haller, D. L. (1974). *The actuarial use of the MMPI with adolescents and adults.* Baltimore: Williams & Wilkins.

Markwardt, F. C. (1989). *Peabody Individual Achievement Test - Revised.* Circle Pines, MN: American Guidance Service.

Martin, H., & Finn, S. E. (2010). *Masculinity and femininity in the MMPI-2 and MMPI-A.* Minneapolis: University of Minnesota Press.

Matarazzo, J. D. (1983). Computerized psychological testing. *Science, 221,* 323.

Matarazzo, J. D. (1986). Computerized clinical psychological test interpretations: Unvalidated plus all mean and no sigma. *American Psychologist, 41,* 14–24.

McCarthy, L., & Archer, R. P. (1998). Factor structure of the MMPI-A content scales: Item-level and scale-level findings. *Journal of Personality Assessment, 7,* 84–97.

McDonald, R. L., & Gynther, M. D. (1962). MMPI norms for southern adolescent Negroes. *Journal of Social Psychology, 58,* 277–282.

McFarland, S. G., & Sparks, C. M. (1985). Age, education, and the internal consistency of personality scales. *Journal of Personality and Social Psychology, 49,* 1692–1702.

McGrath, R. E., Pogge, D. L., & Stokes, J. M. (2002). Incremental validity of selected MMPI-A content scales in an inpatient setting. *Psychological Assessment, 14,* 401–409.

McKinley, J. C., & Hathaway, S. R. (1943). The identification and measurement of the psychoneuroses in medical practice. *Journal of the American Medical Association, 122,* 161–167.

McNulty, J. L., Harkness, A. R., Ben-Porath, Y. S., & Williams, C. L. (1997). Assessing the personality psychopathology five (PSY-5) in adolescents: New MMPI-A scales. *Psychological Assessment, 9,* 250–259.

Meehl, P. E. (1951). *Research results for counselors.* St. Paul, MN: State Department of Education.

Meehl, P. E. (1954). *Clinical versus statistical prediction: A theoretical analysis and a review of the evidence.* Minneapolis: University of Minnesota Press.

Meehl, P. E. (1956). Wanted: A good cookbook. *American Psychologist, 11,* 263–272.

Meehl, P. E. (1986). Causes and effects of my disturbing little book. *Journal of Personality Assessment, 50,* 370–375.

Meehl, P. E., & Dahlstrom, W. G. (1960). Objective configural rules for discriminating psychotic from neurotic MMPI profiles. *Journal of Consulting Psychology, 24,* 375–387.

Meehl, P. E., & Hathaway, S. R. (1946). The K factor as a suppressor variable in the MMPI. *Journal of Applied Psychology, 30,* 525–564.

Meehl, P. E., & Rosen, A. (1955). Antecedent probability and the efficiency of psychometric signs, patterns, or cutting scores. *Psychological Bulletin, 52,* 194–216.

Merydith, E.K., & Phelps, L. (2009). Convergent validity of the MMPI-A and MACI Scales of Depression. *Psychological Reports, 105,* 605–609.

Meunier, G., & Bodkins, M. (2005). Interpretation of MMPI-A Scale 5 with female patients. *Psychological Reports, 96,* 545–546.

Micucci, J. A. (2002). Accuracy of MMPI-A scales ACK, MAC-R and PRO in detecting comorbid substance abuse among psychiatric inpatient. *Assessment, 9,* 111–122.

Miller v. Alabama, 132 S. Ct. 2455, 567 U.S., 183 L. Ed. 2d 407 (2012).

Miller, H. R., & Streiner, D. L. (1985). The Harris–Lingoes subscales: Fact or fiction? *Journal of Clinical Psychology, 41,* 45–51.

Millon, T., Green, C. J., & Meagher, R. B. (1977). *Millon Adolescent Personality Inventory.* Minneapolis, MN: National Computer Systems.

Milne, L. C., & Greenway, P. (1999). Do high scores on the adolescent-school problems and immaturity scales of the MMPI-A have implications for cognitive performance as measured by the WISC-III? *Psychology in the Schools, 36,* 199–203.

Mlott, S. R. (1973). The Mini-Mult and its use with adolescents. *Journal of Clinical Psychology, 29,* 376–377.

Monachesi, E. D. (1948). Some personality characteristics of delinquents and non-delinquents. *Journal of Criminal Law and Criminology, 38,* 487–500.

Monachesi, E. D. (1950). Personality characteristics of institutionalized and non-institutionalized male delinquents. *Journal of Criminal Law and Criminology, 41,* 167–179.

Monachesi, E. D., & Hathaway, S. R. (1969). The personality of delinquents. In J. N. Butcher (Ed.), *MMPI: Research developments and clinical applications* (pp. 207–219). Minneapolis: University of Minnesota Press.

Monroe, L. J., & Marks, P. A. (1977). MMPI differences between adolescent poor and good sleepers. *Journal of Consulting and Clinical Psychology, 45,* 151–152.

Moore, C. D., & Handal, P. J. (1980). Adolescents' MMPI performance, cynicism, estrangement, and personal adjustment as a function of race and sex. *Journal of Clinical Psychology, 36,* 932–936.

Moreland, K. L. (1984, Fall). Intelligent use of automated psychological reports. *Critical Items: A newsletter for the MMPI community, 1,* 4–6.

Moreland, K. L. (1985a). Computer-assisted psychological assessment in 1986: A practical guide. *Computers in Human Behavior, 1,* 221–233.

Moreland, K. L. (1985b). Validation of computer-based test interpretations: Problems and prospects. *Journal of Consulting and Clinical Psychology, 53,* 816–825.

Moreland, K. L. (1990). Computer-assisted assessment of adolescent and child personality: What's available? In C. R. Reynolds & R. W. Kamphaus (Eds.), *Handbook of psychological and educational assessment of children: Personality, behavior, and context* (pp. 395–420). New York: Guilford.

Morrison, T. L., Edwards, D. W., Weissman, H. N., Allen, R., & DeLaCruz, A. (1995). Comparing MMPI and MMPI-2 profiles: Replication and Integration. *Assessment, 2,* 39–46.

National Institute of Mental Health. (1990). *National plan for research on child and adolescent mental disorders* (DHHS Publication No. ADM 90-1683). Washington, DC: U.S. Government Printing Office.

Negy, C., Leal-Puente, L., Trainor, D. J., & Carlson, R. (1997). Mexican-American adolescents' performance on the MMPI-A. *Journal of Personality Assessment, 69,* 205–214.

Nelson, L. D. (1987). Measuring depression in a clinical population using the MMPI. *Journal of Consulting and Clinical Psychology, 55,* 788–790.

Nelson, L. D., & Cicchetti, D. (1991). Validity of the MMPI depression scale for outpatients. *Psychological Assessment: A Journal of Consulting and Clinical Psychology, 3,* 55–59.

Newmark, C. S. (1971). MMPI: Comparison of the oral form presented by a live examiner to the booklet form. *Psychological Reports, 29,* 797–798.

Newmark, C. S., Gentry, L., Whitt, J. K., McKee, D. C., & Wicker, C. (1983). Simulating normal MMPI profiles as a favorable prognostic sign in schizophrenia. *Australian Journal of Psychology, 35,* 433–444.

Newmark, C. S., & Thibodeau, J. R. (1979). Interpretive accuracy and empirical validity of abbreviated forms of the MMPI with hospitalized adolescents. In C. S. Newmark (Ed.), *MMPI: Clinical and research trends* (pp. 248–275). New York: Praeger.

Newsom, C. R., Archer, R. P., Trumbetta, S., & Gottesman, I. I. (2003). Changes in adolescent response patterns on the MMPI/MMPI-A across four decades. *Journal of Personality Assessment, 81,* 74–84.

Newton, C. C. (2008). *MMPI-A structural summary approach: Characteristics of gifted adolescents* (Doctoral dissertation). Available from ProQuest Dissertations & Theses Global. (UMI No. 3303358).

Nichols, D. S. (1987). *Interpreting the Wiggins MMPI content scales* (Clinical Notes on the MMPI, Monograph No. 10). Minneapolis, MN: National Computer Systems.

Nichols, D. S. (1992). Review of the Minnesota Multiphasic Personality Inventory - 2 (MMPI-2). In *The Eleventh Mental Measurements Yearbook* (pp. 562–565). Lincoln: Buros Institute of Mental Measurements, University of Nebraska.

Nichols, D. S. (2001). *Essentials of MMPI-2 Assessment.* New York: John Wiley & Sons.

Offer, D., & Offer, J. B. (1975). *From teenager to young manhood.* New York: Basic Books.

Orr, D. P., Eccles, T., Lawlor, R., & Golden, M. (1986). Surreptitious insulin administration in adolescents with insulin-dependent diabetes mellitus. *Journal of the American Medical Association, 256,* 3227–3230.

Osberg, T. M., & Poland, D. L. (2002). Comparative accuracy of the MMPI-2 and MMPI-A in the diagnosis of psychopathology in 18-year-olds. *Psychological Assessment, 14,* 164–169.

Overall, J. E., & Gomez-Mont, F. (1974). The MMPI-168 for psychiatric screening. *Educational and Psychological Measurement, 34,* 315–319.

Paikoff, R. L., & Brooks-Gunn, J. (1991). Do parent-child relationships change during puberty? *Psychological Bulletin, 110,* 47–66.

Pancoast, D. L., & Archer, R. P. (1988). MMPI adolescent norms: Patterns and trends across 4 decades. *Journal of Personality Assessment, 52,* 691–706.

Pancoast, D. L., & Archer, R. P. (1992). MMPI response patterns of college students: Comparisons to adolescents and adults. *Journal of Clinical Psychology, 48,* 47–53.

Pancoast, D. L., Archer, R. P., & Gordon, R. A. (1988). The MMPI and clinical diagnosis: A comparison of classification system outcomes with discharge diagnoses. *Journal of Personality Assessment, 52,* 81–90.

Paolo, A. M., Ryan, J. J., & Smith, A. J. (1991). Reading difficulty of MMPI-2 subscales. *Journal of Clinical Psychology, 47,* 529–532.

Petersen, A. C. (1985). Pubertal development as a cause of disturbance: Myths, realities, and unanswered questions. *Genetic, Social, and General Psychology Monographs, 111,* 205–232.

Petersen, A. C., & Hamburg, B. A. (1986). Adolescence: A developmental approach to problems and psychopathology. *Behavior Therapy, 17,* 480–499.

Piaget, J. (1975). The intellectual development of the adolescent. In A. H. Esman (Ed.), *The psychology of adolescence: Essential reading* (pp. 104–108). New York: International Universities Press.

Pinsoneault, T. B. (1997). A combined rationally-empirically developed variable response scale for detecting the random response set in the Jesness Inventory. *Journal of Clinical Psychology, 53,* 471–484.

Pinsoneault, T. B. (1999). Efficacy of the three randomness validity scales for the Jesness Inventory. *Journal of Personality Assessment, 73,* 395–406.

Pinsoneault, T. B. (2005). Detecting random, partially random, and nonrandom Minnesota Multiphasic Personality Inventory-Adolescent protocols. *Psychological Assessment, 17,* 476–480.

Pinsoneault, T. B. (2014). Effective cutoffs for detecting random, partially random, and nonrandom 350-item MMPI-A short form protocols. *Psychological Assessment, 26,* 685–690.

Piotrowski, C., & Keller, J. W. (1989). Psychological testing in outpatient mental health facilities: A national study. *Professional Psychology: Research and Practice, 20,* 423–425.

Piotrowski, C., & Keller, J. W. (1992). Psychological testing in applied settings: A literature review from 1982 - 1992. *Journal of Training and Practice in Professional Psychology, 6,* 74–82.

Pogge, D. L., Stokes, J. M., Frank, J., Wong, H., & Harvey, P. D. (1997). Association of MMPI validity scales and therapist ratings of psychopathology in adolescent psychiatric inpatients. *Assessment, 4,* 17–27.

Powers, S. I., Hauser, S. T., & Kilner, L. A. (1989). Adolescent mental health. *American Psychologist, 44,* 200–208.

Pritchard, D. A., & Rosenblatt, A. (1980). Racial bias in the MMPI: A methodological review. *Journal of Consulting and Clinical Psychology, 48,* 263–267.

Rathus, S. A. (1978). Factor structure of the MMPI-168 with and without regression weights. *Psychological Reports, 42,* 643–646.

Rathus, S. A., Fox, J. A., & Ortins, J. B. (1980). The MacAndrew scale as a measure of substance abuse in delinquency among adolescents. *Journal of Clinical Psychology, 36,* 579–583.

Reich, W., & Earls, F. (1987). Rules for making psychiatric diagnoses in children on the basis of multiple sources of information: Preliminary strategies. *Journal of Abnormal Child Psychology, 15,* 601–616.

Rempel, P. P. (1958). The use of multivariate statistical analysis of Minnesota Multiphasic Personality Inventory scores in the classification of delinquent and nondelinquent high school boys. *Journal of Consulting Psychology, 22,* 17–23.

Reyes, A., & Kazdin, A. E. (2005). Informant discrepancies in the assessment of childhood psychopathology: A critical review, theoretical framework, and recommendations for further study. *Psychological Bulliton, 131,* 483–509.

Reynolds, C. R., & Kamphaus, R. W. (2002). *The clinician's guide to the Behavior Assessment System for Children (BASC).* New York: Guilford Press.

Rinaldo, J. C. B., & Baer, R. A. (2003). Incremental validity of the MMPI-A content scales in the prediction of self-reported symptoms. *Journal of Personality Assessment, 80,* 309–318.

Roberts, R. E., Attkisson, C. C., & Rosenblatt, A. (1998). Prevalence of psychopathology among children and adolescents. *American Journal of Psychiatry, 155,* 715–725.

Roberts, R. E., Roberts, C. R., & Chan, W. (2009). One-year incidence of psychiatric disorders and associated risk factors among adolescents in the community. *Journal of Child Psychology and Psychiatry, 50,* 405–415.

Rogers, R., Bagby, R. M., & Chakraborty, D. (1993). Feigning schizophrenic disorders on the MMPI-2: Detection of coached simulators. *Journal of Personality Assessment, 60,* 215–226.

Rogers, R., Hinds, J. D., & Sewell, K. W. (1996). Feigning psychopathology among adolescent offenders: Validation of the SIRS, MMPI-A, and SIMS. *Journal of Personality Assessment, 67,* 244–257.

Rogers, R., Sewell, K. W., & Salekin, R. T. (1994). A meta-analysis of malingering on the MMPI-2. *Assessment, 1,* 227–237.

Rogers, R., Sewell, K. W., & Ustad, K. L. (1995). Feigning among chronic outpatients on the MMPI-2: A systematic examination of fake-bad indicators. *Assessment, 2,* 81–89.

Romano, B., Tremblay, R. E., Vitaro, F., Zoccolillo, M., & Pagani, L. (2001). Prevalence of psychiatric disorders and the role of perceived impairment: Findings from an adolescent community sample. *Journal of Child Psychology and Psychiatry, 42,* 451–461.

Rome, H. P., Swenson, W. M., Mataya, P., McCarthy, C. E., Pearson, J. S., Keating, F. R., & Hathaway, S. R. (1962). Symposium on automation techniques in personality assessment. *Proceedings of the Staff Meetings of the Mayo Clinic, 37,* 61–82.

Roper v. Simmons, 543 U.S. 551, 125 S. Ct. 1183, 161 L. Ed. 2d 1 (2005).

Roper, B. L., Ben-Porath, Y. S., & Butcher, J. N. (1991). Comparability of computerized adaptive and conventional testing with the MMPI-2. *Journal of Personality Assessment, 57,* 278–290.

Roper, B. L., Ben-Porath, Y. S., & Butcher, J. N. (1995). Comparability and validity of computerized adaptive testing with the MMPI-2. *Journal of Personality Assessment, 65,* 358–371.

Rosen, A. (1962). Development of MMPI scales based on a reference group of psychiatric patients. *Psychological Monographs, 76* (8, Whole No. 527).

Rosenberg, L. A., & Joshi, P. (1986). Effect of marital discord on parental reports on the Child Behavior Checklist. *Psychological Reports, 59,* 1255–1259.

Rutter, M., Graham, P., Chadwick, O. F. D., & Yule, W. (1976). Adolescent turmoil: Fact or fiction? *Journal of Child Psychology and Psychiatry, 17,* 35–56.

Schinka, J. A., Elkins, D. E., & Archer, R. P. (1998). Effects of psychopathology and demographic characteristics on MMPI-A scale scores. *Journal of Personality Assessment, 71,* 295–305.

Schuerger, J. M., Foerstner, S. B., Serkownek, K., & Ritz, G. (1987). History and validities of the Serkownek subscales for MMPI Scales 5 and 0. *Psychological Reports, 61,* 227–235.

Scott, R. L., Butcher, J. N., Young, T. L., & Gomez, N. (2002). The Hispanic MMPI-A across five countries. *Journal of Clinical Psychology, 58,* 407–417.

Scott, R. L., Knoth, R. L., Beltran-Quiones, M., & Gomez, N. (2003). Assessment of psychological functioning in adolescent earthquake victims in Columbia using the MMPI-A. *Journal of Traumatic Stress, 16,* 49–57.

Scott, R.L., & Mamani-Pampa, W. (2008). MMPI-A for Peru: Adaptation and normalization. *International Journal of Clinical and Health Psychology, 8,* 719–732.

Serkownek, K. (1975). *Subscales for Scales 5 and 0 of the MMPI.* Unpublished manuscript.

Shaevel, B., & Archer, R. P. (1996). Effects of MMPI-2 and MMPI-A norms on T-score elevations for 18-year-olds. *Journal of Personality Assessment, 67,* 72–78.

Sherwood, N. E., Ben-Porath, Y. S., & Williams, C. L. (1997). The MMPI-A content component scales: Development, psychometric characteristics and clinical application. *MMPI-2/MMPI-A Test Report 3*. Minneapolis: University of Minnesota Press.

Sieber, K. O., & Meyer, L. S. (1992). Validation of the MMPI-2 social introversion subscales. *Psychological Assessment, 4*, 185–189.

Sivec, H. J., Lynn, S. J., & Garske, J. P. (1994). The effect of somatoform disorder and paranoid psychotic role-related dissimulations as a response set on the MMPI-2. *Assessment, 1*, 69–81.

Spielberger, C. D. (1988). *State-Trait Anger Expression Inventory - Research Edition*. Odessa, FL: Psychological Assessment Resources.

Spirito, A., Faust, D., Myers, B., & Bechtel, D. (1988). Clinical utility of the MMPI in the evaluation of adolescent suicide attempters. *Journal of Personality Assessment, 52*, 204–211.

Stehbens, J. A., Ehmke, D. A., & Wilson, B. K. (1982). MMPI profiles of rheumatic fever adolescents and adults. *Journal of Clinical Psychology, 38*, 592–596.

Stein, L.A.R., & Graham, J.R. (2005). Ability of substance abusers to escape detection on the Minnesota Multiphasic Personality Inventory-Adolescent (MMPI-A) in a juvenile correctional facility. *Assessment, 12*, 28–39.

Stein, L. A. R., Graham, J. R., & Williams, C. L. (1995). Detecting fake-bad MMPI-A profiles. *Journal of Personality Assessment, 65*, 415–427.

Stein, L. A. R., McClinton, B. K., & Graham, J. R. (1998). Long-term stability of MMPI-A scales. *Journal of Personality Assessment, 70*, 103–108.

Stokes, J., Pogge, D., Sarnicola, J., & McGrath, R. (2009). Correlates of the MMPI-A Psychopathology Five (PSY-5) facet scales in an adolescent inpatient sample. *Journal of Personality Assessment, 91*, 48–57.

Stone, L. J., & Church, J. (1957). Pubescence, puberty, and physical development. In A. H. Esman (Ed.), *The psychology of adolescence: Essential readings* (pp. 75–85). New York: International Universities Press.

Storm, J., & Graham, J. R. (1998, March). *The effects of validity scale coaching on the ability to malinger psychopathology*. Paper presented at the 33rd Annual Symposium on Research Developments in the Use of the MMPI-2 and MMPI-A. Clearwater Beach, FL.

Strong, E. K., Jr. (1927). Differentiation of certified public accountants from other occupational groups. *Journal of Educational Psychology, 18*, 227–238.

Strong, E. K., Jr. (1943). *Vocational interests of men and women*. Stanford, CA: Stanford University Press.

Super, D. E. (1942). The Bernreuter Personality Inventory: A review of research. *Psychological Bulletin, 39*, 94–125.

Sutker, P. B., Allain, A. N., & Geyer, S. (1980). Female criminal violence and differential MMPI characteristics. *Journal of Consulting and Clinical Psychology, 46*, 1141–1143.

Sutker, P. B., & Archer, R. P. (1979). MMPI characteristics of opiate addicts, alcoholics, and other drug abusers. In C. S. Newmark (Ed.), *MMPI clinical and research trends* (pp. 105–148). New York: Praeger.

Svanum, S., & Ehrmann, L. C. (1992). Alcoholic subtypes and the MacAndrew alcoholism scale. Journal of Personality Assessment, 58, 411–422.

Svanum, S., McGrew, J., & Ehrmann, L. C. (1994). Validity of the substance abuse scales of the MMPI-2 in a college student sample. *Journal of Personality Assessment, 62*, 427–439.

Swenson, W. M., & Pearson, J. S. (1964). Automation techniques in personality assessment: A frontier in behavioral science and medicine. *Methods of Information in Medicine, 3*, 34–36.

Tanner, J. M. (1969). Growth and endocrinology of the adolescent. In L. Gardner (Ed.), *Endocrine and genetic diseases of childhood* (pp. 19–60). Philadelphia: Saunders.

Tanner, J. M., Whitehouse, R. H., & Takaishi, M. (1966). Standards from birth to maturity for height, weight, height velocity, and weight velocity: British children, 1965, Part I. *Archives of Disease in Childhood, 41*, 454–471.

Tellegen, A., & Ben-Porath, Y. S. (1992). The new uniform T-scores for the MMPI-2: Rationale, derivation, and appraisal. *Psychological Assessment, 4*, 145–155.

Tellegen, A., & Ben-Porath, Y. S. (1993). Code-type comparability of the MMPI and MMPI-2: Analysis of recent findings and criticisms. *Journal of Personality Assessment, 61*, 489–500.

Timbrook, R. E., & Graham, J. R. (1994). Ethnic differences on the MMPI-2? *Psychological Assessment, 6*, 212–217.

Timbrook, R. E., Graham, J. R., Keiller, S. W., & Watts, D. (1993). Comparison of the Wiener–Harmon subtle-obvious scales and the standard validity scales in detecting valid and invalid MMPI-2 profiles. *Psychological Assessment, 5*, 53–61.

Tirrell, C. A., Archer, R. P., & Mason, J. (2004). Concurrent validity of the MMPI-A substance abuse scales: MAC-R, ACK, and PRO. Manuscript in preparation.

Todd, A. L., & Gynther, M. D. (1988). Have MMPI Mf scale correlates changed in the past 30 years? *Journal of Clinical Psychology, 44*, 505–510.

Toyer, E. A., & Weed, N. C. (1998). Concurrent validity of the MMPI-A in a counseling program for juvenile offenders. *Journal of Clinical Psychology, 54*, 395–399.

Truscott, D. (1990). Assessment of overcontrolled hostility in adolescence. *Psychological Assessment: A Journal of Consulting and Clinical Psychology, 2*, 145–148.

University of Minnesota Test Division (2014). *Available translations.* [Online]. Available: http://www.upress.umn.edu/test-division/translations-permissions/available-translations.

Veltri, C. O. C., Graham, J. R., Sellbom, M., Ben-Porath, Y. S. Forbey, J. D., O'Connell, C., Rogers, R., & White, R. S. (2009). Correlations of MMPI-A scales in acute psychiatric and forensic samples. *Journal of Personality Assessment, 91*, 288–300.

Veltri, C. O. C., Sellbom, M., Graham., J. R., Ben-Porath, Y. S., Forbey, J. D., & White, R. S. (2014). Distinguishing Personality Psychopathy Five (PSY-5) characteristics associated with violent and nonviolent juvenile delinquency. *Journal of Personality Assessment, 96*, 158–165.

Veltri, C. O. C, & Williams, J. E. (2012). Does the disorder matter? Investigating a moderating effect on coached noncredible overreporting using the MMPI-2 and PAI. *Assessment, 20*, 199–209.

Vondell, N. J., & Cyr, J. J. (1991). MMPI short forms with adolescents: Gender differences and accuracy. *Journal of Personality Assessment, 56*, 254–265.

Walters, G. D. (1983). The MMPI and schizophrenia: A review. *Schizophrenia Bulletin, 9*, 226–246.

Walters, G. D. (1988). Schizophrenia. In R. L. Greene (Ed.), *The MMPI: Use in specific populations* (pp. 50–73). San Antonio, TX: Grune & Stratton.

Ward, L. C., & Ward, J. W. (1980). MMPI readability reconsidered. *Journal of Personality Assessment, 44*, 387–389.

Wasyliw, O. E., Haywood, T. W., Grossman, L. S., & Cavanaugh, J. L. (1993). The psychometric assessment of alcoholism in forensic groups: The MacAndrew scale and response bias. *Journal of Personality Assessment, 60,* 252–266.

Watson, C. G., Thomas, D., & Anderson, P. E. D. (1992). Do computer-administered Minnesota Multiphasic Personality Inventories underestimate booklet-based scores? *Journal of Clinical Psychology, 48,* 744–748.

Weed, N. C., Ben-Porath, Y. S., & Butcher, J. N. (1990). Failure of the Wiener and Harmon Minnesota Multiphasic Personality Inventory (MMPI) subtle scales as personality descriptors and as validity indicators. *Psychological Assessment: A Journal of Consulting and Clinical Psychology, 2,* 281–285.

Weed, N. C., Butcher, J. N., McKenna, T., & Ben-Porath, Y. S. (1992). New measures for assessing alcohol and drug dependence with the MMPI-2: The *APS* and *AAS. Journal of Personality Assessment, 58,* 389–404.

Weed, N. C., Butcher, J. N., & Williams, C. L. (1994). Development of MMPI-A alcohol/drug problems scales. *Journal of Studies on Alcohol, 55(3),* 296–302.

Weiner, I. B., & Del Gaudio, A. C. (1976). Psychopathology in adolescence: An epidemiological study. *Archives of General Psychiatry, 33,* 187–193.

Weissman, M. M., Wickramaratne, P., Warner, V., John, K., Prusoff, B. A., Merikangas, K. R., & Gammon, G. D. (1987). Assessing psychiatric disorders in children: Discrepancies between mothers' and children's reports. *Archives of General Psychiatry, 44,* 747–753.

Welsh, G. S. (1948). An extension of Hathaway's MMPI profile coding system. *Journal of Consulting Psychology, 12,* 343–344.

Welsh, G. S. (1956). Factor dimensions A and R. In G. S. Welsh & W. G. Dahlstrom (Eds.), *Basic reading on the MMPI in psychology and medicine* (pp. 264–281). Minneapolis: University of Minnesota Press.

Wetter, M. W., Baer, R. A., Berry, D. T. R., & Reynolds, S. K. (1994). The effect of symptom information on faking on the MMPI-2. *Assessment, 1,* 199–207.

Wetter, M. W., Baer, R. A., Berry, D. T. R., Robison, L. H., & Sumpter, J. (1993). MMPI-2 profiles of motivated fakers given specific symptom information: A comparison to matched patients. *Psychological Assessment, 3,* 317–323.

Wetter, M. W., Baer, R. A., Berry, D. T. R., Smith, G. T., & Larsen, L. H. (1992). Sensitivity of MMPI-2 validity scales to random responding and malingering. *Psychological Assessment, 4,* 369–374.

Wetter, M. W., & Corrigan, S. K. (1995). Providing information to clients about psychological tests: A survey of attorneys' and law students' attitudes. *Professional Psychology: Research and Practice, 26,* 1–4.

White, A.M. (2009). Understanding adolescent brain development and its implications for the clinician. *Adolescent Medicine, 20,* 73–90.

White, L., & Krishnamurthy, R. (2015, March). *An evaluation of Minnesota Multiphasic Personality Inventory – Adolescent – Restructured Form (MMPI-A-RF) item endorsement frequencies using clinical and non-clinical adolescent samples.* In R. Krishnamurthy (chair), *MMPI research.* Paper presented at the annual convention of the Society for Personality Assessment, Brooklyn, NY.

White, L., & Krishnamurthy, R. (2014, March). *A psychometric evaluation of the MMPI-A-RF using clinical and nonclinical assessment samples.* In R. Krishnamurthy (chair), *MMPI Research I.* Paper presented at the annual convention of the Society for Personality Assessment, Arlington, VA.

Wiederholt, J. L., & Bryant, B. R. (2012). *Gray Oral Reading Tests-Fifth Edition* (GORT-5). Austin, TX: Pro-Ed.

Wiener, D. N. (1948). Subtle and Obvious keys for the MMPI. *Journal of Consulting Psychology, 12,* 164–170.

Wiggins, J. S. (1966). Substantive dimensions of self-report in the MMPI item pool. *Psychological Monographs, 80* (22, Whole No. 630).

Wiggins, J. S. (1969). Content dimensions in the MMPI. In J. N. Butcher (Ed.), *MMPI: Research developments and clinical applications* (pp. 127–180). New York: McGraw-Hill.

Wilkinson, G. S., & Robertson, G. J. (2006). *WRAT 4: Wide Range Achievement Test; professional manual.* Lutz, FL: Psychological Assessment Resources, Incorporated.

Williams, C. L., Ben-Porath, Y. S., & Hevern, B. W. (1994). Item level improvements for use of the MMPI with adolescents. *Journal of Personality Assessment, 63,* 284–293.

Williams, C. L., & Butcher, J. N. (1989a). An MMPI study of adolescents: I. Empirical validity of standard scales. *Psychological Assessment: A Journal of Consulting and Clinical Psychology, 1,* 251–259.

Williams, C. L., & Butcher, J. N. (1989b). An MMPI study of adolescents: II. Verification and limitations of code type classifications. *Psychological Assessment: A Journal of Consulting and Clinical Psychology, 1,* 260–265.

Williams, C. L., & Butcher, J. N. (2011). *Beginner's guide to the MMPI-A.* Washington, DC: American Psychological Association.

Williams, C. L., Butcher, J. N., Ben-Porath, Y. S., & Graham, J. R. (1992). *MMPI-A content scales: Assessing psychopathology in adolescents.* Minneapolis: University of Minnesota Press.

Williams, C. L., Graham, J. R., & Butcher, J. N. (1986, March). *Appropriate MMPI norms for adolescents: An old problem revisited.* Paper presented at the 21st annual Symposium on Recent Developments in the Use of the MMPI, Clearwater, FL.

Williams, C. L., Hearn, M. D., Hostetler, K., & Ben-Porath, Y. S. (1990). *A comparison of several epidemiological measures for adolescents: MMPI, DISC, and YSR.* Unpublished manuscript, University of Minnesota, Minneapolis.

Williams, J. E., & Weed, N. C. (2004). Review of computer-based test interpretation software for the MMPI-2. *Journal of Personality Assessment, 83(1),* 78–83.

Wimbish, L. G. (1984). *The importance of appropriate norms for the computerized interpretations of adolescent MMPI profiles.* Unpublished doctoral dissertation, Ohio State University, Columbus.

Wirt, R. D., & Briggs, P. F. (1959). Personality and environmental factors in the development of delinquency. *Psychological Monographs: General and Applied* (Whole No. 485). 1–47.

Wisniewski, N. M., Glenwick, D. S., & Graham, J. R. (1985). MacAndrew scale and sociodemographic correlates of alcohol and drug use. *Addictive Behaviors, 10,* 55–67.

Wolfson, K. P., & Erbaugh, S. E. (1984). Adolescent responses to the MacAndrew Alcoholism scale. *Journal of Consulting and Clinical Psychology, 52,* 625–630.

Woodworth, R. S. (1920). *Personal data sheet.* Chicago: Stoelting.

Wrobel, N. H. (1991, August). Utility of the Wiggins content scales with an adolescent sample. In R. C. Colligan (Chair), *MMPI and MMPI-2 supplementary scales and profile interpretation - content scales revisited.* Symposium conducted at the annual conference of the American Psychological Association, San Francisco, CA.

Wrobel, N. H., & Gdowski, C. L. (1989, August). *Validation of Wiggins content scales with an adolescent sample.* Paper presented at the annual convention of the American Psychological Association, New Orleans, LA.

Wrobel, N. H., & Lachar, D. (1992). Refining adolescent MMPI interpretations: Moderating effects of gender in prediction of descriptions from parents. *Psychological Assessment, 4,* 375–381.

Wrobel, N. H., & Lachar, D. (1995). Racial differences in adolescent self-report: A comparative validity study using homogeneous MMPI content scales. *Psychological Assessment, 7,* 140–147.

Wrobel, T. A. (1992). Validity of Harris and Lingoes MMPI subscale descriptors in an outpatient sample. *Journal of Personality Assessment, 59,* 14–21.

Yavari, R. (2012). *Examining the Minnesota Multiphasic Personality Inventory-Adolescent: Self-descriptors of the K scale in adolescents* (Doctoral dissertation). Available from ProQuest Dissertations & Theses Global. (UMI No. 3471043).

Zahn-Waxler, C., Shirtcliff, E.A., & Marceau, K. (2008). Disorders of childhood and adolescence: Gender and psychopathology. *Annual Review of Clinical Psychology, 4,* 275–303.

Zinn, S., McCumber, S., & Dahlstrom, W. G. (1999). Cross-validation and extension of the MMPI-A IM scale. *Assessment, 6,* 1–6.

Zubeidat, I., Sierra, J.C., Salinas, J.M., & Rojas-Garcia, A. (2011). Reliability and validity of the Spanish version of the Minnesota Multiphasic Personality Inventory (MMPI-A). *Journal of Personality Assessment, 93,* 26–32.

AUTHOR INDEX

SUBJECT INDEX

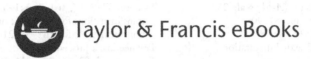